ADVANCES IN

STEROID BIOCHEMISTRY
AND PHARMACOLOGY
VOLUME 4

ADVANCES IN

STEROID BIOCHEMISTRY

AND PHARMACOLOGY

Edited by

M. H. BRIGGS

Biochemistry Department,
Alfred Hospital,
Prahran,
Victoria, Australia

and

G. A. CHRISTIE

Syntex Pharmaceuticals Ltd,
Maidenhead,
Berkshire, England

VOLUME 4

1974

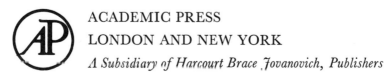

ACADEMIC PRESS
LONDON AND NEW YORK
A Subsidiary of Harcourt Brace Jovanovich, Publishers

ACADEMIC PRESS INC. (LONDON) LTD.
24/28 Oval Road,
London NW1

United States Edition published by
ACADEMIC PRESS INC.
111 Fifth Avenue
New York, New York 10003

Library of Congress Catalog Card Number: 79–109037
ISBN: 0-12-037504-4

Printed in Great Britain by
William Clowes & Sons, Limited
London, Beccles and Colchester

CONTRIBUTORS

F P ALTMAN *Division of Cellular Biology, The Kennedy Institute of Rheumatology, Bute Gardens, London, England.*

LUCILLE BITENSKY *Division of Cellular Biology, The Kennedy Institute of Rheumatology, Bute Gardens, London, England.*

R G BUTCHER *Division of Cellular Biology, The Kennedy Institute of Rheumatology, Bute Gardens, London, England.*

J CHAYEN *Division of Cellular Biology, The Kennedy Institute of Rheumatology, Bute Gardens, London, England.*

J R DALY *Department of Chemical Pathology, Charing Cross Hospital Medical School, London, England.*

H F DeLUCA *Department of Biochemistry, College of Agricultural Life Sciences, University of Wisconsin–Madison, Wisconsin, U.S.A.*

J I EVANS *Sleep Laboratory, Department of Psychiatry, University of Edinburgh, Edinburgh, Scotland.*

P GARZÓN *Depto. Bioquimica, Facultad de Medicina, Universidad de Guadalajara, Guadalajara, Jalisco, Mexico.*

M F HOLICK *Department of Biochemistry, College of Agricultural Life Sciences, University of Wisconsin–Madison, Wisconsin, U.S.A.*

S NACHT *Vick Divisions Research and Development, One Bradford Road, Mount Vernon, New York, U.S.A.*

DENNIS SCHULSTER *School of Biological Sciences, University of Sussex, Falmer, Brighton, Sussex, England.*

JANE E SHAW *ALZA Research, 950 Page Mill Road, Palo Alto, California, U.S.A.*

STEPHEN A TILLSON *ALZA Research, 950 Page Mill Road, Palo Alto, California, U.S.A.*

CONTENTS

Cellular Biochemical Assessment of Steroid Activity

J. CHAYEN, LUCILLE BITENSKY, R. G. BUTCHER and F. P. ALTMAN

Daily Rhythms of Steroid and Associated Pituitary Hormones in Man and Their Relationship to Sleep

J. R. DALY and J. I. EVANS

Chemistry and Biological Activity of Vitamin D, its Metabolites and Analogs

M. F. HOLICK and H. F. DeLUCA

Effects of Corticosteroids on
Connective Tissue and Fibroblasts

S. NACHT and P. GARZÓN

Interactions Between the Prostaglandins and Steroid Hormones

JANE E. SHAW and STEPHEN A. TILLSON

Steroid Hormones and Breast Cancer

D. C. WILLIAMS

Adrenocorticotrophic Hormone and the Control of Adrenal Corticosteroidogenesis

DENNIS SCHULSTER

CELLULAR BIOCHEMICAL ASSESSMENT OF STEROID ACTIVITY

J. CHAYEN, LUCILLE BITENSKY, R. G. BUTCHER AND
F. P. ALTMAN

*Division of Cellular Biology, The Kennedy Institute of Rheumatology,
Bute Gardens, London, England*

1. INTRODUCTION: THE POSSIBLE CELLULAR BIOCHEMICAL EFFECTS OF STEROIDS

Steroids can influence cellular biochemistry in a number of different ways. They may act by influencing gene activity; this aspect has been reviewed by Grant (1969) and will not be discussed further here. They may inhibit particular enzymes by direct action on the enzyme molecule. Or they may alter enzyme activity by interference at the co-enzyme or substrate-level, as appears to be the case in some types of steroid transhydrogenation mechanisms (see Grant, 1969) or by competitive inhibition reactions of the normal type which are not peculiar to steroids. On the other hand, steroids have a particular propensity for altering the chemistry of cells by what amounts predominantly to their physical effects, on cellular and on sub-cellular membranes. These possibilities will be considered

1

briefly before discussing the special methods of cellular biochemistry which have been developed to allow the fuller assessment of these effects to be made.

A. DIRECT EFFECT ON ENZYMES

1. Non-Competitive Inhibition

It now seems quite clear that steroids can have a direct and inhibitory influence on the activity of certain purified enzymes. Marks and Banks (1960) showed that 4.10^{-5} M pregnenolone, dehydroisoandrosterone (dehydroepiandrosterone), epiandrosterone, androstane-3,17-dione and related steroids caused between 75–85% inhibition (depending on the exact steroid used) of the activity of purified human red blood cell glucose -6-phosphate dehydrogenase, and of 73–90% of the activity of a crude glucose 6-phosphate dehydrogenase preparation from rat adrenal. Inhibition (20–30%) was found when the concentrations of these steroids was diminished to 4.10^{-7} M. Other steroids caused some inhibition of this activity, particularly when used at the higher concentrations. The effect of pregnenolone and of dehydroisoandrosterone (dehydroepiandrosterone) on glucose 6-phosphate dehydrogenase from rat and human tissues varied slightly with the tissue; these steroids had no effect on this dehydrogenase isolated from yeast or from spinach. Equally they did not inhibit 6-phosphogluconate dehydrogenase derived from any of these sources or isocitrate dehydrogenase from rat and human tissues. Thus the inhibition appeared to be remarkably selective, and was not due to competitive inhibition with respect either to the co-enzyme or the substrate. They pointed out that all the inhibitory steroids had a ketone group at C_{17} or C_{20}; a hydroxyl group at this position produced little inhibition. Equally, no inhibitory effect was produced if the steroid contained a ketone group or an α or β hydroxyl group at C_3; saturation or unsaturation at C_{4-5} or C_{5-6} had little effect. The significance of these findings has been extended by the application of newer cellular biochemical investigations, as will be discussed below (Section III A 3).

At first sight it seems difficult to understand how steroids can influence the activity of proteins, such as glucose 6-phosphate dehydrogenase. With this enzyme at least, the inhibitory effect of the steroids does not appear to be through competition at the active site of the enzyme; consequently the suggestion is that the steroids produce some effect on the protein molecules akin to the allosteric effects discussed by Monod et al. (1963), and developed further by Monod et al. (1965) more specifically for conformational changes in the protein molecules of enzymes. Levy et al. (1966) confirmed the results of Marks and Banks (1960), namely that dehydroepiandrosterone inhibits mammalian glucose 6-phosphate dehydrogenase in a non-competitive manner. They suggested that this type of inhibition is due to conformational and polymeric change. It is well known that most enzymes occur as macromolecules which are composed of sub-units. Klotz *et al.* (1970) listed about 100 enzymes which appear to fit this rule. Glucose 6-phosphate dehydrogenase in particular has been much studied in this respect. Yoshida (1966) found the molecular weight of the crystalline dehydrogenase from human erythrocytes to be 240,000; it was inactivated if the bound NADP was removed from it. He suggested that the active enzyme was composed of 6 sub-units with 6 molecules of NADP bound to the whole assembly. It readily dissociates into two partially active trimeric assemblies. With glucose 6-phosphate dehydrogenase derived from brewers' yeast, Yue *et al.* (1969) found that the apoenzyme (i.e. lacking bound NADP) had a molecular weight of 101,600 and was made up of two polypeptide sub-units each of molecular weight of 51,000. The addition of NADP caused the sub-units to aggregate into the dimeric active macromolecule (also see Frieden, 1971). Levy *et al.* (1966) suggested that, for glucose 6-phosphate dehydrogenase from the mammary gland, the enzyme exists in two monomeric forms, the X and Y form, which can be in rapid and mobile equilibrium one with the other. The X form can be reversibly dissociated into inactive sub-units and is converted into the active Y form by the presence of NADP or NADPH. They postulated that inhibitory steroids, like dehydroepiandrosterone, can be bound only to the active Y monomer, so that the binding of such steroids can occur only in the presence of NADP. The change from the X to the Y form may be solely a change in the conformation of the protein molecule as Levy *et al.* (1966) indicate (following the views of Monod *et al.*, 1965), or it may involve a greater change in the flexible shape of the enzyme, as favoured by Koshland and Neet (1968).

These results, and the concepts of conformational change and of steroids affecting the quaternary structure of enzymes, have been worked out with purified enzymes. They become of even greater moment when the enzymes are attached to solid surfaces, as are most of the intra-cellular enzymes (and as discussed below). However even these effects may be difficult to analyse completely with isolated enzymes. As Monod *et al.* (1965) pointed out: 'one should note, however, that the capacity to mediate physiologically significant interactions might be more frequent and widespread among proteins than has been realized so far. As we have seen, these properties are frequently very labile and may easily be lost during extraction and purification of an enzyme'.

2. Competitive Inhibition

Steroids can also influence enzymic activity in cells either by fulfilling a co-enzyme function, as in certain transhydrogenation mechanisms (i.e. so stimulating enzymic activity) or by competitive inhibition. An example of steroids functioning as if they were co-enzymes is the well-known case of oestradiol, which appears to be an essential factor in the transhydrogenation reaction $NADPH + NAD^+ \rightleftharpoons NADH + NADP^+$ in placental preparations and for soluble fractions of rat liver (Talalay, 1961; also see Tomkins and Maxwell,

1963; Karavolas and Engel, 1966; Grant, 1969). The reaction appears to take the following form:

$$NADPH + H^+ + \text{ketosteroid} \rightleftharpoons \text{hydroxysteroid} + NADP^+$$
$$NAD^+ + \text{hydroxysteroid} \rightleftharpoons \text{ketosteroid} + NADH + H^+$$

$$NADPH + NAD^+ \rightleftharpoons NADH + NADP^+$$

Oestradiol activates this transhydrogenation at very low (catalytic) concentrations, as if it were acting as a hydrogen carrier or a co-enzyme. It is not inconceivable that other steroids might act competitively in this specific situation.

A different type of competitive inhibition is that described for tryptophan oxygenase in the supernatant fraction of rat liver homogenates (Braidman and Rose, 1970). This enzyme, which has a haem co-factor, was inhibited by deoxycorticosterone and progesterone (10^{-4} M). Other Δ^4-3-oxo steroids, such as cortisol, did not inhibit this enzyme; a double bond in the A ring seems to be essential for inhibitory action. The effect of increasing concentrations of haematin in the assay system, and the Lineweaver–Burk plots indicated that the inhibitory steroids competitively inhibited by involvement with the haem co-factor of the enzyme, as had been postulated by Oelkers and Dulce (1964).

Other aspects of competitive inhibition could involve competition for specific binding sites in the cells, either in the cell membrane and cytoplasm or in chromatin.

B. INDIRECT EFFECTS ON ENZYME ACTIVITIES

1. Physical Effects

Cellular and sub-cellular membranes are constructed of lipids (phospholipids and glycolipids), proteins and steroid. A typical analysis of the lipids of a cell membrane, taken from the erythrocyte, would be: 50–60% phosphatides, 20–30% free cholesterol (Cook, 1968). According to whichever model structure is preferred, for example the Davson and Danielli (1952) bimolecular leaflet or the Lucy (1968) globular micelle structure or any other, steroids are conceded to play a major role at least in the stabilization of the lipid components. Willmer (1961) has reviewed the earlier evidence concerning the significance of steroids in cell surfaces and in lipid monolayers. He drew attention to the fact that the closeness of the packing of the phospholipid components depends on the relative proportion of cholesterol to phospholipid, that is it is strikingly altered by changes in the steroid component. More recent investigations, using artificial thin films or droplets (of the type discussed by Bangham, 1968; Bangham and Haydon, 1968) have largely confirmed the role of steroids in such membranes. Moreover, electron spin resonance studies, with steroid spin labels in biological membranes (Hubbell and McConnell, 1969) and with spin-labelled lipids (Waggoner et al., 1969) have shown decisively that steroids increase the viscosity of lipid membranes. In terms of cellular biochemistry, the physical changes induced in cellular and sub-cellular membranes by different types of steroids could have the following effects:

(1) Alteration in the permeability of the cell membrane. Such a change can alter the water-balance inside and outside the cell, and the flow of ions and of nutrients; it may affect the pinocytotic activity of the cell surface (Holter, 1965; see Chayen and Bitensky, 1973) and may influence cell-to-cell surface interactions.

(2) Alteration in the permeability of sub-cellular organelles and structures. This is an important effect because it controls the flow of substrates into and out of such sub-cellular structures and, in this way, can play a critical part in the control of cellular metabolism.

(3) By changing the physico-chemical characteristics of the solid structures to which most intra-cellular enzymes are attached, steroids can markedly change the activity of the enzymes. This aspect of the control of intra-cellular activity arises from concepts which have become current in biochemistry only relatively recently. Previously biochemistry dealt pre-dominantly with enzyme activities measured on isolated enzymes acting in solution. But it is now apparent that most of the enzymes inside cells occur in or on solid structures. These include not only those enzymes located on, or in, the plasma membrane but also many of the mitochondrial enzymes, distributed on the membranes of the outer surface or of the christae mitochondriales (see Lehninger, 1965); those inside lysosomes and peroxi-somes, in which the nature of the binding of the enzymes to solid surfaces is still not clear; and the enzymes which are bound to the endoplasmic reticulum.

In fact, based on the appearances demonstrated by electron microscopy, Lehninger (1966) has calculated that between 40 and 90% of the mass of cells is composed of membranes, on which—or as part of which—are active enzymes. With the availability of solid matrices, on to which enzymes can be bound (e.g. Hornby et al., 1966; McLaren and Packer, 1970), it has been shown that the physico-chemical properties of matrix-bound enzymes, and their activities generally, may be very different from the physico-chemical properties of the same, purified enzymes when present in solution. From such work in particular has come a great deal of work on the differences between the activity of enzymes in homogeneous phase reactions (i.e. in aqueous solution) as against heterogeneous phase reactions, namely when the enzyme is in a solid matrix, be it an artificial matrix or a natural matrix such as a mitochondrion. These studies, on enzyme reactions in heterogeneous systems, have recently been reviewed by

McLaren and Packer (1970). In particular, changes in enzyme activity can be induced by changing the nature of the charge, and the charge-density, on the matrix around the enzyme molecules (e.g. Hornby *et al.*, 1968; Filip̀usson and Hornby, 1970); by changes in the lipid component of the matrix or membrane in the vicinity of the enzyme (Mazanowska *et al.*, 1966); and by configurational change in the enzyme at an interface (Quarles and Dawson, 1969). Conformational changes in succinate dehydrogenase, associated with substrate (Kearney, 1957) and hypobaric conditions (Aithal and Ramasarma, 1969) have also been reported. All of these can be influenced by steroids if these substances alter the properties of the natural matrix in which the enzymes are embeded.

C. THE ROLE OF CELLULAR (MULTIPHASE) BIOCHEMISTRY

The direct effect of steroids (Section I A), for example their inhibitory effect on enzymes or their interaction with nucleohistone, can be studied by conventional biochemical procedures. These methods generally involve the disruption of the tissue by homogenization and the separation by differential centrifugation of the sub-cellular components into a foreign medium; they frequently require the purification of the enzyme, or the active compound, from other cellular systems. These procedures are liable to alter, sometimes very considerably, the permeability of the membranes of sub-cellular organelles and thus the rate of entry of substrates and other reactants into the organelle; in this way the apparent rate of activity of intra-organelle enzymes will be enhanced. Disruptive biochemical analysis measures the activity of the isolated enzyme, which may be very different from its activity when attached to its natural matrix or when it is able to interact with other cellular systems. Moreover, it is unlikely to be able to record the effect of the more subtle configurational changes which occur in an enzyme, or other active group, when acting as part of a functional, changing membrane system. These are theoretical possibilities. It is now pertinent to see how these arguments are borne out in practice.

1. Effect of Isolating Mitochondria

Lehninger (1951) showed that mitochondria became permeable to NADH after damage such as is produced during homogenization. Bendall and de Duve (1960) subjected mitochondria to increased time of homogenization and found increased activities of glutamate, malate and β-hydroxybutyrate dehydrogenases due to increased permeability of the mitochondrial membranes to the substrates for these enzymes. With prolonged homogenization, these activities approximated to that which they obtained by treating the mitochondria with a surface active agent. Chayen *et al.* (1966) showed that even relatively gentle physical disturbance, which was insufficient to cause the break-down of tissue, produced enhanced mitochondrial glutamate dehydrogenase activity, apparently due to increased permeability of the mitochondrial membranes.

One control of mitochondrial respiratory activity is the permeability of the mitochondrial membrane. If the preparatory methods severely disturb the nature of the membrane, so that it is rendered unduly permeable, it may become impossible to observe whether steroids can influence its natural permeability and so influence mitochondrial respiration. Clearly for this type of work it is necessary to study the mitochondria without isolating them, with the concomitant mechanical trauma, into a foreign medium; the ionic balance, tonicity, pH and lack of colloids, will all tend to alter irrevocably the nature of their membranes. The newer techniques of cellular biochemistry, to be discussed below, have shown that certain steroids can stabilize mitochondrial membranes and make them resistant to the damaging influence of inflammatory amines (Chayen *et al.*, 1970b).

2. Effect of Isolating Lysosomes

The whole concept of enzyme latency, and of the controlling function of organelle membranes, has been established largely by work done on lysosomes. These are sub-cellular organelles, usually about 0.5 μ in diameter, which contain many, if not most, of the hydrolase enzymes of the cell in a fully active state. They cannot express their activity inside the cell because they are sequestered behind a semi-permeable organelle membrane. The subject of lysosomes in biology generally, and in pathology, has been fully reviewed in the three-volume work, edited by Dingle and Fell (1969) and Dingle (1973). Conventional biochemistry would be sufficient to establish the amount and the activity of such lysosomal hydrolases in a sample of tissue. But it is becoming increasingly clear that the function of these organelles, particularly in conditions involving cell injury (Bitensky, 1963a) and inflammation (Weissmann, 1966, 1968, 1969; Chayen and Bitensky, 1971), is related to the condition of the lysosomal membrane. Thus apart from their normal involvement in endocytosis, with the formation of secondary lysosomes and phagosomes, they may also 'leak' inflammatory substances and even degradative enzymes which can act on the extra-cellular matrix. This subject has been extensively investigated by Dingle (e.g. 1968, 1969) who suggested that the 'leakage' of such lysosomal material may be by fusion of the abnormal lysosomal membranes with the cell surface and the ejection of 'packages' of lysosomal contents into the extra-cellular environment. However this may be, the primary consideration is not how much lysosomal activity is present in the cells (as can be determined readily by conventional biochemistry) but how stable is the lysosomal membrane which normally sequesters this activity from the rest of the cell and from the extra-cellular matrix. This question of the state of the lysosomal membrane has also become of some interest in view of the suggestions by Weissmann (1966) and

Glynn (1969) that lysosomes with abnormally labile membranes may not degrade ingested 'self' proteins completely and so may release inadequately degraded polypeptides which could give rise to autoimmune responses.

There is now considerable evidence that steroids can influence the stability of lysosomal membranes. In this way they could modify inflammation and possibly even auto-immunity of this type. Conventional homogenate biochemistry is ill-adapted to this type of analysis because the process of homogenization and isolation into a foreign medium may damage the lysosomal membrane so that it can no longer respond normally to steroids, or show any stabilizing effect which steroids *in vivo* might have had prior to homogenization (e.g. see Allison, 1968 concerning 'free activity' induced by homogenization; Weissmann, 1968, 1969, concerning the different effects of steroids *in vitro* and *in vivo*). Cellular biochemistry, however, can demonstrate the stabilizing effects of certain steroids both *in vitro* and *in vivo* (see below), assumably because it involves none of the trauma of homogenate biochemistry.

3. Effect on Enzymes of the Endoplasmic Reticulum

Superficially it might seem that those enzymes which are found predominantly in the non-sedimentable ('soluble') fraction of homogenates can be fully studied by homogenization procedures. These, at least, would be unaffected by the disturbance to intra-cellular membranes and solid structures induced by the homogenization. The study by Altman and Chayen (1966) suggested that the 'soluble' dehydrogenases of the pentose-shunt (hexose mono-phosphate pathway) might, in fact, be bound in a very labile form to the endoplasmic reticulum; they are 'soluble' because they are readily disjuncted from their sub-cellular structure by mechanical trauma. Moreover, Altman *et al*. (1970) showed that the physico-chemical properties of these enzymes could be drastically altered by quite small changes in the homogenization conditions. The fact that the conditions of isolating enzymes can cause great changes in their physical chemistry has been shown by Mahler (1953), Mahler *et al*. (1953), and has been emphasized by Siekevitz (1962), among others. But here we wish to emphasize the possibility that, in the intact cell, the so-called soluble enzymes which are responsible for much of the NADPH of the cytosol may, in fact, be linked in a labile form to the cytoplasmic microsomal respiratory system which is one of the major pathways for reducing equivalents from cytoplasmic NADPH, and NADH (see Chayen *et al.,* 1973). The significance of the microsomal respiratory system and cytochrome P450 have been discussed in Gillette *et al*. (1969), in which it has been suggested that the attempts to purify the components, from their endoplasmic reticulum matrix, may produce misleading activities and results (Kamin, 1969). Thus steroids can influence all these cytoplasmic enzymes and possibly many other, as yet 'soluble' enzymes, by alteration of the physical matrix to which they are linked. Consequently, increasingly workers are coming to regard activity and cellular structure as inter-linked (see Siekevitz). As Bittar (1964) commented: 'In any case, it is well recognized that a cellular enzyme is a part of structure and that structure and function are inseparable at the molecular level. Since the cell is a multiphase system, and the bulk of the available knowledge is based on enzyme activities in the test tube, the next line of attack is obviously one of charting enzyme and pH relationships in terms of regional distribution in the cell'. It is therefore not surprising that biochemists are turning more to the study of heterogeneous phase chemistry, and finding that it yields more information about the intricacies of cellular biochemistry than could be achieved by the more conventional homogeneous phase biochemistry. In concluding their review, McLaren and Packer (1970) say: 'Clearly, great progress in understanding life processes is emerging as biochemical, biophysical, and structural considerations are treated in an integrated conceptual framework'.

4. Effect on Lipid-Protein Associations

We have seen that most biochemical activities in cells probably take place at surfaces or even inside structures in a micro-environment different from the environment of the 'cell sap' or from that used in conventional biochemistry. The structural matrix to which enzymes are bound, or which affects enzymic activity in other ways, is generally composed of complexes of lipids and proteins, assumably stabilized by steroids. Recently the development of specific fluorescent probes has stimulated interest in determining configurational and other changes which affect both the charge density and the hydrophilic or hydrophobic nature of cellular membranes (see, for example, Radda, 1971). Mazanowska et al. (1966) showed that the activity of certain enzymes depended on the association of these enzymes with phospholipids in the structure to which the enzymes were linked. At the level of molecular organization, Monod et al. (1965) suggested that conformational changes in oligomeric enzymes may function to cover over hydrophobic areas of the monomers, and so to enhance enzyme activity.

Cytochemical methods have shown that one of the most sensitive indicators of cell disturbance, in its widest sense, is a change in the linkage between lipids and proteins of cell and sub-cellular membranes, with concomitant increase in lipophilia (and assumably of hydrophobia). This subject has been reviewed fairly extensively (Chayen, 1968a; Chayen and Bitensky, 1973). The cytochemical methods are highly sensitive and open a promising field of enquiry into the influence of steroids on the membranes of cells and of sub-cellular components.

5. Requirements for the Study of Steroid Pharmacology

From the previous discussion (above) it follows that the study of the mode of action of steroids, and the cellular response to steroid therapy, requires subtle methods of investigation. Homogeneous phase biochemistry on isolated and purified enzymes has given some information concerning the direct effect of steroids, but even for such direct effects the homogenization and isolation procedures may have suppressed some of the effects, as suggested by Monod *et al.* (1965) and by the work of Siekevitz (1962) and of Altman *et al.* (1970). For the indirect effect of steroids, acting on living cells, we require (a) a method of allowing the steroids to be incorporated into active cells; (b) techniques for investigating their effects on the relatively intact heterogeneous phase cellular systems. It was to meet these requirements that the newer methods of cellular biochemistry have been developed. These procedures are fairly recent and therefore require to be explained (below).

II. METHODS OF CELLULAR BIOCHEMISTRY

1. General Considerations

'Cellular biochemistry' and 'Cytochemistry' appear to be synonymous. The reason for using the former title is related to the usages which have become associated with the terms 'histochemistry' and 'cytochemistry'. Some twenty years ago there was a movement, particularly led by Danielli (1953), to make cytochemistry a precise subject dealing with the biochemistry of cells. This trend has been continued by Glick (e.g. 1967) who has developed a very accurate form of quantitative histochemistry, namely the biochemistry of tissue sections. The vast majority of workers in histochemistry, however, have followed Barka and Anderson's (1963) definition of this subject, namely: 'Finite measurement is not the immediate goal of microscopic histochemistry. Deriving its theoretical foundations from chemistry, histochemistry remains essentially a morphological tool . . . Histochemistry is a system of chemical morphology that adds another dimension to histology but which shares the basically static character of the morphological sciences. Its contribution cannot be assessed in the dynamic, physiological terms of biochemistry'. Consequently the term 'histochemistry', and even 'cytochemistry', has come to mean a way of staining tissues, or cells, to demonstrate the location of certain chemical substances or active groups. Because such workers are not concerned with amounts of substances or with activities of enzymes and because they seek the site of the selected substance even with the resolution of electron microscopy, they have to fix their cells chemically and so denature them, with the attendant inhibition of enzyme activity which chemical fixation imposes. In fact, as we shall discuss, enzyme translocation can be stopped without chemical fixation, but the use of colloid stabilizers for this purpose is a relatively recent development. Consequently those workers whose prime interest is the biochemical activity, and functional activity, of cells, have had to refer to their subject as cellular biochemistry rather than histochemistry or cytochemistry which have now developed rigidly morphological connotations unrelated to, and even at times antagonistic to, the quantitative biochemistry and biochemical activity of cells.

A. METHODS OF PREPARING AND REACTING THE SPECIMEN

1. Chilling and Sectioning

Although homogenate biochemistry is very widely practised, the older form of tissue-slice biochemistry is still much used. It has the advantage that the tissue is retained relatively intact. The slices used are often of the order of 200 μ thick and this is too thick to allow us to relate biochemical activity to specific components of the tissue. To achieve this aim, the slices have to be not thicker than 20 μ; they have to be acceptable histological preparations; and yet their preparation must involve no inactivation of the active groups or enzymes, and no treatment with solvents. To cut such sections the tissue must be hardened. It has been known for a very long time that this can be achieved by freezing tissue and cutting frozen sections but such procedures are liable to cause structural and chemical damage by virtue of the ice which forms in the cells during freezing and freeze-sectioning. The ice causes damage both directly, when the ice crystals form inside the cells, and indirectly as a consequence of changes in the tonicity of the extra- and intra-cellular fluids (e.g. Lovelock, 1957). These problems have been fully reviewed by Luyet (1951), Meryman (1957), Asahina (1966) and by Chayen and Bitensky (1968). It was found, however, that if tissue was chilled under precise conditions, the protoplasmic water could be chilled to below $-40°C$ without forming ice crystals; the protoplasm could be super-cooled and solidified (Lynch et al., 1966; also see Luyet, 1951). Consequently the first step in the preparation of tissue sections for cellular biochemistry is to chill the tissue by precipitate immersion, for 30 sec to 1 min in n-hexane (free from aromatic hydrocarbons, boiling range 67-70°C) at $-70°C$. It has been shown that the centre of a specimen of rat liver 5 x 5 x 3 mm taken from the ambient temperature of the laboratory reaches a temperature of $-40°C$ in 9 sec under these conditions. This is twice as rapid as when the tissue is immersed in liquid nitrogen (Moline and Glenner, 1964). The hexane, at this temperature and acting for this period of time, has no solvent action. However, where it is important to localize (for example by autoradiography) soluble, low-molecular-weight compounds, which might be affected by the use of hexane, it is possible to achieve good histological preservation by pressing the specimen gently against the inside of a glass tube which has been cooled to $-70°C$ (Cunningham et al., 1962).

The super-cooled tissue is sectioned in a cryostat, at a cabinet temperature of -25 to $-30°C$ and with the haft of the knife chilled by being packed around with solid CO_2. Under these conditions the heat of sectioning appears to be dissipated into the knife rather than into the tissue (Silcox et al., 1965). The section, lying on the knife at about $-70°C$, is 'flash-dried' by bringing a glass slide, from the ambient temperature of the laboratory, up to it. As the slide approaches the section there is a temperature gradient of at least $90°C$ over a gap of a few millimetres; the tissue water flashes off from the section on to the knife, where it condenses, and the section is ejected from the knife on to the glass slide. It has been shown by double immersion refractometry that such sections are virtually free of water. These methods have been discussed by Chayen and Bitensky (1968) and by Chayen *et al.* (1969a; 1972a).

2. Problems of Incubating Tissue Sections

When dry, undenatured 10μ or 20μ sections of liver are immersed in an aqueous medium to test biochemical activities, they may lose up to 70% of their nitrogenous matter (Jones, 1965) and all their 'soluble' enzymes very rapidly. This is one reason why histochemists have preferred either to fix their sections with chemical fixatives which precipitate or coagulate much of the protoplasm, or to denature the protoplasm with alcohol or acetone. Yet it has been shown that the addition of high concentrations of relatively inert colloid stabilizers can stop this loss both of nitrogenous matter and of 'soluble' enzymes. The most widely used of these stabilizers is one or other of two particular grades of polyvinyl alcohol (PVA; used at 20% w/v), first used by Altman and Chayen (1965; 1966; also Altman, 1971a; 1972a,b); a polypeptide derived from degraded collagen (used at 30% w/v) has proved equally valuable (Stuart *et al.*, 1969; Butcher, 1971a) and Ficoll has also been successfully used (Stuart and Simpson, 1970). It has been shown that such stabilizers do not inhibit enzyme activity but retain full activity of 'soluble' dehydrogenases over reasonably long incubation times, so that the same activity, in absolute terms, can be obtained in sections as in homogenates of the same organ (Altman, 1972b). These techniques were essential if tissue section biochemistry was to be usable as a precise and quantitative form of heterogeneous phase (or multiphase) biochemistry.

In demonstrating dehydrogenating enzyme activity the sections are exposed to the reaction medium, which contains the colloid stabilizer, and which is buffered to the pH which is optimal for the activity to be studied. Hydrogen is removed from the substrate and hydrogen (or hydride ions and protons, i.e. $[H^+ + 2e^-]$ and H^+) is first transmitted to a co-enzyme, like NADP or NAD, or to some similarly functioning receptor, like flavoprotein (which accepts hydrogen) in the case of succinate dehydrogenase. This hydrogen can be transmitted, quantitatively, to a tetrazolium salt such as neotetrazolium, if a suitable intermediate such as phenazine methosulphate (PMS) is present in the reaction medium (Altman, 1972b). In the absence of such an intermediate, the hydrogen can react with a tetrazolium salt, just as it would with methylene blue in the old Thunberg tube studies on tissue respiration, only after it had been passed through a tissue hydrogen-transport system and brought to an electrode potential at which it can react rapidly with the selected tetrazolium salt (Altman, 1972a). Tetrazolium salts with very negative F_0' can react slowly with the NADPH and NADH even in the absence of tissue mediation. In the case of succinate dehydrogenase, the hydrogen-transport system would be that present in mitochondria. Consequently the amount of tetrazolium salt which would be reduced (to be precipitated in the section as a coloured formazan) would depend only partly on the actual potential activity of the dehydrogenase; the factor limiting the rate of production of formazan would be the efficiency of the hydrogen-transport chain. This rate can be measured by excluding PMS from the reaction medium; the efficiency of different parts of the hydrogen-transport chain can be assessed by using tetrazoles which become reduced at different electrode potentials, corresponding to different points in the hydrogen-transport chain. Admittedly the rate of production of formazan from the different tetrazoles depends on kinetic factors as well as on their relative electrode potentials.

In practical terms tissue sections of the supercooled tissue are cut at a defined thickness ($10-20\ \mu$) as described on pp. 11–12. The dried section is taken into a room, maintained at $37°C$ and a ring of Perspex, of diameter just greater than the section, is placed around the section. The reaction medium, adjusted for optimal concentrations of reactants and for pH, which has been saturated with nitrogen and equilibrated to $37°C$, is then poured into the Perspex well. The tissue section, with the reaction medium, is maintained in an atmosphere of nitrogen at 100% humidity. An atmosphere of nitrogen is required when the tetrazolium salt has a more electropositive standard electrode potential. Such tetrazoles, e.g. neotetrazolium, are unable to compete adequately with atmospheric oxygen as hydrogen acceptors in normal tissues (Altman, 1970); in this respect they are comparable to methylene blue, as used in the Thunberg respiration systems.

3. The Assessment of Lysosomal Membrane Function

The study of hydrolytic enzymes present in lysosomes requires a more subtle approach because it is only rarely of interest to know if there has been net change in the total activity of these enzymes. According to our present understanding, these enzymes are peculiar in cellular chemistry in that they are fully active and are not apparently bound to a complex matrix, as are the enzymes of mitochondria. It may be that this view will change as more detailed studies are made of these hydrolases. But, at present, it seems that they are present in a fully active state but sequestered from the cytoplasm—and incidentally from substrates used for testing their activity—by a semi-permeable lysosomal membrane. This membrane fuses with endocytotic and phagocytotic vacuoles to form secondary lysosomes, or to form large phagosomes, in which hydrolysis of phagocytosed matter takes place, still sequestered from the rest of the cell inside the vacuolar system, which is analogous to the digestive tract. Moreover, parts of the cell itself, such as fragments of endoplasmic reticulum or even mitochondria, can be engulfed by lysosomes and degraded inside cytolysomes (or autophagosomes). This process is enhanced in certain disease conditions. It may also happen that the lysosomes may fuse with the cell membrane and eject either separate hydrolases, or packets of lysosomal contents (Dingle, 1968) into the extra-cellular environment. These processes may also involve the 'processing of antigen' (Weissmann, 1966) and there is some suggestion that unstable lysosomes, that is lysosomes with abnormally fragile membranes, may be inefficient in this process and give rise to new antigenic material which can maintain a chronic inflammatory state (as discussed above, and by Chayen and Bitensky, 1971; see also Dingle and Fell (1969) and Dingle (1973)). All these effects, which can profoundly affect cellular and extra-cellular metabolism, depend on the state of the lysosomal membrane rather than on fluctuations in total content of lysosomal enzymes. Hence the study of lysosomal intervention in cellular biochemistry requires a measure of lysosomal membrane function; this function can be markedly affected by steroids (Weissmann, 1968, 1969). The same arguments may also apply when considering the function of peroxisomes.

Cellular biochemical methods are ideally suited for such investigations, partly because the lysosomes are retained inside their cytoplasm during the tests. These can be done in one of two ways. The older, now well established technique, involves Bitensky's (1962, 1963a,b) fragility test. This depends on the cytochemical demonstration of acid phosphatase activity. The substrate, β-glycerophosphate, does not readily penetrate intact, normal lysosomal membranes; consequently no reaction would be produced. But lysosomal membranes are altered by acetate buffer, at 37°C, at pH 5.0 so that, with time, they become permeable to the substrate and a reaction product forms. The time taken to obtain a just discernable reaction product in relatively normal cells is found and compared with the time taken to obtain this amount of reaction in the abnormal or treated cells. Thus the reaction depends on the time required, in acidic acetate, to bring the lysosomal membranes to a standard level of permeability to β-glycerophosphate. A more kinetic approach is that described by Chayen (1968b).

The second technique depends on the demonstration of lysosomal naphthylamidases (e.g. Tappel, 1969) in which the substrate is leucine-2-naphthylamide the hydrolysis of which yields naphthylamine which is coupled to Fast blue B to form a precipitated dye. This method, by Nachlas et al. (1957) was used by Sylvén and Bois-Svensson (1964) and by McCabe and Chayen (1965) for demonstrating lysosomal activity. Its validity, and the measurement of the reaction product, have been discussed by Bitensky et al. (1973). In brief, normal lysosomal membranes are somewhat permeable to this substrate but they do impose a restriction on the rate of lysosomal naphthylamidase activity. This restriction is changed, by acetate buffer even at the higher pH of pH 6.5, and the latency of the naphthylamidase can be demonstrated either by plotting activity against time of incubation (Fig. 1) or measuring the activity directly and comparing it with the maximum activity which can be produced by pre-incubation at 37°C in acetate buffer at pH 5.0 (see for example Chayen et al., 1971a). Such measurements give the proportion between the activity which is readily manifest to this substrate and that which is latent, or 'bound' and not available until the lysosomal membranes are rendered fully permeable to this

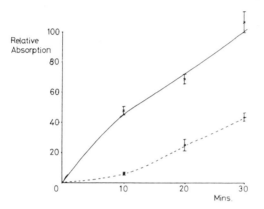

Fig. 1. Naphthylamidase activity (relative absorption/unit field, measured by a scanning and integrating micro-densitometer) against increasing time of incubation, in human synovial lining cells. In non-rheumatoid cells (broken line) there is no appreciable activity for the first 10 min during which time the enzyme activity is latent. Thereafter the activity rises linearly with time, showing that this lysosomal enzyme is now manifest. In contrast, in the synovial lining cells from rheumatoid tissue (solid line) there is no latency, the activity rising steeply with time of incubation. (Reproduced with permission from Chayen et al., 1971a).

substrate. This 'manifest: latent' activity is, in many ways, comparable to the 'free : bound' ratio used by biochemists who study lysosomal activity in homogenates. The proportion of 'latent', or 'bound', activity, as a percentage of the total (maximum) activity, is a measure of the functional state of the lysosomal membranes; these activities can be measured accurately by scanning and integrating microdensitometry.

4. The Assessment of Mitochondrial Activity

Even in the absence of increase or decrease in the enzyme content, mitochondrial activity is governed by many factors. These include the permeability of the mitochondrial outer membrane, for which monoamine oxidase activity is often a useful parameter; changes in permeability into the body of the mitochondrion; and the efficiency of the hydrogen-transport system. The last mentioned factor can be measured by testing the mitochondrial oxidation of a suitable substrate, such as glutamate or succinate, in the presence of PMS (for testing the dehydrogenase activity directly) or in its absence, with a tetrazole such as neotetrazolium which accepts hydrogen late in the hydrogen-transport chain. Studies of this type, and the problems related to them, have been discussed by Butcher (1970, 1972a; also see Altman, 1972b). Up to the present, the investigations which have proved of most value in assessing the effect of steroids have been concerned with the enhanced monoamine oxidase activity which occurs when the mitochondrial membranes are rendered more permeable to the substrate, which may be tryptamine or adrenaline (e.g. Diengdoh, 1965; Chayen *et al.*, 1970b). Some care must be exercised with this assessment, however, unless a test of maximal activity is also made. Otherwise this labile enzyme can readily be lost from mitochondria when the mito-chondrial membrane is over-permeable. For all that, the effect of stabilizers of mitochondrial membranes, such as promethazine (Chayen and Bitensky, 1973) and steroids (Chayen *et al.*, 1970b), acting on tissue maintained *in vitro*, can be readily demonstrated by this test.

B. QUANTITATION

The aim of quantitative histochemical, or cellular biochemical, techniques is to precipitate a coloured end-product of the reaction in the cell in which the activity occurs. This facilitates relating the activity to a particular region of the tissue, or to a particular cell type, or even to a specified cell. The method selected for measuring the activity depends on the information required. Elution methods alone give the amount of activity of the whole section. This frequently is sufficient information, particularly when the tissue may be considered as a relatively homogeneous population of similar cells. This assumption is used in homogenate biochemistry of the liver; in so far as it is valid, the same assumption can be used for sections of liver. However, it is obvious that not even liver should be regarded, rigorously, as a homogenous population of hepatocytes. The contribution made by bile duct, connective and littoral cells, which together constitute some 40% of the total number of cells (Daoust and Cantero, 1959), is appreciable. Changes in the relative proportions of these cells to the hepatocytes have led to erroneous conclusions concerning the metabolic changes which occur in the liver subjected to toxic or carcinogenic agents (Chayen *et al.*, 1961; Jones *et al.*, 1961; Jones, 1963). But even among the hepatocytes, those in the periportal regions have different metabolic activities from those in the centrilobular sites (Fig. 3, on p. 19); this may be the basis of the different sites of necrosis found with different toxic agents (Chayen *et al.*, 1973). This type of information, namely the variation of activity in the different histological sites, can be obtained by double-beam recording microdensitometry of the reacted sections; this technique does not exclude the possibility of also eluting the coloured end-product. Finally, the activity in each selected cell, especially in those reactions where the reaction product is not evenly dispersed throughout the cell (as with lysosomal activities), can be measured accurately only by scanning the integrating microdensitometry.

1. Elution techniques

The idea that the amount of an enzyme reaction in a tissue section can be quantified is not new. Kun and Abood (1949) measured succinate dehydrogenase activity in sections by eluting the formazan produced by the reduction of triphenyltetrazolium. Defendi and Pearson (1955) and Jardetsky and Glick (1956) measured the activity of the same enzyme when neotetrazolium was the sole hydrogen acceptor. In all these studies (also Jones et al., 1963) the activity was expressed as weight (μg) of formazan produced (and measured spectrophotometrically), per unit of tissue section. Such investigations measure the amount of hydrogen which, generated by the oxidation of succinate, is processed by the hydrogen-transport system of the mitochondria. The use of tetrazolium salts which are reduced at higher electrode potentials, and with greater kinetic efficiency, allows a closer assessment of the primary dehydrogenase activity, which is more relatable to more biochemical estimations; the use of phenazine methosulphate as an intermediate hydrogen carrier is even more beneficial. The elution of the formazans from the more electro-negative and more efficient tetrazoles is more difficult than when neotetrazolium is used; methods for the quantitative elution of all commonly used tetrazolium salts have now been described (Altman, 1969a,b; 1972a,b). Moreover Altman (1969c, 1972b) has shown that the amount of hydrogen liberated in unit time by pentose-shunt dehydrogenases in tissue sections, calculated from the amount of formazan precipitated, and eluted and measured spectrophotometrically, is comparable to the amount measured in homogenates of the same organ (and estimated by the change NADP $\rightarrow$ NADPH, measured spectrophotometrically). Similarly, Butcher (1970) found that the K_m/K_i (using malonate as inhibitor) for succinate dehydrogenase, in the presence of PMS, was 48 when measured in tissue sections of rat liver, as against the value of 50 found by Potter and Du Bois (1943) in homogenates. Thus it appears that the elution methods can give the same quantitative data as can be obtained by more conventional, larger-scale biochemical analysis.

In practice the section, with the coloured reaction product (which may be a formazan, but could equally be the reaction product of any chromogenic enzyme reaction), is washed free of reactants and dried. The area of the section is measured by planimetry of its image magnified by projection through a photographic enlarger. The section, on the glass support is cut out of the glass slide and the fragment of glass plus section is dropped into a test tube and covered with the solvent most suitable for the particular reaction product (Altman, 1969a,b; 1972a). Normally 0.5 ml of solvent is sufficient. The coloured solution is then measured in a micro-cell of a standard spectrophotometer and the amount of formazan, and thus the μmoles of hydrogen which this represents, can be calculated. These procedures give the enzyme activity in terms of μmoles of hydrogen/unit area of tissue/unit time of reaction (see Altman, 1972a,b). Normally, 4-6 sections are taken for each estimation and the standard deviation should not be more than ±10%. Under ideal conditions the reproducibility can be ±1%.

To calculate the activity per unit volume of tissue either one has to assume the thickness of the sections to be equal to the setting of the microtome, or one has to have some parameter of thickness. For any one experienced worker, particularly if he uses an automatic sectioning device as is fitted to Bright's cryostats, the thickness will probably be constant throughout his studies (see Butcher, 1971b). But the actual thickness will vary according to the speed at which the sections are cut, and this may vary from one worker to the next. It may therefore be advisable to use the nucleic acid content of the section as the tissue-mass parameter, that is to give the activity as μmoles of hydrogen/unit nucleic acid/unit time. This is recommended because, particularly if the collagen polypeptide (Butcher, 1971a) is used as colloid stabilizer, it is relatively simple to

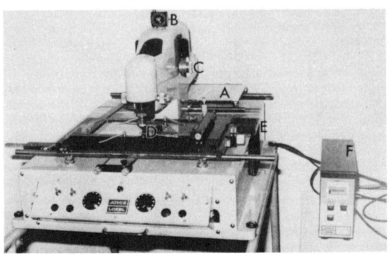

Fig. 2. The Joyce–Loebl double-beam recording micro-densitometer (reproduced with permission from Altman, 1971b). This instrument is used for microdensitometry of sections and of negatives of interference images (as in Figs 5 and 6). A: the moving recording table, geared to the moving specimen table (D) on which a pen traces the changes in absorption. B and C: controls for determining the height and width of the scanning slit. E: lamp housing. F: integrator, which integrates the area under the trace.

measure the nucleic acid content of the sections after the formazan has been eluted from them (Butcher, 1968, 1971b). Alternatively, the estimation of the amount of nitrogen in these sections can be made (Sloane–Stanley, 1967), but these estimations are not easy to do and may be liable to more error than the estimation of nucleic acids.

2. Microdensitometry

Elution methods give the amount of reaction product, and hence of activity (assuming that stoichiometry has been proven), in the whole section. To obtain a measure of how this activity is distributed in the histologically distinct regions of

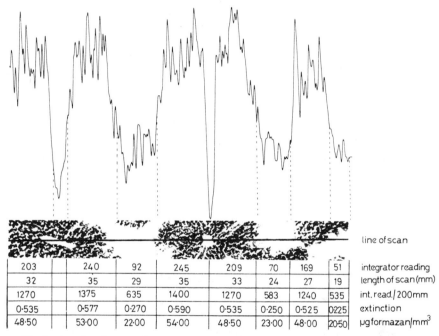

203		240	92	245	209	70	169	51	integrator reading
32		35	29	35	33	24	27	19	length of scan (mm)
1270		1375	635	1400	1270	583	1240	535	int. read./200mm
0·535		0·577	0·270	0·590	0·535	0·250	0·525	0225	extinction
48·50		53·00	22·00	54·00	48·50	23·00	48·00	2050	µg formazan/mm³

line of scan

Fig. 3. A strip of the section of rat liver reacted for glucose 6-phosphate dehydrogenase activity, shows the line of the scan (magnification x57). Above it is shown the microdensitometric trace, obtained for that scan, by the Joyce–Loebl microdensitometer. The steps needed to calculate the amount of formazan in each region are shown. (Reproduced with permission from Altman, 1971b.)

the section, recourse is made to microdensitometry (Altman, 1971b). After the reaction is complete, the reacted (coloured) section is placed on the stage of a Joyce–Loebl double-beam recording microdensitometer (Fig. 2). The section is then traversed across the objective (x20 magnification is often sufficient) and the image is projected on to a photocell. The amount of light impinging on the photocell is balanced by light passing through a movable graded density wedge and the movement of this wedge is reflected by the movement of a recording pen. This pen thus traces out changes in absorption while the section is moved, by motor, across the objective. Inspection of the regions scanned allows correlation to be made of histological detail and absorption (Fig. 3). The trace of absorption can be calibrated in terms of μg formazan/cm^2 from suitable calibration curves and by using a device for integrating the area under each region of the trace. Calibration curves (Altman, 1971b) are obtained by eluting the coloured reaction-product from sections in which the colour is reasonably homogeneously distributed and plotting μg formazan/cm^2 (from elution studies) against absolute extinction; similarly the integrated readings on the micro-densitometer are calibrated against absolute units of extinction by tracing across neutral density filters of known extinction (see Altman, 1971b).

3. Scanning and Integrating Microdensitometry

There are now a number of cytochemical reactions which are stoichiometric provided, of course, they are done under precise conditions. Almost invariably they produce an inhomogeneously distributed coloured precipitated reaction product. The inhomogeneity may be a reflection of the nature of the precipitate, as in the case of the formazan produced by the reduction of neotetrazolium in measuring oxidative metabolism, or it may reflect the nature and distribution of the active sites inside the cell. This inhomogeneous distribution of the coloured matter which is to be measured is the major problem in applying normal spectrophotometric procedures to cellular biochemistry (see Chayen and Denby, 1968 for discussion of inhomogeneity errors and the use of this form of microdensitometry). It is readily overcome by the use of a scanning and integrating microdensitometer such as the Barr and Stroud GN2 (Fig. 4) or the Vickers M85. In principle these instruments scan the cell or groups of cells, selected in a conventional microscope, with a scanning spot which can be made to be as small as 0.25 μ, this being the limit of resolution of the microscope, so that each spot is optically homogeneous as far as the microscope optics can discern. The light from each spot is transmitted to a photomultiplier and the amount of light from all the spots of the selected field is integrated. By beginning with a value for 100% transmission, the amount of light in each field is converted, instrumentally, into the amount of absorption. This absorption, given instrumentally in relative absorption units, is directly proportional to extinction; this can be converted into absolute units of extinction by calibrating the instrumental response against graded neutral density filters of known absolute extinction values. Thus it is possible to measure enzyme activity in single cells, whether isolated naturally or by optical means, in terms of extinction (equivalent to amount of coloured reaction product) measured at the absorption maximum of the colour (selected by the monochromating system of the microdensitometer). The details of such measurements, for hydrolytic as well as for oxidative enzyme activity, have been discussed recently (Bitensky *et al.*, 1973).

To convert integrated extinction/cell to the amount of dye present per cell requires knowledge of the extinction coefficient of the dye as it occurs in the

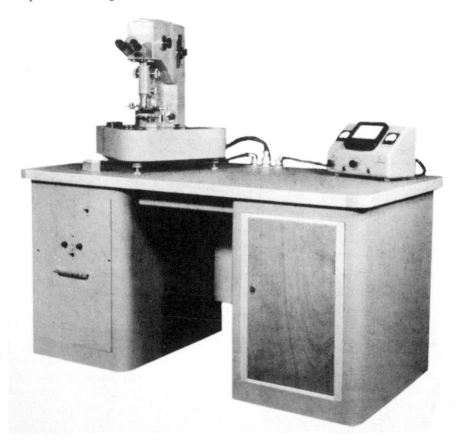

Fig. 4. A scanning and integrating microdensitometer (the Barr and Stroud GN2, reproduced by permission of Barr and Stroud Ltd.). This consists of a conventional microscope with a scanning system and photomultiplier in the top and back of the microscope casing. The electronics are in the cabinet at the left. The meter, showing relative absorption, is on the bench-top, on the right.

solid state in the cell. Generally this step is not required if relative activities only are to be measured. But the extinction coefficient can be calculated, as has been done by Butcher (1972b), and highly accurate measurements of the amount of dye can be made taking into account the changes in the extinction coefficient which occur when the dye becomes bound to different sub-cellular surfaces and when the dye-molecules aggregate (see Butcher, 1972b). This involves finding the isobestic point for the different absorption curves and calculating the extinction coefficient at that point. From such studies it is possible to calculate oxidative activity in terms of μmoles hydrogen/cell/unit time and hydrolytic activity as the number of bonds hydrolysed/cell/unit time.

4. The Measurement of Tissue Water

In general chemistry, particularly in protein chemistry, it is known that when light passes through a solution, it is retarded in direct proportion to the weight of solute present per 100 ml of solvent. This means that for every gramme of protein in 100 ml of water, the refractive index of the solution will increase by a particular value, known as the specific refractive increment. Thus the refractive index of water is 1.334; the refractive index of a solution containing 1 g of protein in 100 ml of water will be 1.334 plus the specific refractive increment of protein (which is about 0.0018), giving a refractive index of 1.3358. This property is used in quantitative interference microscopy which measures changes in refractive index and thus the absolute concentration of dry matter (Davies *et al.,* 1954; Ross, 1967; Chayen, 1967; Chayen and Denby, 1968). From this parameter, changes in water content can be calculated.

Measurement of water content both inside each cell and in the inter-cellular environment is of great significance in many studies. It is obviously important where it is necessary to quantify the extent of oedema, whether this occurs primarily inside or outside cells, and so to assess the anti-oedema action of drugs or steroids. The intra-cellular water balance gives a measure of how well the cell membrane acts as a semi-permeable membrane and how effective is the osmotic work done by the cells. Extra-cellular oedema, especially in the vicinity of small capillaries and lymphatics, is a measure of the permeability or over-permeability of these vessels and hence of how effective steroids may be in restoring their normal permeability properties (e.g. Chayen *et al.*, 1970b; 1971b). In the newer developments of this technique sections of the tissue, for example skin, are examined before and after treatment with a substance (such as histamine) which induces oedema. The tissue is photographed by interference microscopy in monochromatic light; under these conditions variations in mass are seen as variations in density in the photographic negative. These variations are recorded by means of a Joyce–Loebl double-beam recording microdensitometer and the effect of the oedema can be quantified by integrating the amount of mass per unit area of selected regions (Figs 5 and 6). If the tissue is treated with an anti-oedema agent, the efficacy of this agent in reducing the histamine-induced oedema can be measured.

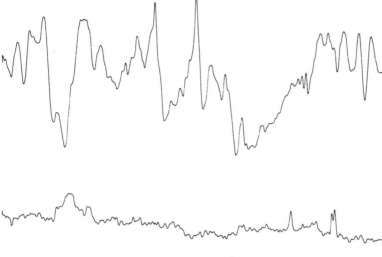

INTEGRATED READING/ CM. = 83·3

Fig. 5.

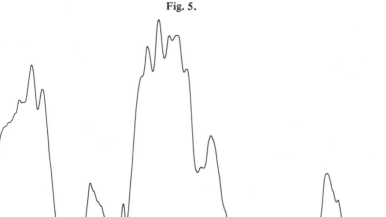

INTEGRATED READING/ CM. = 51·5

Figs 5 and 6. Microdensitometer traces through the interferometric image of the dermis, parallel to the epidermis, in photographic negatives of human skin, photographed with monochromatic light. Both samples of skin have been maintained *in vitro*. That in Fig. 5 was not subjected to any further treatment; that shown in Fig. 6 had been exposed to 10^{-7} M histamine. The mass/unit area in Fig. 5 is obviously greater than in Fig. 6, as shown qualitatively by the general height of the trace above the base line and quantitatively by the integrated reading per unit length of trace. The extensive oedema, induced by histamine, is seen as the regions of the trace, in Fig. 6, which approximate to the base line (i.e. equal to the field outside the specimen). This oedema has caused redistribution of mass, as evidenced by the greater height of some parts of the trace in Fig. 6.

C. CULTURE METHODS

1. Methodology

We have said that the biochemical and pharmacological effect of steroids can be due to either a direct or an indirect action; in the latter the molecules, possibly modified by the cells, are actively incorporated into structural components of the living cells. Consequently, to test the indirect effect it is necessary to apply the steroids to living cells and to test the biochemical changes subsequently by the methods of cellular biochemistry which have already been discussed. There is some dichotomy of view as to what type of living cells should be used for such studies. Prompted largely, in all probability, by the need for a large bulk (milligramme amounts) of tissue of homogeneous cell type, many biochemists have used proliferative cell culture of a particular cell type. We do not advocate this course of action for a number of reasons. Firstly it is well known that cells in proliferative culture do not behave in the same way as do the cells, from which these came, in organized tissue; in brief, fibroblasts in culture are not identical, structurally or chemically, with fibrocytes in the heart or skin. This is obvious in proliferating cell culture because a mitotically active cell suppresses many of the activities that it requires in its non-mitotic, specialized state, and calls into play many other activities which are specifically required for cell division. But it also applies albeit less obviously to the cells in a tissue culture which has ceased to proliferate (e.g. Fell, 1969). But the most serious objection lies in the fact that the effect of drugs and steroids may apply differently to the different cell types in an organized tissue, and that cells in organized tissue, embedded in the inter-cellular material that is so important for the integrity of the tissue, interact with one another and with the extra-cellular environment. For example, Lever (1967) has suggested that the major lesion in psoriasis is in the dermis and that this influences the epidermal changes; the beneficial effect of topical steroids (fluclorolone acetonide and betamethasone-17-valerate) has been linked with their action on the dermis (Chayen et al., 1971b). Not all workers agree with Lever, but the controversy is raised in order to show how misleading it may be to study only one cell type in the response of a complex tissue to injury, disease and to steroid action.

For these reasons we have preferred to study adult tissue maintained in non-proliferative culture. The methods were fully described by Trowell (1959, 1965); they have been used to maintain various human and animal tissues, as will be discussed below. In this system small pieces of the adult tissue are placed on a defatted lens tissue which lies on a table made of expanded metal grid. This table is stood in a vitreosil dish in a larger container (now made of glass) which has entry and exit leads for the gas supply; this container acts as a gas reservoir. The lid of the container is pierced with a number of holes, which can be sealed, to facilitate removal and replacement of the culture medium which is pipetted into the vitreosil dish up to the level of the top of the table (Fig. 7). Thus the tissue is fed from below; it stands in the moist gas phase (95% oxygen : 5% carbon dioxide). The culture medium basically is Trowell's T8 synthetic medium; to it is added such particular additives as are found necessary for the maintenance of the full structure and biochemical activity of the particular tissue to be maintained. In general the tissue is left for 5 hr to recover from the trauma involved in its removal from the body and in cutting the small pieces for culture. From then onwards it can be subjected to precisely known concentrations of pharmacologically active agents, acting for defined periods of time. Tissue is not usually kept for more than 1-2 days in this system, although other workers have

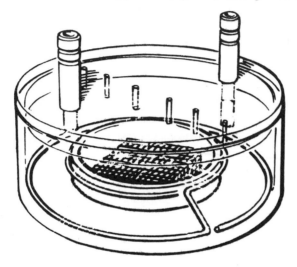

Fig. 7. Drawing of the chamber used for Trowell culture. (By permission of Frost Instruments Ltd.)

maintained tissue for weeks in this way. This maintenance of adult tissue has not achieved widespread acceptance in the past because the pieces which can be cultured (e.g. 3-mm strips of human skin, 3 mm long) are too small for the more conventional methods of biochemical analysis; they are ideal for the techniques of cellular biochemistry which have been outlined above.

2. Use of Culture Procedure for Assessing the Effect of Steroids in Breast Cancers

The clearest illustration of the cellular biological type of information which can be obtained simply by maintaining tissue *in vitro*, comes from studies designed to test whether it was possible to distinguish between steroid-dependent and steroid-independent breast cancers (Altman and Chayen, 1968;

Altman *et al.*, 1968; Chayen *et al.*, 1970a). The question which was posed was very simple: if some breast cancers require oestrogen to maintain their existence they should die if kept in maintenance culture *in vitro* with no added oestrogen; those which are not so dependent on oestrogen should survive under these conditions. To test this question, samples taken at operation were put into maintenance culture with Trowell's T8 medium, fortified with ascorbate and glutathione (both at 10^{-4} M) which gave better maintenance of the stroma. Times of culture varied from 5 hr to 24 hr. Sixteen specimens of carcinoma (adenocarcinoma of different degrees of differentiation and scirrhous adeno-carcinoma) were tested; specimens from seven patients with benign cystic fibroepithelial hyperplasia were tested as controls. All the latter were not influenced by the presence or absence of oestradiol. Seven of the sixteen malignant tissues died in the absence of oestradiol; they survived well, as seen histologically, if sufficient oestradiol was included in the culture medium (10^{-4}–10^{-6} M) but this beneficial effect of oestradiol was lost if an equi-molar concentration of drostanolone (10^{-5} M drostanolone : 10^{-5} M oestradiol) was included with the oestradiol in the culture medium. Drostanolone (2α-methyl-17β-hydroxy-5α-androstan-3-one) was selected because it appears to be an effective oestradiol antagonist, in some experiments testosterone was used. Thus there was a distinct difference in the ability of about half the cancers to survive without added oestradiol; this could be seen by sectioning the tissue after maintenance *in vitro*, and staining the sections with haematoxylin and eosin. Supplementary information could be obtained by testing the cancer cells for glucose 6-phosphate dehydrogenase activity (Altman and Chayen, 1968; Altman *et al.*, 1968; also see Altman *et al.*, 1970a,b). These results have been fully confirmed by Salih *et al.* (1972). It is too early yet to say whether the oestrogen dependence of the cells of the primary cancer *in vitro* can be equated with the behaviour of hormone-dependent secondary growths in the body.

3. Maintenance Culture in a Highly Sensitive Bio-assay for ACTH

The new bio-assay for ACTH can be used as an indication of the precision which can be attained when quantitative cellular biochemical methods are applied to the analysis of chemical changes induced by pharmacologically active substances acting on tissue maintained *in vitro*. It is based on the well-established diminution of reductive potency, mainly by depletion of ascorbate, of the adrenal cortex under the influence of adrenocorticotrophic hormone (ACTH). This has been studied extensively and has been the basis of one of the main methods for assaying this hormone (Sayers *et al.*, 1948).

The new bio-assay is based on the following findings. The adrenal glands are removed from one guinea pig and each is cut into three roughly equal segments. Each segment is maintained for 5 hr in the Trowell tissue maintenance system, with the T8 medium reinforced with 10^{-3} M ascorbate. During this period the adrenal tissue recovers from the trauma of removal from the animal and of being cut into segments. It escapes from the effects of the hormonal influence of the animal and it becomes replenished, if need be, with ascorbate. The T8 ascorbate medium is then replaced by the same medium, containing graded concentrations of ACTH and the tissue is left for only 4 min before it is chilled. Later it is

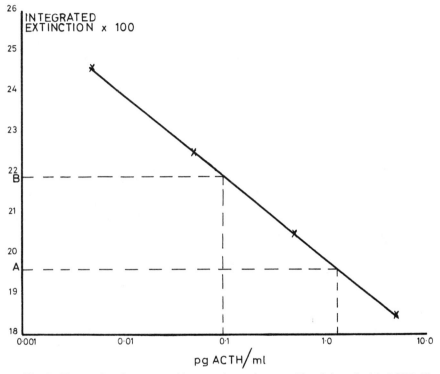

Fig. 8. The results of an assay of human plasma from a subject injected with ACTH. The four points obtained with the graded standard concentrations of ACTH (3rd International Working Standard) fall on the straight regression line. The two dilutions of the plasma (diluted 1 : 100 and 1 : 1,000) are plotted on to this line (A and B). The two dilutions gave values of 95 and 103 pg/ml; mean: 99 pg/ml.

sectioned and tested with a cytochemical method for reducing potency (reduction of ferricyanide, in the presence of ferric ions to yield ferric ferrocyanide, i.e. Prussian blue). The amount of Prussian blue in the zona reticularis is measured by scanning and integrating microdensitometry. It was first found that there was a linear inverse relationship between the amount of Prussian blue per unit area of the zona reticularis and the logarithmic concentration (to the base 10) of ACTH added over the range 0.0025–2.5 pg/ml (Chayen *et al.*, 1971c). It has now been shown that this phenomenon can be used to measure the concentration of ACTH in human plasma (Daly *et al.*, 1972;

Chayen *et al.*, 1972b). Again six segments are taken from the two adrenal glands of a guinea pig and each is placed separately in Trowell maintenance culture for 5 hr with the T8 medium reinforced with 10^{-3} M ascorbate. Four of these are then treated for 4 min with the T8-ascorbate medium which contains one of a graded concentration of the Third International Working Standard for ACTH; the other two are treated with human plasma, usually diluted 1/100 and 1/1,000. These dilutions are suitable for the range of concentrations normally found in humans during the course of the diurnal cycle. The amount of Prussian blue in the zona reticularis in the segments treated with the known concentrations of ACTH is measured and plotted on 5-cycle semi-log graph paper; the intensity of stain, measured in the sections of the tissue which has been treated with the diluted human plasma is read on this calibration graph (Fig. 8). The results of the two dilutions should agree to ±15%; they are usually considerably better than this.

This method assays 0.005–2.5 pg of ACTH ml; the index of precision on a 4 min assay is 0.05; the fiducial limits ($p = 0.95$) of a number of two-by-two assays have varied from ±15% to ±4%. In studies (Rees *et al.*, 1972) in which ACTH has been added to plasma, it has been shown that this new bio-assay gave the same results as did the Lipscomb–Nelson bio-assay (based on steroido-genesis) and the radio-immunoassay (using antibody to both the C-terminal and the N-terminal moiety) at concentrations of 2000 and 500 pg of ACTH/ml and with the radio-immunoassays at 50 pg/ml; only the new bio-assay could detect the lowest level used in this study (approximately 5 pg/ml). Moreover, it was able to measure the decline in plasma ACTH following the intravenous administration of 100 mg of cortisol to a normal male subject; the concentration of ACTH reached 34 femto-gramme/ml (34×10^{-15} g/ml) 4 hr after the steroid had been administered.

III. CELLULAR BIOCHEMICAL MEASUREMENT OF DIRECT EFFECTS OF STEROIDS

A. TYPES 1 AND 2 NADPH PATHWAYS IN SECTIONS

1. Concepts

As discussed above, NADP-dependent oxidative systems, particularly the two dehydrogenase enzymes of the pentose-shunt (hexose monophosphate pathway), can be studied accurately in tissue sections. It has been shown by Altman (1972a,b) that, if phenazine methosulphate (PMS) is used as the intermediate hydrogen carrier, the amount of NADPH generated in a reaction, such as Eq. 1 (involving glucose 6-phosphate dehydrogenase, G6PD), can be measured quantitatively:

$$\text{Glucose 6-phosphate} + \text{NADP} \xrightarrow[-2H]{\text{G6PD}} \text{6-phosphogluconate} + \text{NADPH} + \text{H}^+ \qquad (1)$$

Certain tetrazolium salts, of sufficiently electro-negative standard electrode potentials and with suitable kinetic properties, such as MTT give an almost quantitative measure of the production of NADPH even in the absence of PMS However, neotetrazolium will not react readily with NADPH if the two are added together in a test-tube (i.e. there is no reduction at all after 30 min at 37°C). On the other hand, the reaction

$$\text{NADPH} + \text{neotetrazolium} \rightarrow \text{NADP} + \text{coloured formazan} \qquad (2)$$

does occur if the NADPH and the neotetrazolium are added to a tissue section. Equally, the coloured formazan is produced when glucose 6-phosphate and NADP are used to provide an endogenous source of NADPH in the section, and neotetrazolium is used alone as the final hydrogen acceptor [i.e. Eqs (1) + (2)]. Thus, on one hand it is possible to measure the amount of NADPH generated by the selected dehydrogenase [Eq. (1)] provided PMS and neotetrazolium are used; on the other hand it is possible to measure how much of the NADPH, generated by the dehydrogenase, is oxidized by some tissue enzymatic system to a stage at which the hydrogen can reduce neotetrazolium. It is convenient to designate this tissue-bound enzymatic system (e.g. Altman and Chayen, 1966) as a diaphorase system. It is also convenient to refer to this hydrogen, or these reducing equivalents, derived from NADPH and transmitted to neotetrazolium through the tissue-bound diaphorase as Type 1 hydrogen (i.e. that NADPH-hydrogen which passes through a Type 1 pathway). The total potential production of NADPH by the selected dehydrogenase is measured in the presence of PMS. The difference between this amount of NADPH-hydrogen, and Type 1 NADPH hydrogen, is referred to as Type 2 NADPH-hydrogen (or Type 2 hydrogen, or that amount of potential NADPH-hydrogen which does not pass along the Type 1 pathway).

2. Type 1 and Type 2 Hydrogen in Various Tissues

At first sight it would be reasonable to explain the difference between the activity in the absence and presence of PMS (i.e. why Type 1 + 2 is often so much greater than Type 1), by the following type of argument.

Glucose 6-phosphate dehydrogenase is inhibited by NADPH. Moreover in the absence of PMS, the tissue diaphorase system is rate-limiting and only relatively slowly reoxidizes NADPH and passes the hydrogen to neotetrazolium. Phenazine methosulphate rapidly re-oxidizes NADPH as it is formed, so removing this inhibitory factor; it also short-circuits the slow diaphorase pathway and so drives the dehydrogenase reaction away from equilibrium towards completion.

This argument would be reasonable as regards studies in homogenates (Gumaa and McLean, 1969). The following evidence, from studies with tissue sections, tends to indicate that it is unlikely to be the complete explanation; this evidence

Table 1. *The activity of NADPH-generating dehydrogenases in various tissues, analysed for Type 1 and Type 2 hydrogen (as μg neotetrazolium formazan/mm³/10 min, unless specified otherwise) and their related diaphorase system.*

Tissue	Enzyme	Maximum activity	Type 1	Type 2	Type 1/Type 2 (%)	Ref.
Female rat liver	G6PD	28.7	15.8	12.9	122	1
Female rat liver	NADPH diaphorase	33.5	—	—	—	1
Female rat liver (normal)	G6PD	32.0	17.9	14.1	127	2
Female rat liver with secondary hepatoma	G6PD	30.8	8.45	21.55	39	2
Female rat liver with secondary hepatoma	G6PD	47.8	11.0	36.8	30	2
Human breast cancer	G6PD	7.1	0.55	6.45	9	3
Human breast cancer	6PGD	1.5	0.13	1.37	9	3

Rat adipose tissue	G6PD	56.0	2.0	54.0	3.7	1
Guinea pig adrenal cortex (zona fasciculata)	G6PD*	161*	144*	17	847	4
Guinea pig adrenal cortex (zona reticularis)	G6PD*	290*	279*	11	2536	4
Human synovial lining cells (rheumatoid and non-rheumatoid)	NADPH diaphorase	36–42†	—	—	—	5
Human non-rheumatoid synovial lining cells	G6PD	108†	18†	90	20	5
Human rheumatoid synovial lining cells	G6PD	440†	34†	406	8.4	5

1. Altman, 1972b; 2. Altman et al., 1970; 3. Altman et al., 1968; 4. Chayen and Loveridge, unpublished data; 5. Butcher and Chayen, 1971, also in 1.

* Units of relative absorption/3 min measured in the tissue by microdensitometry. Menadione has been used as the intermediate hydrogen acceptor in place of PMS which may be inhibitory in this tissue.

† Integrated extinction x 10^3/10 min, by microdensitometry.

suggests that the Type 1 and Type 2 hydrogen, measured in the cellular biochemical system, are functions of two distinct physiological pathways.

Table 1 shows the amount of Type 1 and Type 2 hydrogen from NADPH generated either from glucose 6-phosphate (G6PD) or from 6-phosphogluconate dehydrogenase (6PGD) activity in various tissues. In some tissues the rate of activity of the diaphorase system, acting on exogenously added NADPH, has also been determined. It will be seen that the proportions of Type 1 to Type 2 hydrogen, or the proportion of the maximal production of NADPH (by the dehydrogenase) which can pass through the diaphorase system (as Type 1 hydrogen) varies very widely in the different tissues. Clearly there is no kinetic relationship between the potential activity of the dehydrogenase and the amount which is used in the diaphorase system. For example, in the rheumatoid synovial lining cells there is a four-fold increase in the maximal activity of glucose 6-phosphate dehydrogenase, as compared with non-rheumatoid synovial lining cells, but no change in that of the diaphorase, acting on exogenous NADPH. Thus in the non-rheumatoid cells the latter could produce 36 units of activity, but actually produces only 18; in contrast, in the rheumatoid the NADPH-diaphorase activity does appear to be the rate-limiting factor for Type 1 hydrogen.

The results with normal rat liver, as against experimentally induced secondary hepatomas indicate that this analysis of NADPH-hydrogen into the two types (or two pathways) may be significant in cellular physiology. Consider the two situations, namely where the normal and the malignant tissue both produce the same over-all amount of NADPH-hydrogen from the activity of glucose 6-phosphate dehydrogenase (32.0 as against 30.8 μg formazan/mm^3/10 min). In the normal tissue there is roughly the same amount of Type 1 and Type 2 hydrogen, with a slight preponderance of the former. In the invasive malignant tissue there is almost three times as much Type 2 as Type 1. This tendency for NADPH-hydrogen, from this enzyme or from 6-phosphogluconate dehydrogenase, to be predominantly of Type 2 has been found in other tumours (including human cervical carcinoma); in the example of human breast cancer (in Table 1) Type 1 is almost suppressed. The extreme example of this condition is seen in adipose tissue (Table 1). These findings lead us to suggest that Type 2 hydrogen, from NADPH, is involved mainly in biosynthetic mechanisms. They indicate that at least some of the NADPH-hydrogen which cannot be detected by neotetrazolium (which has a positive standard electrode potential, probably about +170 mV) is in fact used by the cells at a relatively high negative electrode potential (the standard electrode potential for the NADP$^+$/NADPH couple is −320 mV). Some of this NADPH may be used in various biosyntheses, such as in the biosynthesis of fatty acids, of steroids and in forming tetrahydrofolate for the synthesis of nucleic acids. The importance of NADPH for lipid synthesis in the mammary gland (Walters and McLean, 1967) and for fat in adipose tissue

(Saggerson and Greenbaum, 1970a,b) is well known, and these data fit well with those in Table 1. It has been suggested (Chayen *et al.*, 1973) that some of the Type 2 hydrogen may also be involved in the other reductive systems in the cytoplasm, including the glutathione reductase pathway which may be related to steroid metabolism (Pinto and Bartley, 1969; Fig. 9).

In contrast, Type 1 hydrogen is that NADPH-hydrogen which is processed by the tissue in such a way so that it can reduce neotetrazolium. Assumably this 'processing' involves a cytoplasmic hydrogen transport system such as occurs in

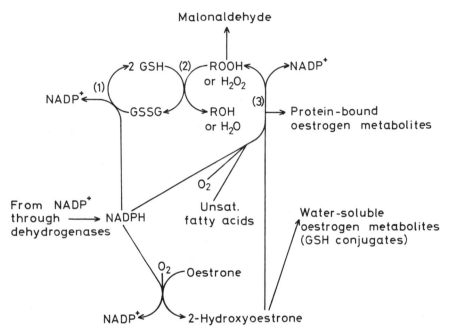

Fig. 9. The scheme of Pinto and Bartley (1969) relating NADPH with glutathione reductase (1) glutathione peroxidase (2) and lipid peroxidation (3).

the cytochrome P450 respiratory chain (Estabrook and Cohen, 1969; Sato *et al.*, 1969). This system (Sih, 1969) involves two routes for NADPH (Fig. 10). Some of the NADPH passes along this respiratory chain and assumably reaches a low negative, or even positive, electrode potential. Other molecules of NADPH react directly with the haem iron of cytochrome P-450, which is said to have a very negative standard electrode potential (Schleyer *et al.*, 1971). Possibly some Type 2 hydrogen may be required for this direct reaction with cytochrome P-450. The whole respiratory system is involved in hydroxylation mechanisms, particularly of steroids and in mixed function oxidase reactions, all of which are important in drug detoxicating mechanisms (as discussed in Gillette *et al.*, 1969). It is noticeable that Type 1 hydrogen predominates in the adrenal cortex, almost to the exclusion of Type 2, and it is in this tissue (particularly in the zona reticularis) that steroid hydroxylation is a major activity.

The concept that Type 1 hydrogen is a function of the cytochrome P-450 respiratory chain gained some cofirmation from studies made to enhance the activity of this pathway. Phenobarbitone, fed to male rats, causes proliferation of the endoplasmic reticulum, particularly of the smooth endoplasmic reticulum, and induction of the enzymes and components of the cytochrome P-450

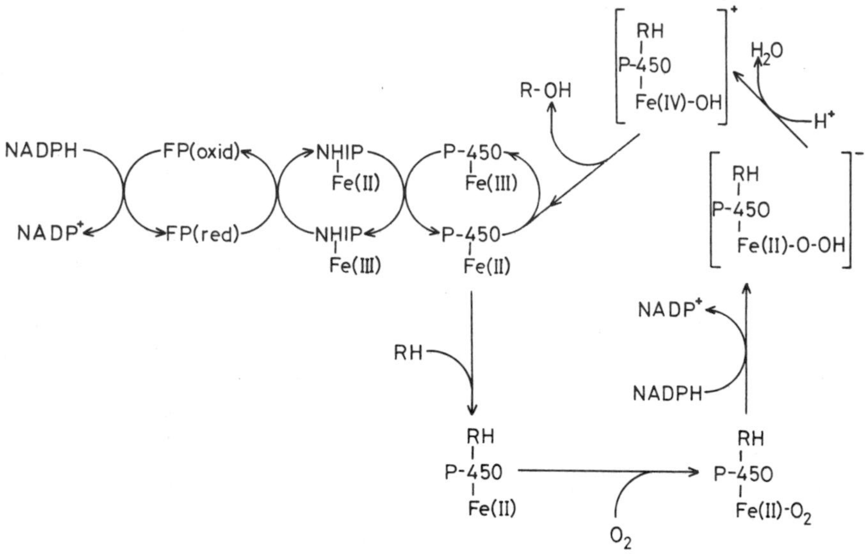

Fig. 10. The scheme suggested by Sih (1969) for steroid hydroxylation in the adrenal cortex. FP and NHIP are two carriers in the chain. P-450: cytochrome P-450. RH: steroid. The point to be emphasized here is that NADPH acts at two points: at the beginning of the hydrogen-transport chain, so that its hydrogen passes down the chain to P-450, and also on cytochrome P-450 directly. The latter may therefore act at a very electro-negative electrode potential. (Copyright 1969 by the American Association for the Advancement of Science.)

respiratory chain (e.g. Smuckler and Arcasoy, 1969). When the livers of such rats were investigated by these methods of cellular biochemistry, increases in total activity of glucose 6-phosphate dehydrogenase and of the NADPH-diaphorase system were observed (Table 2). But when the NADPH-production was analysed, it was found that this increase was due solely to an increase in Type 1 hydrogen, as would be expected if Type 1 hydrogen were a function of the cytochrome P-450 respiratory chain. In contrast, thyroxine injected over 10 days (0.25 mg/day) produced an even greater increase in the glucose 6-phosphate dehydrogenase activity but this was equally distributed between Type 1 and

Table 2. *The activity of glucose 6-phosphate dehydrogenase and of the NADPH-diaphorase system in the liver of male rats treated with phenobarbitone or with thyroxine. Activities expressed as μg of formazan/mm^3/10 min*

Treatment	Substrate	Maximum rate of production of NADPH	Maximum rate of oxidation of NADPH	Type 1	Type 2	Type 1/Type 2 (%)	Ref.
None	G6P + NADP	34.56 ± 3.28	—	6.4 ± 0.63	28.16 ± 3.59	23	1
None	Exogenous NADPH		27.09 ± 1.55				1
Phenobarbitone	G6P + NADP	47.44 ± 1.41		14.7 ± 1.71	32.73 ± 2.11	45	1
Phenobarbitone	Exogenous NADPH		36.03 ± 3.93				
None	G6P + NADP	22.1 ± 1.1		5.3 ± 0.5	14.8	36	2
Thyroxine	G6P + NADP	66.4 ± 2.5		18.7 ± 0.9	47.7	39	2

1. Altman, unpublished data.
2. Butcher, unpublished data.

Type 2 hydrogen (Table 2). It is readily seen from these two examples how this type of analysis gives more information than could have otherwise been obtained. It is known that phenobarbitone increases the detoxicating hydroxylating mechanisms and that thyroxine increases the activity of many enzymes, acting apparently by a completely different mechanism. Normal chemical analysis shows that both increase the activity of glucose 6-phosphate dehydrogenase. The cellular biochemical analysis shows that this increase is related, in the one case, to increased microsomal respiration alone and in the other case to a general increase in activity (Type 1 and Type 2).

3. The Effect of Steroids on Type 1 and 2 Hydrogen

When the activity of purified or isolated glucose 6-phosphate dehydrogenase is tested in the presence of certain steroids, there is an appreciable inhibition of activity (e.g. Marks and Banks, 1960; as discussed above). This was shown to

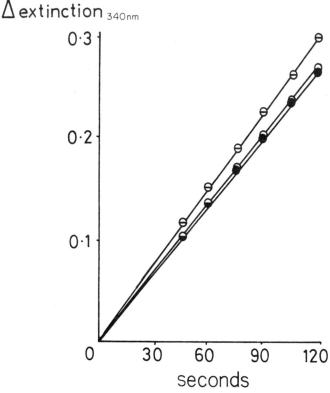

Fig. 11. Progress curves of pure yeast glucose 6-phosphate dehydrogenase measured by following the change in extinction at 340 nm against time. ⊖: control. ○: with 10^{-4} M progesterone in the reaction medium. ●: with 10^{-4} M dehydroepiandrosterone. Both steroids produce about 10% inhibition.

occur when progesterone or dehydroepiandrosterone acted on this dehydrogenase obtained from a yeast (*Candida utilis*) (Sigma Chemical Company, Missouri, U.S.A. Type XI); it was not found when 6-phosphogluconate (from the same source) was tested under the same conditions (Figs 11 and 12).

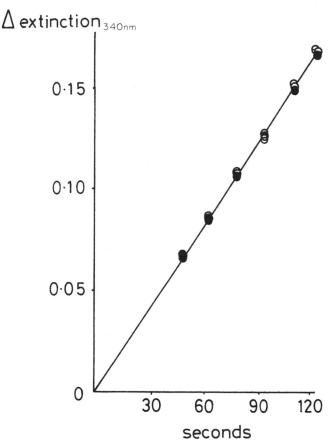

Fig. 12. Progress curve for pure yeast 6-phosphogluconate dehydrogenase (as for Fig. 11). The steroids produce no inhibition.

Such results can show only that a certain steroid has an effect, or no effect, on the production of NADPH by a particular enzyme. When such tests are done on sections of rat liver, incubated with neotetrazolium (with and without phenazine methosulphate), similar inhibitory effects can be measured, namely that certain steroids can inhibit glucose 6-phosphate dehydrogenase activity but have little or no effect on that of 6-phosphogluconate dehydrogenase (Table 3). Although for convenience these tests are done with the steroid at 10^{-4} M

Table 3. *The effect of the five classes of steroids on glucose 6-phosphate dehydrogenase and 6-phosphogluconate dehydrogenase. Activities are expressed as μg formazan/mm^3/15 min*

Steroid	Glucose 6-phosphate dehydrogenase		6-Phosphogluconate dehydrogenase	
	Type 1 hydrogen	Type 2 hydrogen	Type 1 hydrogen	Type 2 hydrogen
Control	23.00 ± 0.80	42.60 ± 1.20	23.60 ± 0.30	38.10 ± 2.10
1. Oestriol (0/0)	21.10 ± 1.50	45.30 ± 1.70	20.00 ± 2.00	41.40 ± 1.40
2. Progesterone (−/+)	14.00 ± 0.30	49.80 ± 2.30	24.30 ± 1.50	35.30 ± 2.00
3. Pregnenolone (−/−)	15.00 ± 0.40	37.30 ± 0.30	26.30 ± 1.50	35.10 ± 1.30
4. Cortisone (0/−)	23.60 ± 1.40	33.70 ± 2.00	24.70 ± 1.50	37.30 ± 1.70
5. Aetiocholan-3αol-17-one (−/0)	15.80 ± 1.30	43.90 ± 2.10	23.50 ± 1.70	36.80 ± 1.90

concentration, these effects can be found down to 10^{-9} M (Fig. 13), there being a linear relationship between the logarithm of the concentration of the steroid and the amount of inhibition. But when the effect of the steroids is analysed according to the two types of NADPH, five classes of response are found:

Class 1: no inhibition and no effect on either Type (class 0/0).
Class 2: no overall inhibition, but Type 2 is increased at the expense of Type 1 (class −/+, i.e. Type 1: −; Type 2: +).
Class 3: inhibition of Type 1 and Type 2 (class −/−).
Class 4: inhibition of Type 2 but little or no effect on Type 1 (class 0/−).
Class 5: inhibition of Type 1 with no effect on Type 2 (class −/0).

Examples of these classes (2–5 inclusive) are shown in Table 3.

From a study of 21 steroids, acting on sections of rat liver, some rules seem to be emerging. Care must be exercised in generalizing, however, both because steroids may have different effects in different tissues and because the effect of steroids, and of pharmacologically active molecules in general, may be very different when they act in living cells over periods of several hours or days, than when they act for a matter of minutes in an incubation medium. But there is significance in the fact that there seems to be some relationship between structure and function even when the steroids act in the incubation medium; it is particularly relevant that the effect of these molecules, or their substituents, may be selectively for one or other type of hydrogen.

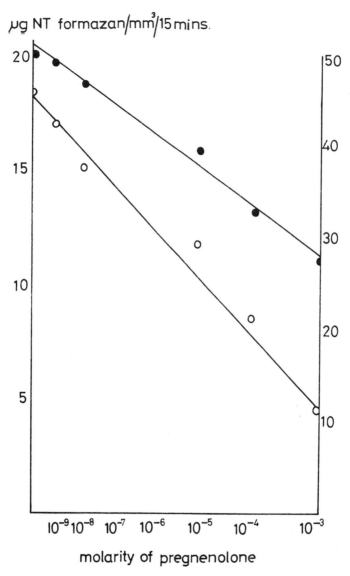

Fig. 13. The effect of pregnenolone (10^{-3} to 10^{-9} M) on glucose 6-phosphate dehydrogenase activity in sections of rat liver (female). o: Type 1 hydrogen. •: Type 2 hydrogen. (Reproduced with permission from Altman, 1972b.)

Two major divisions must be defined. Some steroids inhibit the overall production of NADPH by glucose 6-phosphate dehydrogenase in sections of female rat liver. We will analyse this inhibitory effect in terms of the two pathways for NADPH. But some steroids cause little over-all change in the production of NADPH and act by channelling the hydrogen into one or other pathway. This effect is different from the first and will need to be considered separately.

If we first consider the inhibitory effects, the following generalizations seem to apply in the small number of steroids examined up to the present.

(a) An α or β hydroxy group on a normal steroid A ring (i.e. not an aromatic ring as in oestriol) causes depression of Type 1 hydrogen (i.e. $-/0$ or $-/-$). Examples of this are: pregnenolone, dehydroepiandrosterone, 5β-pregnane-3α,20α-diol, 5α-pregnane-3β,20α-diol, 3α-aetiocholanolone and 17α-hydroxy-pregnenolone. Of these only the first two are $-/-$.

(b) An α or β hydroxy- or keto- group on C_{11} decreases Type 2 hydrogen. This effect may produce a diminution of Type 2, i.e. $0/-$ or $-/-$ class, or it may show itself as a diminution of Type 2 activity in an otherwise Type 2-stimulating steroid.

The first effect, namely a direct diminution of Type 2 hydrogen, occurs with cortisone, corticosterone, hydrocortisone and prednisolone. All are of class $0/-$. The fact that they reduce Type 2 hydrogen is of considerable value in the cellular physiology of certain diseases, particularly in rheumatoid arthritis, as will be discussed later.

The second effect, i.e. of modifying an otherwise Type 2-stimulating molecule, is found with 11α-hydroxyprogesterone. Progesterone itself causes stimulation of Type 2 hydrogen ($-/+$); 11α-hydroxyprogesterone does not cause any change in this hydrogen ($-/0$).

(c) The presence of a 3α keto group and a double bond between C_4 and C_5 will influence Type 2 hydrogen. If there is a β-hydroxy or a keto group at C_{11} it will depress Type 2 hydrogen (as discussed for b, above). If these substituents are not present at C_{11}, then Type 2 will be stimulated at the expense of Type 1.

The steroids which produce redistribution of the NADPH hydrogen, that is a diminution of Type 1 but concomitant increase in Type 2 (class $-/+$) are the following: 11-deoxy-17-hydroxycorticosterone, testosterone and progesterone, all of which have the C_{4-5} double-bond structure with a 3α keto group but no substituent on C_{11} as discussed in (c) above, and androsterone and pregnenolone-3-acetate. Of the last two, androsterone has a hydroxy at C_3 which could account for the depression of Type 1 hydrogen (a, above) and an α hydrogen at C_5; pregnenolone-3-acetate has RO— at C_3, which might account for its depression of Type 1 hydrogen, but its effect on Type 2 cannot be explained on the basis of the generalizations which have been made.

Of the steroids which have been studied, 17β-oestradiol and oestriol have not fitted readily into the scheme, possibly because the A ring is truly aromatic; fluorinated or chlorinated molecules have also been excluded because of the very strong effect these atoms are likely to exert.

It is too early yet to propose these generalizations for anything more than indications. In any complete analysis, the precise three-dimensional structural form of the various steroid molecules would have to be taken into account. But these results may be considered of some significance in that they demonstrate that effects can occur in relation to one or other type or pathway of NADPH-hydrogen. The results therefore strengthen the view that the difference between the amount of hydrogen detected by neotetrazolium in the presence and absence of PMS is not due solely to kinetic causes but may represent different, physiologically meaningful, pools or pathways for hydrogen derived from NADPH.

4. Cell Physiological Effects of Type 1 and Type 2 Hydrogen

We have suggested that the physiological significance of Type 1 hydrogen is in relation to hydroxylation reactions related to cytochrome P-450; that of Type 2 may be for biosynthetic mechanisms. It was shown (Table 2) that phenobarbitone, which increases the microsomal cytochrome P-450 system in rat liver, increases the Type 1 system selectively. The evidence that Type 2 hydrogen is related to biosynthesis is based mainly on circumstantial evidence, namely that it is exceptionally elevated over Type 1 in those tissues which are engaged actively in the synthesis of lipids and proteins. Additional confirmatory evidence comes from studies on human breast cancers. We have discussed (above) how human breast cancers, maintained *in vitro*, can be divided into two types, one which survives in the normal culture medium and the other which will not survive unless 17β-oestradiol was included in the medium. Moreover, the latter type died if an oestrogen antagonist, drostanolone (2α-methyl-17β-hydroxy-5α-androstan-3-one), was added to the oestradiol-enriched culture medium. When tested on rat liver, 17β-oestradiol was $-/+$, that is it enhanced Type 2 hydrogen at the expense of Type 1. It was found to have this effect also in the oestrogen-requiring breast cancers maintained *in vitro* (Altman and Chayen, 1968). Drostanolone, acting on liver sections, was found to be a $0/-$ steroid. (This is additional to the 21 steroids discussed above; the effect is in keeping with the idea that a 3α keto group influences Type 2 hydrogen.) In human oestrogen-requiring breast cancers, maintained *in vitro*, it reversed the inhibitory effect of oestradiol on Type 1 hydrogen (Altman and Chayen, 1968) and appeared to inhibit Type 2 hydrogen (Altman *et al.*, 1968). Thus both oestradiol and drostanolone appeared to act on oestrogen-requiring human breast tissue, maintained *in vitro*, as they did in our test system, i.e. when included in the reaction medium for testing glucose 6-phosphate dehydrogenase activity in slices of rat liver. But of greater interest was the fact that, in the responsive breast cancers, drostanolone appeared to inhibit Type 2 hydrogen which we interpret as indicating that it suppressed the disposition of NADPH into biosynthetic pathways. It seems possible that this could account for its efficacy in killing oestrogen-requiring breast cancers maintained *in vitro* in the presence of oestrogen.

5. Concerning the Theoretical Basis of the Two Types of NADPH-Hydrogen

We have adduced some evidence to support the contention that the difference between the amount of neotetrazolium formazan produced by dehydrogenase activity in the presence and absence of phenazine methosulphate is not solely due to the different kinetics of the reaction in the presence and absence of PMS. We have suggested that there are two types of NADPH-hydrogen, Type 1 which passes through the cytochrome respiratory pathway to a more positive electrode potential at which it reacts readily with neotetrazolium, and Type 2 which is retained at a more negative electrode potential so that it cannot react with neotetrazolium but will reduce PMS which, in turn, reduces the tetrazole. Some evidence has been presented to indicate that this analysis of NADPH-hydrogen may yield useful results in distinguishing between NADPH used in the cytochrome P-450 respiratory chain (hydroxylation; mixed function oxidases) and that used in biosynthetic reactions. However, some of the concepts and results require further clarification.

The NADPH produced from both glucose 6-phosphate and 6-phospho-gluconate dehydrogenases can be analysed in terms of Type 1 and Type 2 hydrogen. Steroids have little or no effect on the hydrogen from 6-phospho-gluconate dehydrogenase but many affect the NADPH-hydrogen derived from glucose 6-phosphate dehydrogenase. These findings make it unlikely that Type 1 and Type 2 NADPH-hydrogen merely represent the two pathways, i.e. the cytochrome P-450 and the biosynthetic pathways, assuming that these are common to all NADPH-hydrogen (Fig. 14). A steroid which depresses Type 1 hydrogen (a −/0 or −/+ steroid) would have to act at A (or later, at B or C) and so would depress Type 1 hydrogen from 6-phosphogluconate dehydrogenase as well (but see Section 6). The same type of argument applies to suppression of Type 2 hydrogen. This argument leaves two alternatives: either the NADPH-hydrogen derived from 6-phosphogluconate dehydrogenase enters the pathways at a different point, for example at B and Y respectively (the steroids acting only at A and X) or the bifurcation into Type 1 and Type 2 NADPH-hydrogen is a property of the enzyme itself. There is no evidence as yet of the first of these alternatives which may or may not be correct. For the present therefore, we will consider only the second.

The first point which this line of speculation emphasizes is that it would not be correct to speak of two pathways for the NADPH-hydrogen; the pathways, equivalent to A–B–C and X–Y–Z in Fig. 14, are believed to be common to NADPH-hydrogen from both dehydrogenases yet only NADPH-hydrogen from glucose 6-phosphate dehydrogenase is affected by steroids. Yet calling the two entities Type 1 and Type 2 suggests they are different forms of hydrogen, or of

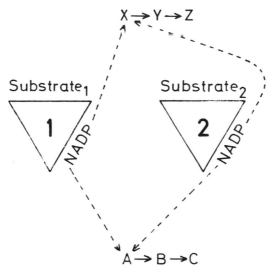

Fig. 14. A schematic representation of the two pentose-shunt dehydrogenase enzymes in relation to the flow of hydrogen into the microsomal respiratory pathway, or diaphorase system (A, B, C, etc.) or into reductive pathways (X, Y, Z, etc.) which may be biosynthetic or may be involved with other systems such as the glutathione reductase pathway (Fig. 9). The flow of hydrogen is indicated by the broken line. 1: glucose 6-phosphate dehydrogenase. 2: 6-phosphogluconate dehydrogenase. Substrate 1: glucose 6-phosphate. Substrate 2: 6-phosphogluconate.

NADPH. This may be unfortunate even though it is true that two forms of NADPH do exist, namely the A and B form. In the formula

Nicotinamide moiety of NADP$^+$ → Nicotinamide moiety of NADPH

$H^+ + 2e^-$

the A form has the incoming hydrogen atom (marked by an asterisk) situated above the plane of the nicotinamide ring and the B form has it situated below the plane (see Dixon and Webb, 1964, p. 267 referring to the work of Cornforth *et al.*, 1962). There has been much recent work on the stereospecificity of NAD- and NADP-dependent oxidoreductases (e.g. see in Wilton *et al.*, 1970; Davies *et al.*, 1972) but it appears that both glucose 6-phosphate and 6-phosphogluconate dehydrogenases show the same B-stereospecificity, so making it unlikely that Type 1 and Type 2 hydrogen refers to a stereochemical difference. For all that it is conceivable that this specificity is incomplete or even variable, depending on the configuration of the enzyme. If the Type 1 and Type 2 phenomenon were to depend on such a stereochemical effect, then the effect of steroids on glucose 6-phosphate dehydrogenase but not on 6-phosphogluconate dehydrogenase might be related to the fact that the co-enzyme binds only loosely to the latter but strongly with the former (Glock and McLean, 1953). However, it is more likely that this specific effect of steroids is related more to the actual

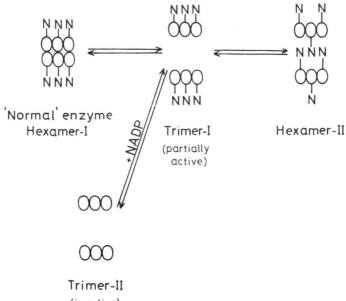

Fig. 15. The multi-meric structure of glucose 6-phosphate dehydrogenase as proposed by Yoshida (1966). ○ represents the sub-unit. N represents NADP. It will be seen that there are two different locations for NADP in the hexamer-II form, one on the outside of the hexamer and one inside the hexamer. It will be noted that the change from the inactive trimeric form to the active trimer-I and hexameric forms depends on the presence of NADP.

structure of the enzymes concerned, because only glucose 6-phosphate dehydrogenase occurs in a multi-meric form. The implications of this, and of allosteric effects in an enzyme composed of more than one sub-unit, have already been discussed (Section I A 1). Some of the possibilities will be readily appreciated by reference (Fig. 15) to some of the structures proposed by Yoshida (1966). This, however, is far into the realm of speculation. The essential findings are that steroids seem to be capable of diverting the NADPH-hydrogen associated with glucose 6-phosphate dehydrogenase, which is the first step in the hexose–mono-phosphate shunt, out of, or into, biosynthetic pathways. This may have considerable implications in biochemical pharmacology; some will be considered later in relation to rheumatoid arthritis.

6. Steroidal Effect on Cytoplasmic–Mitochondrial Interactions

One of the particular benefits of the cellular biochemical analysis of biochemical activity in intact tissue sections is that the spatial relationships of the different components of the cells are retained. Under these conditions it is possible to show that, in rat liver, there is a synergistic effect between oxidation occurring in the cytosol (e.g. glucose 6-phosphate or 6-phosphogluconate dehydrogenation, or NADPH-diaphorase) and in the mitochondria (glutamate or succinate oxidation). Some of this synergism is concerned with a transhydrogenation mechanism between cytoplasmic NADPH and mitochondrial NAD (Butcher and Chayen, 1968). Of possibly greater interest is the synergism between cytoplasmic NADPH and mitochondrial oxidation of succinate. Butcher

Table 4. *The synergistic effects of cytoplasmic oxidation on mitochondrial succinate oxidation and the effect of steroids. Activity measured as µg neotetrazolium formazan/mm³ of rat liver/hr, in an atmosphere of air*

Additions	1 Succinate	2 G6P + NADP	3 Succinate + G6P + NADP	4 3 − 2 synergistic enhancement of succinate oxidation
0	2.2 ± 0.3	37.8 ± 2.0	76.8 ± 6.6	39.0
10^{-4}M progesterone	2.2 ± 0.2	28.2 ± 2.0	33.0 ± 1.0	4.8
0	2.9 ± 0.4	44.6 ± 2.2	80.0 ± 3.0	35.4
10^{-4}M cortisone	2.6 ± 0.4	45.0 ± 2.6	76.0 ± 6.0	31.0
0	1.5 ± 0.1	41.2 ± 3.4	73.0 ± 5.4	31.8
10^{-4}M pregnenolone	1.4 ± 0.1	23.2 ± 3.4	28.6 ± 2.4	5.4

(1970) has made a detailed study of succinate dehydrogenase activity in sections of rat liver and showed that this enzyme, in sections, behaved very much as it did in isolated mitochondria. He showed, however, that its apparent activity was greatly enhanced if pentose-shunt dehydrogenation, or NADPH-diaphorase activity, was allowed to continue while the succinate dehydrogenation was being tested (Butcher, 1972a). This synergistic effect is shown in Table 4. When sections were tested with succinate as the substrate they gave values of, for example, 2.2 µg formazan/mm³/hr. Serial sections, given glucose 6-phosphate and NADP as substrate, gave activities of 37.8. When both succinate and glucose 6-phosphate plus NADP were given as substrates simultaneously, it was to be expected that both systems, one in the cytosol and the other in the mitochondria, would maintain their own levels of activity to yield 40 µg formazan/mm³/hr. In fact they produced 76.8 µg formazan/mm³/hr, namely almost double what should have been expected. The amount of activity in the medium containing both substrates was 39 units (column $3 - 2$) in excess of the amount found with only glucose 6-phosphate and NADP (column 2) as substrate and it was malonate-sensitive so showing it to be an enhancement of succinate dehydrogenation (and mitochondrial hydrogen transport). This is the synergistic effect of cytoplasmic oxidation on mitochondrial (malonate-sensitive) succinate dehydrogenase activity (2.2 to 39.0 units).

Both progesterone and pregnenolone had no effect on the production of neotetrazolium formazan from succinate alone (column 1). Both had an inhibitory effect on the activity against glucose 6-phosphate and NADP. Both had already been shown to inhibit Type 1 hydrogen and it is only this which was being tested in this study, progesterone being a $-/+$ steroid and pregnenolone a $-/-$ steroid. But the startling effect of both these steroids was that they almost

Table 5. *The effect of pregnenolone on the synergistic effect of NADPH oxidation and mitochondrial succinate oxidation in sections of rat liver. Activity in air measured as µg of neotetrazolium formazan/mm³/hr*

Addition	1 Succinate	2 Exogenous NADPH	3 Succinate + NADPH	4 $(3 - 2)$ Enhanced succinate oxidation
0	1.5 ± 0.1	40.4 ± 3.0	72.0 ± 5.2	31.6
10^{-4}M pregnenolone	1.4 ± 0.1	42.0 ± 3.4	70.4 ± 5.6	28.4

completely inhibited the enhanced succinate dehydrogenase activity normally induced by cytoplasmic pentose-shunt activity (column 4). In contrast cortisone, a $0/-$ steroid, had no effect on any of these systems. It is also noteworthy that pregnenolone had no effect directly on the NADPH-diaphorase system (column 2 Table 5) even though it normally depresses Type 1 hydrogen which in fact passes along the diaphorase pathway. Similarly it had no effect on the interaction between cytoplasmic and mitochondrial oxidation (columns 3 and 4, Table 5) even though it has such a markedly inhibitory effect on this interaction when the NADPH is generated endogenously in the section by the action of glucose 6-phosphate dehydrogenase (Table 4). In these studies the level of activity of the diaphorase system, acting on exogenously added or endogenously produced NADPH has been adjusted to be almost the same.

The fact that steroids which affect this cytoplasmic–mitochondrial interaction can act only on NADPH generated from glucose 6-phosphate dehydrogenase but not on NADPH added exogenously or produced endogenously by

6-phosphogluconate dehydrogenase raises interesting speculations. It seems to indicate that NADPH is handled differently according to how it is produced in the sections, and that certain steroids can influence the amount and the disposition of NADPH generated by glucose 6-phosphate dehydrogenase. Since this dehydrogenase is the first step in the hexose–monophosphate pathway these steroids can exercise some control over this pathway. But they may also control whether this NADPH-hydrogen is transmitted into biosynthetic or hydroxylating mechanisms. However the fact that NADPH from different sources is handled differently indicates either that it may be fed in at different points, A or B, in the scheme in Fig. 14, or that there may be two different diaphorase systems, one for NADPH produced by glucose 6-phosphate dehydrogenase and the other for NADPH from 6-phosphogluconate dehydrogenase or for exogenous NADPH.

In this context it is very pertinent that Katz and Wals (1972) have shown that different proportions of ^3H from C_1 and C_3 of glucose 6-phosphate, utilized by the pentose shunt, are incorporated into fat and water. The greater proportion of ^3H from C_3 that is incorporated into fat might correspond to the greater amount of Type 2 hydrogen produced by 6-phosphogluconate dehydrogenase, which acts on the hydrogen on C_3, than is produced by glucose 6-phosphate dehydrogenase (which acts on the hydrogen on C_1). Moreover this evidence, that hydrogen from the different carbon atoms of the glucose ring, is found mainly either in water, or in fat, or is distributed between these end-products in different proportions, emphasizes that not all NADPH-hydrogen is treated similarly. (For example, 35% of ^3H from C_3 and 25% from C_1 were incorporated into fatty acids; 45% and 50%, respectively, were found in water. It must be assumed that half the hydrogen from any reaction with NADP will be the proton which is not accepted by the co-enzyme.)

Whatever the mechanisms which ensure that NADPH from different sources behaves differently, it will be apparent that these cellular biochemical methods allow a more detailed analysis of the effect of steroids on NADPH-associated systems and on cytoplasmic–mitochondrial interactions, than could hitherto have been made.

IV. INDIRECT EFFECTS

In this section we will discuss the effects of steroids acting on whole living cells in an organized tissue. Some of these effects will be direct effects of steroids, as have been discussed in the previous section; it will be pertinent to see to what extent steroids do exert the same direct effects in living cells as they have been shown to produce on sections, and to what extent living cells may modify these direct effects. But to a large degree, these indirect effects will be those produced typically by living cells, for example by incorporation of the steroid into organelle-membranes and so influencing the enzyme activity either by altering the properties of the membrane on which the enzyme is situated, or by changing the permeability of the membrane which controls the rate of enzyme activity (as in the case of lysosomal enzymes).

Generally for this work the tissue is maintained in non-proliferative organ culture and the steroids are allowed to act on the living tissue *in vitro* for periods of a few hours up to one day. The tissue is then chilled, sectioned and tested for the cellular biochemical effects of the selected steroid by the micro-biochemical methods described above. We will now review our investigations on how steroids affect the cellular biochemistry of each major component of the cytoplasm in turn.

A. ENDOPLASMIC RETICULUM

The enzyme systems of the endoplasmic reticulum which have been most studied are glucose 6-phosphate dehydrogenase, which is a 'soluble' or very loosely bound enzyme of the endoplasmic reticulum, and the NADPH-diaphorase system which is firmly bound to the endoplasmic reticulum. Particular attention has been given to the analysis of the effects on Type 1 and Type 2 hydrogen (as defined above).

1. Human Skin

We have seen (above) that hydrocortisone is a $0/-$ steroid when tested in the reaction medium for measuring the glucose 6-phosphate oxidative activity of sections of rat liver. When applied to human skin in maintenance culture it has a similar effect (Table 6) in that it diminishes the amount of Type 2 hydrogen.

Table 6. *The effect of $10^{-4}M$ hydrocortisone on human skin maintained* in vitro *for 4 hr. (Glucose 6-phosphate dehydrogenase activity measured as µg neotetra-zolium formazan/mm³/hr in the epidermis)*

	Type 1	Type 2
Normal culture	10.60 ± 2.50	122.60 ± 5.00
Hydrocortisone culture	8.10 ± 2.00	77.20 ± 4.00

2. Human Rheumatoid and Non-Rheumatoid Synovial Lining Cells

Two of the striking chemical phenomena associated with rheumatoid arthritis are the chemical changes in the lysosomal membranes and the generation of NADPH in the synovial lining cells. The first of these will be considered later, but it has been suggested (e.g. Chayen and Bitensky, 1971) that the two phenomena are related. In brief, the results are as follows. Rheumatoid arthritis involves a chronic inflammatory condition of the synovium, associated with erosion of the cartilage which begins at the junction between the cartilage and the synovium (Ball, 1968). Both the chronic inflammatory condition and the erosion could be induced by lysosomal contents which could be released from synovial lining cells if the lysosomal membranes became fully permeable. It was shown (Chayen et al., 1969b; 1971a) that the lysosomal membranes in these cells were non-functional in the rheumatoid tissue; this lack of function was related to an imbalance of the redox equilibrium in the cytoplasm (as measured by $-SH : -S-S-$ ratios). It was then shown that the synovial lining cells in the rheumatoid tissue were capable of generating four times as much NADPH as were the non-rheumatoid cells, even though the rate of oxidation of NADPH (Type 1 hydrogen) was the same in both rheumatoid and non-rheumatoid cells (Butcher and Chayen, 1971). It was suggested (e.g. Chayen et al., 1973) that this over-production of Type 2 hydrogen might explain at least some of the excessively reductive state of the rheumatoid synovial lining cells (as shown by the $-SH : -S-S-$ ratio).

In view of the benefit obtained from hydrocortisone by rheumatoid patients it was of interest to investigate whether such steroids, which are classed as $0/-$ in our system (i.e. they depress Type 2 hydrogen), might have some of their effect by diminishing this excessive production of Type 2 hydrogen. Human synovial tissue was therefore maintained for up to 24 hr in maintenance culture in the absence or presence of various concentrations of hydrocortisone or prednisolone. The steroid was dissolved in alcohol and dispersed into the culture medium to achieve a determined final concentration of the steroid; the concentration of alcohol in the culture medium was 1% and the same concentration of alcohol was added to the normal culture medium (lacking steroid).

In both the rheumatoid and the non-rheumatoid synovial lining cells the alcohol-soluble hydrocortisone and prednisolone produced a diminution of Type 2 hydrogen when the steroid was present in sufficiently high concentration. The diminution was particularly noticeable in the rheumatoid cells. In general the rate of production of Type 2 hydrogen in these cells, both in the biopsy and in the normal culture, was about 400 units/cell/10 min (1 unit = relative extinction $\times 10^3$) in contrast to about 50–90 units/cell/10 min in the non-rheumatoid cells. This rate of production of Type 2 NADPH-hydrogen was not affected by 10^{-6} M prednisolone or hydrocortisone; in the rheumatoid cells it was diminished towards normality by 10^{-4} M of either steroid (Table 7). In other specimens appreciable diminution was observed when the tissue was exposed to 10^{-5} M hydrocortisone.

It follows that the depressive effect of $0/-$ steroids, as found by their direct effects on sections, occurs also when these substances act on living cells in vitro. Similar results have been found in synovial biopsies taken at synovectomy from joints of patients with rheumatoid arthritis who had been treated with such steroids. Provided they had received 6 mg of prednisolone (occasionally 5 mg) a day, the rate of production of Type 2 hydrogen by the synovial lining cells was between 84 and 146 units/cell/10 min, which is close to the range found in non-rheumatoid synovial lining cells. On lower doses of prednisolone (1 mg/day) the rate of production of Type 2 NADPH-hydrogen was 430 units/cell/10 min, that is within the values found for untreated patients. For comparison of *in vitro* and *in vivo* effects, we may use the data of Peterson (1959) for oral hydrocortisone, which suggest it goes into 10–20 litres of body fluid, i.e. into the space of extra-cellular fluid volume. This implies that the maximum concentration of hydrocortisone in the body, given 6 mg/day, will be 1–2 x 10^{-6} M.

Table 7. *The effect of prednisolone on NADPH-hydrogen in human rheumatoid synovial lining cells. Activities expressed as integrated extinction x1000 (by microdensitometry) per cell for 10 min reaction*

Treatment	Type 1 (against exogenous NADPH)	Type 2
Normal culture	34	368
+10^{-6} M prednisolone	45	322
+10^{-5} M prednisolone	29	399
+10^{-4} M prednisolone	30	210

It seems, therefore, that one of the effects of hydrocortisone, and its related substances, in improving the rheumatoid condition may be its depression of the over-production of NADPH-hydrogen. This depression will diminish the redox imbalance which has been implicated as a factor in the disease.

B. EFFECTS ON MITOCHONDRIA

Two possible points of action have been investigated in relation to the effects of steroids on mitochondria. These are (a) in the interaction between the cytoplasmic and mitochondrial oxidative activities, as discussed above; (b) in effects on the permeability of mitochondrial membranes.

1. The Interaction between Cytoplasmic and Mitochondrial Oxidation

As had been shown above, more neotetrazolium formazan is produced by the mitochondrial oxidation of succinate if cytoplasmic oxidation proceeds at the same time. This increased reduction of the tetrazole is derived from the dehydrogenation of succinate as shown by the fact that it is malonate-sensitive. It is probably due primarily to enhanced flow of hydrogen through the mitochondrial hydrogen-transport system rather than to increased dehydrogenase activity, although the latter will be rate-limited by the former (see Butcher, 1970, 1972a). Thus the cytoplasmic production of NADPH appears to affect the efficiency of the mitochondrial hydrogen-transport system. When this was tested in sections of rat liver, oestradiol (10^{-4} M) had no effect on the amount of hydrogen (measured as neotetrazolium formazan) produced by the dehydrogenation of succinate or of glucose 6-phosphate (Table 8); it only slightly diminished the interaction (3 − 2 in Table 8). However when the oestradiol was added at even lower concentration (10^{-6} M) to rat liver maintained *in vitro*, it obliterated the interaction (column D in Fig. 16). Thus *in vitro*, the activity for succinate dehydrogenase in the presence of glucose 6-phosphate dehydrogenation was only equal to the sum of each activity. There

Table 8. *The effects of 10^{-4} M oestradiol in the incubation medium (incubation in an atmosphere of air for 30 min)*

	μg formazan/mm^3/hr	
	No oestradiol	+10^{-4} M oestradiol
1. Succinate	2.9 ± 0.4	3.6 ± 0.4
2. G6P + NADP	44.6 ± 2.2	41.2 ± 1.7
3. Succinate + G6P + NADP	80.0 ± 3.0	69.0 ± 6.6
4. 3 − 2	35.4	27.8

was no synergistic effect (that is, the activity in the presence of both activities minus the glucose 6-phosphate dehydrogenase activity, i.e. C − B, was equal only to the original succinate dehydrogenase activity, i.e. D = A in Fig. 16).

Thus on living cells, oestradiol can influence the degree of interaction between cytoplasmic and mitochondrial oxidative activities. This is a truly indirect effect of the steroid. It may imply that the steroid must be converted into an active molecule by the cells, or that it (or its active derivative) has to be actively incorporated into the system, as yet unknown, which controls such interactions. But of greater significance is the possibility that steroids may influence cellular metabolism and physiology by affecting systems which can be investigated only in relatively intact cells, in which the sub-cellular organelles are retained in their normal spatial relationships. This is one of the particular advantages of this form of cellular biochemistry.

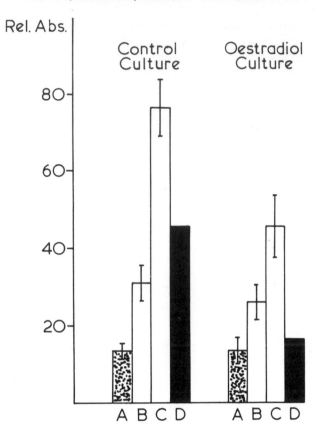

Fig. 16. The effect of 10^{-6} M oestradiol on the cytoplasmic–mitochondrial oxidative activity of rat liver maintained *in vitro* for 5 hr. A: succinate as substrate. B: glucose 6-phosphate + NADP as substrate. C: succinate + glucose 6-phosphate + NADP as substrate. D: C − B, enhanced succinate oxidation. Activities recorded by microdensitometry as relative absorption/unit field/unit time.

2. The Permeability of Mitochondrial Membranes

When mouse skin is treated with crotonaldehyde in life, to produce a brisk inflammation, it was noted that the activity of mitochondrial monoamine oxidase in sections of the skin was increased (Diengdoh, 1965). This increased activity was due, apparently, to increased permeability of the mitochondrial membranes which otherwise restrict the rate of entry of reactants. A similar increase in activity occurs when human skin, maintained *in vitro* in non-proliferative culture, is treated with histamine which also causes other cellular parameters of acute inflammation (as will be discussed later). This increase in mitochondrial permeability is inhibited if the human skin is maintained *in vitro* in the presence of such anti-inflammatory steroids as fluclorolone acetonide and betamethasone-17-valerate (Chayen *et al.*, 1970b). It is also inhibited by some other anti-inflammatory drugs. This test of mitochondrial permeability and resistance to the labilizing influence of histamine is one of the factors now used in the objective and quantitative assessment of anti-inflammatory drugs. It is of some interest that some steroids may stabilize mitochondrial membranes while having less protective effect on lysosomal membranes (Chayen *et al.*, 1970b).

C. EFFECT ON LYSOSOMES

Cellular biochemical methods have confirmed the findings of Weissmann (e.g. 1968; also Allison, 1968) that hydrocortisone-like steroids, when incorporated into living cells, stabilize lysosomes. Human rheumatoid synovial tissue was maintained in the Trowell system (as described above) either in the presence or absence of such steroids. At the end of 24 hr the tissue was chilled, sectioned, and tested for lysosomal membrane activity, using either the naphthylamidase method (Chayen *et al.*, 1970c, 1971) or the acid phosphatase method (Section II A 3, above). The test of lysosomal membrane function, by the naphthylamidase method, is the latent ('bound') activity as a percentage of the maximal activity. In the rheumatoid synovial lining cells, both in the biopsy and in the tissue maintained *in vitro*, there was no latent activity, i.e. the lysosomal membranes were apparently functionless with regard to impeding entry of reactants; after treatment *in vitro* with 10^{-5} M and 10^{-4} M hydrocortisone or prednisolone there was 16–20% latent activity, implying that the membranes were somewhat stabilized. (In non-rheumatoid cells the latent activity varies between 35–50%). When the steroids were added at a concentration of 10^{-6} M, there was only slight effect, e.g. 5% latent activity.

Weissmann (1969) has shown that cortisone and its analogues stabilized isolated lysosomes when added at concentrations of $10^{-3} - 10^{-4}$ M. If dimethyl-sulphoxide was used as the solvent for the steroids, enzyme release from isolated rabbit liver lysosomes was retarded with as little as 10^{-6} M of the steroid. These findings represent a direct action of the steroid on the lysosomal membranes. The greater sensitivity of response shown by living cells (in the absence of dimethyl-sulphoxide) probably represents an active incorporation into the lysosomal membranes, but it may also be related to the fact that these cortisone-like steroids partially correct the redox imbalance (as discussed above).

Patients, with active rheumatoid arthritis, who have been treated with 6 mg/day of prednisolone (equivalent to $1-2 \times 10^{-6}$ M; see above) have shown 15–20% latent activity in the lysosomes of the synovial lining cells (tested at biopsy); there was virtually no latent activity in the lysosomes of synovial lining cells in a patient treated with 1 mg/day. Thus the results in life reduplicate those found *in vitro*; the tissue in the patient appears to be slightly more responsive than when it is maintained *in vitro*.

The anti-inflammatory effect of steroids, normally used as topical application to the skin, has also been tested. Fluclorolone acetonide (10^{-4} M) was shown to stabilize lysosomes in human skin, maintained *in vitro*, against the labilizing effect of histamine (Chayen *et al.*, 1970b). Betamethasone-17-valerate was less effective at equimolar concentration although it was a slightly better stabilizer of mitochondrial membranes (see above). These results emphasize that steroids can influence cellular events, such as inflammation, by their ability to stabilize sub-cellular membranes, and that different steroids may be relatively selective as regards the membranes of different cellular organelles.

D. EFFECT ON PLASMA MEMBRANE AND OEDEMA

The balance between intra-cellular and extra-cellular water is of considerable importance in cellular biochemical pathology. It is of particular significance in inflammatory conditions such as the various inflammatory disorders of the skin (including psoriasis) and in the chronic inflammation of rheumatoid arthritis. Direct measurement of the water content of each cell, and of each extra-cellular space, can be made by quantitative interferometry of sections of tissue, prepared as described above (Section II B 4).

Changes in activity of the plasma membrane can be followed by investigating the activity of the enzyme 5-nucleotidase. This enzyme is now widely considered to be a marker of the plasma membrane in homogenate studies (e.g. see Fleischer *et al.*, 1969; Cheetham *et al.*, 1970). In recent investigations we have shown that this enzyme activity increases in human skin which has been subjected, *in vitro*, to the histamine-induced inflammation (described above) and the activity is related directly to the extent of cellular and intra-cellular oedema, as measured by interferometry. This enzyme is also very active at the cell surfaces, particularly of small blood vessels, in the synovium of human rheumatoid joints and in the dermal papillae of psoriatic plaques.

When human psoriatic skin was maintained *in vitro*, the most striking effect of tropical steroids, used in the treatment of psoriasis, was their effect in reducing the 5-nucleotidase activity in the dermal papillae, especially in the small capillaries. Both betamethasone-17-valerate and fluclorolone acetonide reduced this activity and reduced the amount of cellular and extra-cellular oedema, as measured by interferometry (Chayen *et al.*, 1971b). This is another example of how steroids can influence cellular pathology by their action on cellular membranes. Assumably they exert this influence both by a physical effect on the structure of the plasma membrane and by modulating the activity of enzymes in the cell membrane.

V. CONCLUSIONS

From the evidence cited in this review it seems clear that steroids have many potential effects on cellular biochemistry. These include:

(1) An influence on the gene itself, affecting the degree of repression of the gene and transcription from it. This aspect has been reviewed elsewhere.
(2) A direct influence on enzymatic activity, which may be due to the steroid partaking in the activity, as in steroid transhydrogenation mechanisms, or to effects more akin to allosteric phenomena.
(3) An indirect influence on enzymatic activity, as is found when the steroids alter the physical properties of the membranes which either control enzymatic activity (as in the endoplasmic reticulum) or which control the entry of reactants to the enzymes (as in mitochondria and lysosomes).
(4) An effect on membrane permeability, as in (3) and as shown by the way steroids may affect plasma membranes and so alter tissue water balance.
(5) A subtle switch mechanism by which hydrogen, from cytoplasmic NADPH, can be diverted from, or into, more biosynthetic reductive or more hydroxylating pathways.
(6) An influence on the synergistic interactions which take place between cytoplasmic and mitochondrial oxidations.

It will be appreciated that most of these effects [apart from (1) and possibly (2)] involve structural chemical phenomena. The conventional procedures of biochemistry, which involve the isolation of the sub-cellular components, are likely to alter to some degree the physical state of these components and so will obscure some of these structural chemical effects. Once isolated, the components may not respond to added steroids in the way they can when in intact cells. Effects like (5) and (6) cannot readily be discerned if the spatial relationships within cells are dislocated. The methods of cellular biochemistry discussed in this review are particularly suited for investigating this type of spatially determined interaction. The steroids are allowed to act on living cells, maintained in their normal relationships with other cells and with stroma in the fully differentiated tissue. Their effects are studied chemically in intact sections of that tissue. The membranes of sub-cellular organelles, and even of the cells themselves, are studied while they are embedded in their natural cytoplasmic or extra-cellular medium, without the trauma of isolation into a foreign medium. This has been made possible by the quantification of enzyme activity per cell by biophysical techniques. Finally these methods have particular relevance to pharmacology because they are applied to human tissue so obviating the need for extrapolation from rodents, or other animals, to man.

ACKNOWLEDGEMENT

We are grateful to the Medical Research Council and the Arthritis and Rheumatism Council for Research for their support for this work.

REFERENCES

Aithal, H. N. and Ramasarma, T. (1969). *Biochem. J.* **115**, 77-83.
Allison, A. C. (1968). *In* 'The Biological Basis of Medicine' (E. E. Bittar and N. Bittar, eds), Vol. 1, pp. 209-333. Academic Press, New York and London
Altman, F. P. (1969a). *Histochemie* **17**, 319-326.
Altman, F. P. (1969b). *Histochemie* **19**, 363-374.
Altman, F. P. (1970). *Histochemie* **22**, 256-261.
Altman, F. P. (1971a). *Histochemie* **28**, 236-242.
Altman, F. P. (1971b). *Histochemie* **27**, 125-136.
Altman, F. P. (1972a). 'An Introduction to the Use of Tetrazolium Salts in Quantitative Enzyme Cytochemistry'. Koch-Light Laboratories, Colnbrook.
Altman, F. P. (1972b). 'Quantitative Dehydrogenase Histochemistry with special reference to the Pentose Shunt Dehydrogenases'. Progress in Histochemistry and Cytochemistry, Fischer, Stuttgart.
Altman, F. P. and Chayen, J. (1965). *Nature, Lond.* **207**, 1205-1206.
Altman, F. P. and Chayen, J. (1966). *J. Roy. micr. Soc.* **85**, 175-180.
Altman, F. P. and Chayen, J. (1968). *In* 'The Treatment of Carcinoma of the Breast' (A. S. Jarrett, ed.), pp. 56-63. Excerpta Medical Foundation.
Altman, F. P., Bitensky, L., Butcher, R. G. and Chayen, J. (1970). *In* 'Cytology Automation' (D. M. D. Evans, ed.), pp. 82-97. Livingstone, Edinburgh.
Altman, F. P., Bitensky, L., Chayen, J. and Daly, J. R. (1968). *Proc. Assoc. clin. Biochem.* **5**, 119-120.
Asahina, E. (1966). *In* 'Cryobiology' (H. T. Meryman, ed.), pp. 451-486. Academic Press, New York and London.
Ball, J. (1968). *In* 'Rheumatic Diseases' (J. R. Duthie and W. R. M. Alexander, eds), pp. 124-126. University Press, Edinburgh.
Bangham, A. D. (1968). *Prog. Biophys. molec. Biol.* **18**, 29-95.
Bangham, A. D. and Haydon, D. A. (1968). *Brit. Med. Bull.* **24**, 124-126.
Barka, T. and Anderson, P. J. (1963). 'Histochemistry'. Harper and Row, New York.
Bendall, D. S. and Duve, C. de. (1960). *Biochem. J.* **74**, 444-450.
Bitensky, L. (1962). *Quart. J. Micros. Sci.* **103**, 205-209.
Bitensky, L. (1963a). *In* 'Ciba Symposium on Lysosomes' (A. V. S. de Reuck and M. P. Cameron, eds), pp. 362-375. Churchill, London.
Bitensky, L. (1963b). *Quart. J. micros. Sci.* **104**, 193-196.
Bitensky, L., Butcher, R. G. and Chayen, J. (1973). *In* 'Lysosomes in Biology and Pathology' (J. T. Dingle, ed.), Vol. 3. North Holland, Amsterdam.
Bittar, E. E. (1964). 'Cell pH'. Butterworths, London.
Braidman, I. P. and Rose, D. P. (1970). *Biochem. J.* **118**, 7-8P.

Butcher, R. G. (1968). *Histochemie* 13, 263-275.
Butcher, R. G. (1970), *Exp. Cell Res.* 60, 54-60.
Butcher, R. G. (1971a). *Histochemie,* 28, 231 235.
Butcher, R. G. (1971b). *Histochemie,* 28, 131-136.
Butcher, R. G. (1972a) *Histochemie,* 32, 369-378.
Butcher, R. G. (1972b) *Histochemie,* 32, 171-190.
Butcher, R. G. and Chayen, J. (1968). *Exp. Cell. Res.* 49, 656-665.
Butcher, R. G. and Chayen, J. (1971). *Biochem. J.* 124, 19P.
Chayen, J. (1967). *In 'In vivo* Techniques in Histology' (G. H. Bourne, ed.), pp. 40-68. Williams and Wilkins, Baltimore.
Chayen, J. (1968a). *In* 'Cell Structure and its interpretation' (S. M. McGee-Russell and K. F. A. Ross, eds), pp. 149-156. Arnold, London.
Chayen, J. (1968b). *In* 'Cell Structure and Its Interpretation' (S. M. McGee-Russell and K. F. A. Ross, eds), pp. 265-274. Arnold, London.
Chayen, J. and Bitensky, L. (1968). *In* 'The Biological Basis of Medicine' (E. E. Bittar and N. Bittar, eds), Vol. 1, pp. 337-368. Academic Press, London and New York.
Chayen, J. and Bitensky, L. (1971). *Ann. rheum. Dis.* 30, 522-536.
Chayen, J. and Bitensky, L. (1973) *In* 'Cell Biology in Medicine' (E. E. Bittar, ed.), Wiley, New York.
Chayen, J. and Denby, E. F. (1968). 'Biophysical Technique as applied to Cell Biology'. Methuen, London.
Chayen, J., Jones, G. R. N., Bitensky, L. and Cunningham, G. J. (1961). *Biochem. J.* 79, 34P.
Chayen, J., Bitensky, L. and Wells, P. J. (1966). *J. Roy. micr. Soc.,* 86, 69-74.
Chayen, J., Bitensky, L., Butcher, R. G. and Poulter, L. W. (1969a). 'A Guide to Practical Histochemistry'. Oliver and Boyd, Edinburgh.
Chayen, J., Bitensky, L., Butcher, R. G. and Poulter, L. W. (1969b). *Nature, Lond.* 222, 281-282.
Chayen, J., Altman, F. P., Bitensky, L. and Daly, J. R. (1970a). *Lancet* i, 868-870.
Chayen, J., Bitensky, L., Butcher, R. G., Poulter, L. W. and Ubhi, G. S. (1970b). *Br. J. Derm.* 82, suppl. 6, 62–81.
Chayen, J., Bitensky, L. and Poulter, L. W. (1970c). *Nature, Lond.* 225, 1050-1051.
Chayen, J., Bitensky, L., Butcher, R. G. and Cashman, B. (1971a). *Beitr. Path.* 142, 137-149.
Chayen, J., Bitensky, L. and Ubhi, G. S. (1971b). *Clin. Trials J.* 8, 35-44.
Chayen, J., Loveridge, N. and Daly, J. R. (1971c). *Clin. Sci.* 41, 2-3P.
Chayen, J., Bitensky, L. and Butcher, R. G. (1972a). 'Practical Histochemistry'. Wiley, London.
Chayen, J., Loveridge, N. and Daly, J. R. (1972b). *Clin. Endocrinol.* 1, 219-233.
Chayen, J., Altman, F. P. and Butcher, R. G. (1973). *In* 'Fundamentals of Cell Pharmacology' (S. Dikstein, ed.). Thomas, Illinois.
Cheetham, R. D., Morré, D. J. and Yunghans, W. N. (1970). *J. Cell Biol.* 44, 492-500.
Cook, G. M. W. (1968). *Brit. Med. Bull.* 24, 118-123.
Cornforth, J. W., Ryback, G., Popjak, G., Donninger, C. and Schroepfer, G. (1962). *Biochem. biophys. res. Comm.* 9, 371-375 (quoted by Dixon and Webb, 1964).

Cunningham, G. J., Bitensky, L., Chayen, J. and Silcox, A. A. (1962). *Ann. Histochim.* 7, 433-435.

Daly, J. R., Loveridge, N., Bitensky, L. and Chayen, J. (1972). *Ann. clin. Biochem.* 9, 81-84.

Danielli, J. F. (1953). 'Cytochemistry, a Critical Approach'. Wiley, New York.

Daoust, R. and Cantero, A. (1959). *Canc. Res.* 19, 757-762.

Davies, D. D., Teixeira, A. and Kenworthy, P. (1972). *Biochem. J.* 127, 335-343.

Davies, H. G., Wilkins, M. H. F., Chayen, J. and La Cour, L. F. (1954). *Quart. J. micr. Sci.* 95, 271-304.

Davson, H. and Danielli, J. F. (1952). 'The Permeability of Natural Membranes', 2nd Edn. Cambridge University Press.

Defendi, V. and Pearson, B. (1955). *J. Histochem. Cytochem.* 3, 61-69.

Diengdoh, J. V. (1965). *J. Roy. micr. Soc.* 85, 103-109.

Dingle, J. T. (1968). *Brit. Med. Bull.* 24, 141-145.

Dingle, J. T. (1969). *In* 'Lysosomes in Biology and Pathology' (J. T. Dingle and H. B. Fell, eds), Vol. 2, pp. 421-436. North Holland, Amsterdam.

Dingle, J. T. (ed.) (1973). 'Lysosomes in Biology and Pathology', Vol. 3. North Holland, Amsterdam.

Dingle, J. T. and Fell, H. B. (eds). (1969). 'Lysosomes in Biology and Pathology', Vols 1 and 2. North Holland, Amsterdam.

Dixon, M. and Webb, E. C. (1964). 'Enzymes' 2nd Edn. Longmans Green, London.

Estabrook, R. W. and Cohen, B. (1969). *In* 'Microsomes and Drug Oxidations' (J. R. Gillette, A. H. Conney, G. J. Cosmides, R. W. Estabrook, J. R. Fouts and G. J. Mannering, eds), pp. 95-105. Academic Press, New York and London.

Fell, H. B. (1969). *Ann. rheum. Dis.* 28, 213-227.

Filippusson, H. and Hornby, W. E. (1970). *Biochem. J.* 120, 215-219.

Fleischer, B., Fleischer, S. and Ozawa, H. (1969) *J. Cell Biol.* 43, 59-77.

Frieden, C. (1971). *Ann. Rev. Biochem.* 40, 653-696.

Gillette, J. R., Conney, A. H., Cosmides, G. J., Estabrook, R. W. Fouts, J. R. and Mannering, G. J. (1969). 'Microsomes and Drug Oxidations'. Academic Press, New York and London.

Glick, D. (1967). *J. Histochem. Cytochem.* 15, 299.

Glock, G. E. and McLean, P. (1953). *Biochem. J.* 55, 400-408.

Glynn, L. E. (1969). *Vox. Sang.* 16, 356-358.

Grant, J. K. (1969). *In* 'Essays in Biochemistry' (P. N. Campbell and G. D. Greville, eds), Vol. 5, pp. 2-58. Academic Press, New York and London.

Gumaa, K. A. and McLean, P. (1969). *Biochem. J.* 115, 1009-1029.

Holter, H. (1965). *Symp. Soc. Gen. Microbiol.* 15, 89-114.

Hornby, W. E., Lilly, M. D. and Crook, E. M. (1966). *Biochem. J.* 98, 420-425.

Hornby, W. E., Lilly, M. D. and Crook, E. M. (1968). *Biochem. J.* 107, 669-674.

Hubbell, W. L. and McConnell, H. M. (1969). *Proc. Natl. Acad. Sci.* 63, 16-22.

Jardetsky, C. D. and Glick, D. (1956). *J. biol. Chem.* 216, 283-292.

Jones, G. R. N. (1963). *Br. J. Canc.* 17, 153-161.

Jones, G. R. N. (1965). *Biochem. J.* 96, 10P.

Jones, G. R. N., Bitensky, L., Chayen, J. and Cunningham, G. J. (1961). *Nature, Lond.* 191, 1203.

Jones, G. R. N., Maple, A. J., Aves, E. K., Chayen, J. and Cunningham, G. J. (1963). *Nature, Lond.* 197, 568-570.

Kamin, H. (1969). *In* 'Microsomes and Drug Oxidations' (J. R. Gillette, A, H. Conney, G. I. Cosmides, R. W. Estabrook, J. R. Fouts, and G. J. Mannering, eds), p. 105. Academic Press, New York and London

Karavolas, H. J. and Engel, L. L. (1966). *J. biol. Chem.* **241**, 3454-3456.

Katz, J. and Wals, P. A. (1972). *Biochem. J.* **128**, 879-899.

Kearney, E. B. (1957). *J. biol. Chem.* **229**, 363-375.

Klotz, I., Langerman, N. R. and Darnall, D. W. (1970). *Ann. Rev. Biochem.* **39**, 25-62.

Koshland, D. E. and Neet, K. E. (1968). *Ann. Rev. Biochem.* **37**, 359-410.

Kun, E. and Abood, L. G. (1949). *Science, N.Y.* **109**, 144-146.

Lehninger, A. L. (1951). *J. biol. Chem.* **190**, 345-359.

Lehninger, A. L. (1965). 'The Mitochondrion'. Benjamin, New York.

Lehninger, A. L. (1966). *Naturwiss.* **53**, 57-100.

Lever, W. F. (1967). 'Histopathology of the Skin , 4th Edn. Pitman, London.

Levy, H. R., Raineri, R. R. and Nevaldine, B. H. (1966). *J. biol. Chem.* **241**, 2181-2187.

Lovelock, J. E. (1957). *Proc. Roy. Soc. B.* **147**, 427-433.

Lucy, J. A. (1968). *Brit. Med. Bull.* **24**, 127-129.

Luyet, B. J. (1951). *In* 'Freezing and Drying' (R. J. C. Harris, ed.), pp. 77-98. Institute of Biology, London.

Lynch, R., Bitensky, L. and Chayen, J. (1966). *J. Roy. micr. Soc.* **85** 213-222.

Mahler, H. R. (1953). *Int. Rev. Cytol.* **2**, 201-230.

Mahler, H. R., Tomisek, A. and Huennekens, F. M. (1953). *Exp. Cell Res.* **4**, 208-221.

Marks, P. A. and Banks, J. (1960). *Proc. Natl. Acad. Sci.* **46**, 447-452.

Mazanowska, A. M., Neuberger, A. and Tait, G. H. (1966). *Biochem. J.* **98**, 117-127.

McCabe, M. and Chayen, J. (1965). *J. Roy. micr. Soc.* **84**, 361-371.

McLaren, A. D. and Packer, L. (1970). *Advs. Enzymol.* **33**, 245-308.

Meryman, H. T. (1957). *Proc. Roy. Soc. B.* **147**, 452-459.

Moline, S. W. and Glenner, G. G. (1964). *J. Histochem. Cytochem.* **12**, 777-783.

Monod, J., Changeux, J.-P. and Jacob, F. (1963). *J. Mol. Biol.* **6**, 306-329.

Monod, J., Wyman, J. and Changeux, J.-P. (1965). *J. Mol. Biol.* **12**, 88-118.

Nachlas, M. M., Crawford, D. T. and Seligman, A. M. (1957). *J. Histochem. Cytochem.* **5**, 264-278.

Oelkers, W. and Dulce, H. J. (1964). *Hoppe-Seyler's Z. physiol. Chem.* **337**, 150-158.

Peterson, R. E. (1959). *In* 'Recent Progress in Hormone Research' (G. Pincus, ed.), Vol. 15, pp. 231-261. Academic Press, New York and London.

Pinto, R. E. and Bartley, W. (1969). *Biochem. J.* **115**, 449-456.

Potter, V. R. and Du Bois, K. P. (1943). *J. gen. Physiol.* **26**, 391-404.

Quarles, R. H. and Dawson, R. M. C. (1969). *Biochem. J.* **112**, 795-799.

Radda, G. K. (1971). *Biochem. J.* **122**, 385-396.

Rees, L. H., Ratcliffe, J. G., Besser, G. M., Kramer, R. and Chayen, J. (1972). *Nature, Lond.* **241**, 84-85.

Ross. K. F. A. (1967). 'Phase Contrast and Interference Microscopy for Cell Biologists'. Arnold, London.

Saggerson, E. D. and Greenbaum, A. L. (1970a). *Biochem. J.* **119**, 193-219.

Saggerson, E. D. and Greenbaum, A. L. (1970b). *Biochem. J.* **119**, 221-242.

Salih, H., Flax, H. and Hobbs, J. R. (1972). *Lancet* i, 1198-1202.

Sato, R., Nishibayashi, H. and Ito, A. (1969). In 'Microsomes and Drug Oxidations' (J. R. Gillette, A. H. Conney, G. J. Cosmides, R. W. Estabrook, J. R. Fouts and G. J. Mannering, eds), pp. 111-128. Academic Press, New York and London.

Sayers, M. A., Sayers, G. and Woodbury, L. A. (1948). Endocrinology 42, 379-393.

Schleyer, H., Cooper, D. Y., Levin, S. S. and Rosenthal, O. (1971). Biochem. J. 125, 10-11P.

Siekevitz, P. (1962). In 'The Molecular Control of Cellular Activity' (J. M. Allen, ed.), pp. 143-166. McGraw-Hill, New York.

Sih, C. J. (1969). Science, N.Y. 163, 1297-1300.

Silcox, A. A., Poulter, L. W., Bitensky, L. and Chayen, J. (1965). J. Roy. micr. Soc. 84, 559-564.

Sloane-Stanley, G. H. (1967). Biochem. J. 104, 293-295.

Smuckler, E. A. and Arcasoy, M. (1969). Int. Rev. Exp. Path. 7, 305-418.

Stuart, J. and Simpson, J. S. (1970). J. clin. Path. 23, 517-521.

Stuart, J., Bitensky, L. and Chayen, J. (1969). J. clin. Path. 22, 563-566.

Sylvén, B. and Bois-Svensson, I. (1964). Histochemie 4, 135-149.

Talalay, P. (1961). In 'Biochemists' Handbook' (C. Long, ed.), pp. 350-352. Spon, London.

Tappel, A. L. (1969). In 'Lysosomes in Biology and Pathology' (J. T. Dingle and H. B. Fell, eds), Vol. 2, pp. 207-244. North-Holland, Amsterdam.

Tomkins, G. M. and Maxwell, E. S. (1963). Ann. Rev. Biochem. 32, 677-708.

Trowell, O. A. (1959). Exp. Cell Res. 16, 118-147.

Trowell, O. A. (1965). In 'Cells and tissues in Culture' (E. N. Willmer, ed.), Vol. 2, pp. 96-172. Academic Press, New York and London.

Waggoner, A. S., Kingzett, T. J., Rottschaefer, S., Griffith, O. H. and Keith, A. D. (1969). Chem. Phys. Lipids 3, 245-253.

Walters, E. and McLean, P. (1967). Biochem. J. 105, 615-623.

Weissmann, G. (1966). Arth. and Rheum. 9, 834-840.

Weissmann, G. (1968). In 'The Interaction of Drugs and Sub-cellular Components in Animal Cells' (P. N. Campbell, ed.), pp. 203-212. Churchill, London.

Weissmann, G. (1969). In 'Lysosomes in Biology and Pathology' (J. T. Dingle and H. B. Fell, eds), Vol. 1, pp. 276-295. North-Holland, Amsterdam.

Willmer, E. N. (1961). Biol. Rev. 36, 368-398.

Wilton, D. C., Watkinson, I. A. and Akhtar, M. (1970). Biochem. J. 119, 673-675.

Yoshida, A. (1966). J. biol. Chem. 241, 4966-4976.

Yue, R. H., Noltmann, E. A. and Kurby, S. A. (1969). J. biol. Chem. 244, 1353-1364.

DAILY RHYTHMS OF STEROID AND ASSOCIATED PITUITARY HORMONES IN MAN AND THEIR RELATIONSHIP TO SLEEP

J. R. DALY and J. I. EVANS

Department of Chemical Pathology,
Charing Cross Hospital Medical School, London, W6 8RF
and the Sleep Laboratory, Department of Psychiatry,
University of Edinburgh, Edinburgh, EH10 5HF.

I. INTRODUCTION

That many natural phenomena occur in cycles is among the oldest of biological observations. During the past 25 years there has been growing recognition of physiological cycles whose period is roughly 24 hr long, and which have therefore been named circadian (Halberg, 1959). Many physiological, biochemical and psychological functions show circadian rhythmicity, and Aschoff (1965) has tabulated about fifty of these.

Such rhythms may be exogenous or endogenous. Exogenous rhythms are direct responses to an environmental periodicity, and fade when the environmental factor becomes constant. Endogenous rhythms, on the other hand, have their own inherent period, but this can be modified by stimulation from a rhythmic environmental variable such as the alternation of light/darkness. In this case the environmental variable is said to entrain the biological rhythm. Sollberger (1969) has suggested that endogenous circadian rhythms were originally acquired by an adaptation to the 24 hr environment and have now been inherited through evolutionary selection. It has been pointed out by Aschoff (1965) that the adaptive significance of such a rhythm, giving it survival value, might be that it helps the organism to master the changing conditions of a temporally programmed world. In other words, it enables it to do the right thing at the right time. By developing a self sustained oscillation with approximately the same frequency as a major environmental rhythm the organism is to some extent prepared in advance for the variable conditions it may meet.

For general discussion of circadian rhythms the reader is referred to Aschoff (1965), Mills (1966), Sollberger (1969), Halberg (1969) and Hastings (1970).

It is apparent that the secretion of certain pituitary and steroid hormones shows distinct circadian rhythms. These are probably endogenous, but the precise nature of their environmental or internal synchronizers remains uncertain. What is clear, however, is that the secretion of these hormones is greatly influenced by the alternation of sleep and wakefulness. The complexity of this relationship has become more obvious since the realization that sleep itself is no simple amorphous period of unconsciousness, but is highly structured in time.

In considering the relationship to sleep of the secretion of the hormones of the hypothalamo-pituitary-adrenal (HPA) axis, and of growth hormone (GH), this review will first outline what is at present understood about the structure of sleep. The circadian rhythm of the HPA axis will then be described, together with a review of experiments which have been carried out in an attempt to identify the synchronizers of the rhythm, including certain elements of sleep, and also the rhythm's alteration in certain disease states. The rhythm of GH will then be described, together with its relation to sleep structure, and this relationship contrasted with that of the rhythm of the HPA axis. Finally what little is known of the rhythm of the hypothalamo-pituitary-gonadal (HPG) axis will be briefly reviewed.

II. SLEEP

A. HISTORICAL INTRODUCTION

In the past decade there has been a change in the traditional view of sleep from that of a state of relative inertia and unresponsiveness associated with some basic restorative function, to one of sleep as an active physiological process which can subserve several functions (Oswald, 1969, 1970).

Early observations were in accord with the traditional view. In the 4th century B.C., Aristotle noted that respiration slowed with the onset of sleep, and Galen, in the 2nd century A.D., described the diminished heart action and fall in pulse rate. Fontana (1765) observed that in sleep the pupil became constricted, and Tarchanoff (1894) demonstrated that blood pressure fell as sleep developed.

These reports depended on observations made soon after the onset of sleep. Curiously, the results of overnight studies made little impact on this traditional view of passive sleep. Kohlschütter (1862) described arousal thresholds in sleepers, and found that arousal was more difficult to achieve in the first 2–3 hr of the sleep period. Howell (1897) after training himself to sleep with his arm in a plethysmograph, described vasodilation in sleep and also periodic variations in arm volume at approximately hourly intervals. The most significant overnight studies were those of MacWilliam (1923). He observed that while blood pressure and pulse rates declined at sleep onset, there were periods during the night of 'disturbed' sleep in which blood pressure could rise dramatically, and pulse and respiration rates increased. He related these changes to dreaming, and suggested that in an active dream adrenaline was pumped into the blood stream and brought about the physiological changes of disturbed sleep.

Other workers described cycles of physiological changes in sleep. Denisova and Figurin (1926) noted that the pulse rate and breathing of sleeping infants were alternately accelerated and slowed over periods of 50 min. Magnussen in 1944, found cycles in the variation of respiratory rate in sleep; and Ohlmeyer *et al.* (1944) described periodic episodes of penile tumescence during sleep at approximately 85 minute intervals.

The electroencephalogram (EEG) was described by Berger in 1929, and the behaviour of the EEG in sleep was investigated by Loomis *et al.* (1937), Blake and Gerard (1937) and Blake *et al.* (1939). These workers described the development of increasing slow waves in the EEG with sleep, and also runs of fast activity—the sleep spindles. Loomis developed a five point scale, which depended on the amount and appearance of EEG wave forms, and allowed him to present the physiological changes of sleep as a series of cycles waxing and waning over the sleep period. Blake *et al.* (1939) also noted that most of the large slow waves occurred in the first few hours of sleep.

Unfortunately, monitoring the EEG alone during sleep proved insufficient as a basic measurement to stimulate research, as the paper of Brooks *et al.* (1956) illustrates when compared with those of Aserinsky and Kleitman (1953, 1955). Aserinsky and Kleitman began by attempting to measure the blinks and eye movements of sleeping babies. They described periods of intense eye activity associated with small body movements, facial grimaces and sucking movements. These active periods occurred at mean intervals of 50 min. Next, they examined the sleep of an older child and of some students by monitoring the EEG and the electro-oculogram (the field created by the choric-retinal potential as the eyes moved). They found that while there were slow rolling movements of the eyes during drowsiness and early sleep, bursts of active synchronous movements— which they termed *rapid eye movement* (REM) occurred at intervals of 80-90 min, and lasted from 10 to 50 min. They woke subjects when eye movements were occurring and in periods of ocular inactivity, and showed that dreaming was significantly associated with REM activity.

This work proved to be the basic stimulus to modern sleep research, and within a decade workers were recognizing the presence of two sorts of sleep (Oswald, 1962).

B. METHODS OF STUDYING SLEEP

The technique of continuous monitoring of the EEG and electro-oculogram as a basis for sleep studies has proved to be most useful. However, other variables have been successfully used to study sleep. Hinton and Marley (1959) and Samuel (1964) used body movement as a means of studying the effects of hypnotic and tranquillizing drugs, and in recording the sleep of depressed patients. Other physiological measurements have been added to the basic monitoring procedure when appropriate. Blood pressure, pulse rate, muscle tone and penile changes have been recorded in many studies (Hartmann, 1967).

The normal recording procedure is as follows (Fig. 1):

At bedtime, electrodes (small silver discs) are stuck to the face and around the eyes with adhesive strapping, and to the scalp in the midline with collodion. The skin is previously cleaned with spirit to lower skin resistance. A pair of electrodes is placed over the submental muscles near the lower margin of the mandible (Evans *et al.,* 1968). Leads, often 8 or 10 ft in length, connect these electrodes to the headbox at the bed head so that subjects have a free range of movement in sleep. Appropriate transducers, mercury enclosed in silicone rubber tubing, or carbon filament resistors, are used to monitor respiration or penile circumference.

The headbox leads to an encephalograph, usually sited at a distance. This machine records variation in electrical potentials as a moving graph and therefore runs throughout the sleep period.

Microphones and television cameras may be used to allow direct observations of the subject, and to record on tape any disturbed behaviour or verbal material.

Levels of metabolites in blood, urine or exhaled breath have been monitored successfully. Urine has been collected via a catheter into small tubes rotated at intervals during sleep, so that collections of 5 or 10 min duration can be made (Mandell *et al.,* 1966a). Blood samples have been taken at intervals during sleep through an indwelling catheter (Weitzman *et al.,* 1966), and masks and appropriate connections were used by Robin *et al.* (1958) to measure CO_2 and oxygen in expired air. A more recent sampling procedure (Vankirk and Sassin,

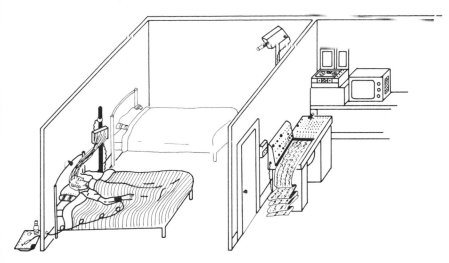

Fig. 1. Diagram of the sleep laboratory at Edinburgh. The subject is connected by a leash of electrodes to a headbox which conducts the electrical signals to the encephalograph in the adjacent room. Tape recording is available to record material such as dreams, and closed circuit television is used for direct observation. An intravenous catheter in the (R) arm is connected to an extension which runs through the wall to the outside so that blood samples can be taken remotely.

1969) involved connecting a 10 ft nylon catheter extension to a standard intravenous polythene catheter, the system being filled with heparin saline to prevent clotting. Samples are taken remotely after the heparin saline is removed, and under favourable circumstances 10 ml of blood can be taken within 2 min without significant disturbance of the subject's sleep. Removal of heparin saline, aspiration of the blood samples and replacing the fresh heparin saline generally takes 2-3 min.

C. THE MEASUREMENT OF SLEEP

Sleep consists of two distinct states which can readily be measured (Snyder, 1971). In normal subjects the initial 60-90 min are occupied by a cycle of orthodox or slow wave sleep. During orthodox sleep the EEG contains a varying amount of slow wave activity together with runs of fast waves—the sleep spindles. In orthodox sleep most physiological variables decline towards basal levels, but coincident with body movement small increases occur in pulse rate, respiratory rate and blood pressure, so that an overnight profile of any of these variables shows an irregular spiked appearance. Since the pioneering studies of Loomis *et al.* (1935) it has proved logical to divide this type of sleep into contiguous stages (Dement and Kleitman, 1957). Stage 1 or drowsiness is characterized by low voltage fast activity and lack of continuous alpha (10 Hz)

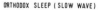

ORTHODOX SLEEP (SLOW WAVE)

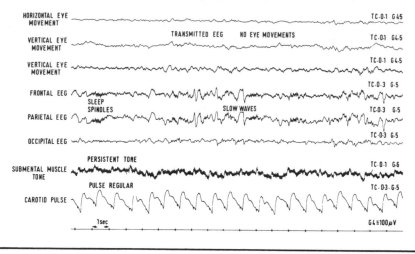

PARADOXICAL SLEEP (R.E.M.)

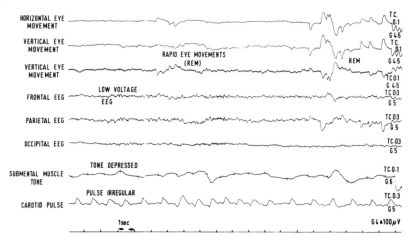

Fig. 2. Two types of sleep. Orthodox sleep (upper section) consists of sleep spindles (14 Hz) and slow waves in the electroencephalogram, but muscle tone is persistent and other physiological variables regular. Paradoxical (REM) sleep, is characterized by large jerking eye movements, while muscle tone is minimal or absent. Physiological variables show irregularity and an overall increase.

activity in the EEG, and persists until evidence of sleep spindles (14 Hz) activity occurs. Sleep spindles indicate transition to Stage 2 orthodox sleep, and thereafter Stage 3 and 4 sleep depend on the amount of large slow waves present (Stage 3: 20%+; Stage 4: 50%+) in a 20 sec scoring epoch. Transition from stage to stage creates a rather irregular cycle of 90 min mean duration. Overnight, there are 4 or 5 such cycles, but as Blake *et al.* (1939) noted, the bulk of Stage 4 sleep is contained in the first 2-3 hr.

Between these cycles periods of paradoxical or REM sleep occur. In REM sleep there are bursts of rapid jerking synchronous eye movements. The EEG contains a mixture of relatively low voltage activity but is devoid of sleep spindles (Dement and Kleitman, 1957). Tone in muscle groups of the head and neck falls to zero level at, or occasionally prior to, the start of REM sleep

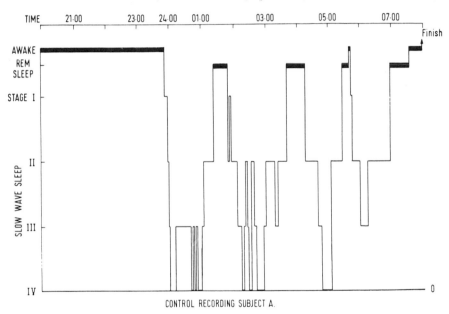

CONTROL RECORDING SUBJECT A.

Fig. 3. Histogram of sleep. The stages of orthodox sleep may be seen to form a series of cycles (usually 4 or 5) in an 8 hr period. Interdigitating episodes of REM sleep lasting from 10 to 50 min occur at mean intervals of 90 min during sleep.

(Berger, 1961), and there is a redistribution of tone in many muscle groups (Jacobson *et al.*, 1964). Overall, there is a rise in pulse rate, respiration rate and blood pressure, but of greater significance is the variability of these physiological parameters (Snyder, 1967). Penile tumescence, frequently to the point of erection, accompanies 75–85% of REM sleep periods (Karacan *et al.,* 1966, 1972).

REM sleep periods vary from 10–50 min, and tend to increase in length as the night proceeds, so there is more REM sleep in the second four hours. Four or five REM sleep periods contribute a total of over a 100 min a night—a mean of about 24% of total sleep. The association of REM sleep with dreaming has been confirmed many times (Hartmann, 1967), but present concepts suggest that mental activity is seldom in abeyance during sleep, and dreams may be recalled after awakening from orthodox sleep. Nevertheless, mental activity in which fantasy and disorientation are prominent, usually occurs during REM sleep.

Many workers have shown that sleep is related to age (Roffwarg *et al.*, 1966). High levels of REM sleep occur in premature babies and neonates, but during the

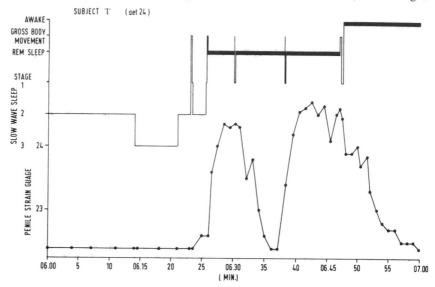

Fig. 4. Penile tumescence during sleep. This part of an overnight record shows the last cycle of orthodox sleep and last REM sleep period between 0600 and 0700. Penile tumescence occurs during REM sleep and is fluctuant. The tumescence persists to form the morning rise which was formerly attributed to a full bladder!

bulk of childhood and adult life REM sleep values are consistent in the healthy subject. In extreme old age some fall in REM sleep occurs. Orthodox sleep changes during adult life. Aged 60 years, the individual obtains approximately 50% of the Stage 4 sleep present at 20.

D. PHYSIOLOGICAL BASIS OF SLEEP

The physiological basis of sleep is relatively well established in animal studies (Jouvet, 1961, 1965). At first the role of the ascending reticular formation in the production of cortical desynchronization and arousal (Moruzzi and Magoun, 1949) made sleep appear as a passive state due to the withdrawal of the ascending activating influence. This passive theory did not accord with Hess' observations (1933) of sleep induction by electrical stimulation of the central midline nuclei of the thalamus and mass intermedia. Further work had demonstrated several brain sites which appeared to depress reticular arousal effects and promote cortical synchrony and the development of sleep. A site in the caudal reticular formation was demonstrated by Magnes *et al.* (1961), who produced sleep by electrical stimulation in the region of the nucleus of the tractus solitarius. Jouvet (1961) demonstrated that sleep spindles originated in the cerebral cortex. Orthodox sleep can therefore be seen as a neuro-physiological event associated with a decline in the activation due to the reticular formation under the influence of a number of cerebral 'centres'—in the hypothalamus, reticular formation and cerebral cortex. The decline in many peripheral physiological variables may be due to a decreased sensitivity in the medullary centres, closely associated with the reticular formation (Smyth *et al.*, 1969).

Paradoxical (REM) sleep has a less well defined physiological basis. It is generally agreed (Jouvet, 1961, 1965; Snyder, 1971), that this sleep is initiated by a nuclear centre in the mid pons—the locus coeruleus; the superior connections are apparently multiple. There is a pathway via the lateral geniculate bodies to the occipital cortex—the ponto-geniculate occipital system from which electrical spikes can be defined in animals (Pompeiano and Morrison, 1965), and this system may be responsible for rapid eye movements. Cortical connections via the limbic system, suggested by Jouvet (1961) have not been clearly identified (Carli *et al.*, 1965), and it is possible that some part of the ascending reticular pathway is involved (Parmeggiani and Zancocco, 1963). Peripheral connections via the extra pyramidal system have also been described (Pompeiano, 1967). The anatomical relations of the brain stem nuclei involved in cardiac and respiratory reflexes suggests that connections exist which affect the centres during REM sleep; an effect which can be demonstrated (Smyth *et al.*, 1969) through altered cardiac reflexes.

Currently research has focussed on the neurochemistry of the state of sleep (Jouvet, 1969; Hartmann, 1967), and the changes during sleep of circulating metabolites and hormones have also attracted much attention. The development of sleep research is illustrated by the fact that in 1950 there were only a few papers about sleep in the current journals, while in 1970 papers exceeded 60 a month (Williams, 1971). Sleep is an active state which may subserve many functions; there is no evidence that it has yet been fully or adequately explored.

III. CIRCADIAN RHYTHM OF THE HPA AXIS

A. GENERAL FEATURES OF THE RHYTHM

Pincus (1943) was the first to observe a circadian rhythm in adrenal activity. He collected urine in 6 hourly specimens from 7 young men over a period of from 5 to 9 days, and found that night values for 17-oxosteroid output were consistently lower than the day values in all subjects. The maximum values tended to occur in specimens taken during the morning hours. Pincus concluded that, as 17-oxosteroid excretion was probably an index of adrenal steroid secretion, his findings offered an interesting basis for suggesting a neuroendocrine mechanism. The circadian rhythm of adrenal activity was subsequently confirmed by many workers, and was apparent whether plasma or urinary corticosteroids were measured (Bliss *et al.*, 1953; Laidlaw *et al.*, 1954; Tyler *et al.*, 1954; Doe *et al.*, 1956; Migeon *et al.*, 1956; Perkoff *et al.*, 1959). In these early studies plasma sampling was relatively infrequent, with intervals of three hours or more between specimens, and the analytical methods employed were based on the Porter-Silber reaction (Silber and Porter, 1954) which shows a reasonable, but by no means absolute, specificity for cortisol. Peterson (1957) measured cortisol by a Porter-Silber based method and corticosterone by an isotope dilution method, and showed that the rhythms of corticosterone and cortisol were parallel. This has been confirmed by Gordon *et al.* (1968) and Williams *et al.* (1972). Most studies in which the rhythm of urinary excretion of steroids was investigated likewise employed the Porter-Silber reagent, and as this reacts with compounds having a dihydroxy-acetone side chain on carbon 17 of the steroid molecule, the substances determined were mostly the tetra-hydro derivatives of cortisol. Gordon *et al.* (1968) specifically measured tetra-hydrocortisol and tetrahydrocorticosterone in urine, and found a rhythm similar to that described using the group-specific methods.

Although there were some variations in the results reported by different research groups, a clear picture of the circadian rhythm of adrenal steroids emerged from these studies. The plasma cortisol level reaches a peak of 15-25 μg/100 ml between 0600 and 0800 hr and falls more or less steadily to a nadir of less than 5 μg/100 ml at around midnight. The rise to the morning peak is apparent by about 0400 hr. The mean peak urinary excretion of corti-costeroids is seen between 0600 and 1200, with a trough between midnight and 0600. It seems there is rather more variability in the rhythm found in the urine than in the plasma, but there are obviously greater difficulties in sampling. In general the urine peak values seem to lag about three hours behind those of plasma (Doe *et al.*, 1960; Gordon *et al.*, 1968).

The levels of plasma corticosterone found by Williams *et al.* (1972) ranged from 0.66 ± 0.09 μg/100 ml at 0800 to 0.19 ± 0.04 μg/100 ml at 2300 hr.

There have been few studies of the circadian rhythm of aldosterone secretion. This is no doubt due in part to the difficulty of its determination. Bartter *et al.* (1962) found the timing of the peak excretion of aldosterone in the urine to be very similar to that of the 17-hydroxycorticosteroids (17-OHCS). The plasma level of aldosterone is subject to many variables, including dietary intake of sodium and potassium, and posture; however, when these were maintained constant, with the subject supine, Williams et al. (1972) found plasma aldosterone to have a circadian rhythm identical in shape with that of cortisol and corticosterone. The levels were 88 ± 7 ng/100 ml at 0800 and 31 ± 5 ng/100 ml at 2300 hr on a low sodium diet (100 mEq/day) and 28 ± 3 ng/100 ml at 0800 and 6 ± 1 ng/100 ml at 2300 hr on a high sodium diet (200 mEq/day).

A review of the work on the circadian rhythm of adrenal steroids up to mid 1966 has been published by Nichols and Tyler (1967).

There is remarkable regularity in the rhythm of plasma cortisol both from subject to subject and from time to time in the same subject provided sampling is relatively infrequent (Fig. 5 (a) and (b)). Although a sex difference in circadian rhythm of adrenal steroids has been reported in the mouse (Halberg and Haus, 1960) and the rat (Critchlow et al., 1963), this has not generally been found in man, but Asfeldt (1971) reported a difference in plasma cortisol between the sexes at 0700 hr, at which time he found a higher level in females, but at no other time was there a significant difference. However, during oestrogen therapy, for example oral contraception with oestrogen-progestogen combinations, there is a marked increase in the amplitude of the circadian oscillation of the plasma cortisol, but the shape of the rhythm is unaltered (Grant et al., 1965; Daly and Elstein, 1972).

Silverberg et al. (1968) showed that there was a normal circadian rhythm in most elderly subjects, although a small proportion (two out of eighteen) showed a peak at noon rather than at around 0800, and one out of eighteen had a rather high value at midnight.

The circadian rhythm of plasma cortisol is not apparent at birth. Franks (1967) showed that it appeared during the second year of life, but it was not until three years old that all children showed a rhythm of the same phase and amplitude as adults.

Recently there have been several studies of the circadian rhythm of plasma cortisol in man in which very frequent sampling has been employed. Pointing out that there had been a wide variety of sampling times in previous studies of the rhythm, Krieger et al. (1971) carried out a very detailed investigation using a fluorimetric technique for plasma cortisol (Braunsberg and James, 1960). Three healthy male and one female subjects on a normal diet and with normal day/night, activity/sleep cycles had blood sampled at 30 min intervals throughout the 24 hr for corticosteroid and corticotrophin (ACTH) determinations. The circadian pattern was of 5 to 10 peaks per 24 hr and 75% of these occurred between midnight and 0900. All subjects showed a progressive rise in plasma corticosteroid levels beginning from $2\frac{1}{2}$ to 5 hr following the onset of sleep. Maximum levels were achieved from $\frac{1}{2}$ to 2 hr after awakening, corresponding to 0800 to 0900 clock-time. There was then a gradual downward trend with some peaking between 1130 and 1400 hr and 1630 and 1800 hr. These latter peaks

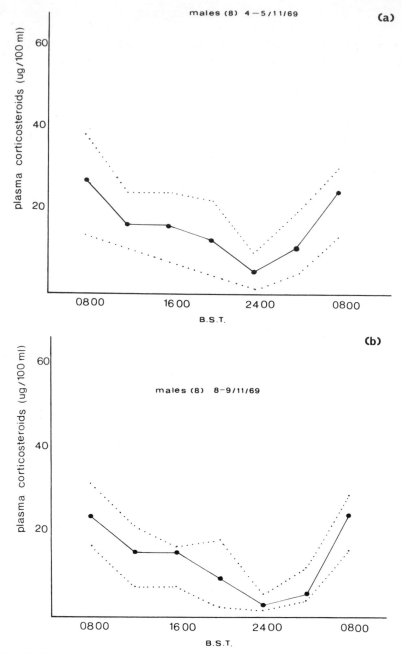

Fig. 5. Mean (●——●) and limits (. . . .) of the plasma corticosteroids in 8 healthy men, with 4 hourly sampling from 0800 on one day to 0800 on the next, and repeated 4 days later. The similarity of the pattern on the two days is marked. Copied, with permission, from Daly (1970).

were not so high as the morning peak, except in two instances where the midday peak was greater. The three male subjects were similarly studied on a subsequent occasion with small half hourly feedings instead of normal meals. This did not significantly alter the rhythm.

Krieger *et al.* (1971) also studied 44 normal female and 35 normal male subjects with 4 hourly sampling. These showed patterns similar to those previously described. Considerable variation was noted in the absolute levels at any given time from subject to subject, the variances being greatest at the periods of peaking between 0400 and 0800 hr. Different individuals followed the same general pattern of change, but displayed very different absolute plasma levels at any given clock hour. Nevertheless all the subjects tested revealed the general shape of their circadian pattern to be reproducible from one day to another. The highest level was usually at 0800, but in about 5% at midday. There was no difference due to age and sex.

On the basis of these data the authors defined a normal rhythm as one in which all values after 0800 are less than 75% of the 0800 value. Presumably this means with 4 hourly sampling. The noon value however may be an exception to this, but should not exceed the 0800 value by more than 15%.

Hellman *et al.* (1970a), studying two healthy subjects, sampled blood every 15 min and determined plasma cortisol by competitive protein binding (Murphy *et al.*, 1963). They showed that between 2300 and 0700 hr there were at least 5 episodes of evident secretory activity. No cortisol was secreted between 0245 and 0300 hr. Thereafter there was a brisk rise, followed by no secretion between 0415 and 0445 hr, a further rise to 0500, then no secretion till 0515, further secretion until 0530 hr, when the level became steady again. Over the whole 24 hr there were 8 episodes of secretory activity. Five of these were during the night—representing over half the total daily secretion of cortisol. Total secretory episodes occupied around 6 hr of the 24, i.e. the adrenals were quiescent during 75% of the day.

In a subsequent study the same group (Weitzman *et al.*, 1971), investigated 6 healthy subjects, and took blood samples every 20 min for 24 hr. All subjects showed sharp rises and slow falls throughout the 24 hr period; the cortisol level was never constant except when it was nearly zero at the time of sleep onset. The intervals between each period of cortisol elevation were irregular, ranging from 40 min to 4 hr and 40 min. There were from 7-13 secretory episodes during the 24 hr. It was the number and duration of these periods, rather than a change in the secretion rate, that determined the amount of cortisol secreted during any given time period. Since the individual secretory episodes occurred irregularly, when averaged they tended to cancel each other, and this may account for the smooth curves described in previous studies (e.g. see Fig. 5). Cortisol did not begin its fall towards the nadir until the fourth hour before sleep was anticipated.

These studies led the authors to suggest that there are 4 unequal temporal phases during each 24 hr period:

1. A 6 hr period starting 4 hr before and continuing for 2 hr after sleep onset, when secretion is negligible.
2. A single isolated episode around midsleep.
3. The main phase, during the last 3 hr of sleep to wakefulness. Nearly half the total cortisol produced during the 24 hr is secreted during this period.

In these last 3 studies great care was taken to avoid disturbing the subject during sleep when taking the blood sample, by the use of techniques similar to those described in II.B above.

B. REGULATION OF THE CIRCADIAN RHYTHM OF THE HPA AXIS

The production of cortisol by the normal adrenal cortex is controlled by a most elaborate mechanism. Synthesis and secretion of cortisol occur only when the adrenal is stimulated by adrenocorticotrophic hormone (corticotrophin, ACTH) from the anterior pituitary, and it appears that secretion of cortisol in the absence of ACTH is negligible.

ACTH is produced by the anterior pituitary under the stimulus of another hormone, corticotrophin releasing factor (CRF) from the hypothalamus. Hypothalamus, anterior pituitary and adrenal cortex thus form a hormonally-linked functional unit known as the hypothalamo-pituitary-adrenal (HPA) axis.

Apart from the circadian rhythm there are two major determinants of adrenal activity, viz. a negative feedback mechanism and responsiveness to stress. The level of the plasma cortisol exerts an effect on the secretion of ACTH in such a way that an increase in the former causes a decrease in secretion of the latter, and conversely a fall in plasma cortisol causes increased secretion of ACTH. A mechanism such as this whereby a change in the level of the hormone from a target gland produces an opposite change in the secretion of the corresponding trophic hormone from the anterior pituitary is known as a negative feedback mechanism. It is now doubtful, however, whether this mechanism plays any role in the minute to minute regulation of HPA function (Weitzman *et al.,* 1971).

One of the most striking attributes of the HPA axis is its ability to respond to stress by greatly increased activity. Stress is a term which is used to describe a very wide variety of stimuli. These include emotional states, such as excitement or fear, nervous stimuli such as pain or injury, and altered metabolic states, such as pyrexia or hypoglycaemia. The brisk rise of plasma cortisol, sometimes to several times the basal level, which follows any of these stimuli is perhaps the most extensively documented of all aspects of HPA function, yet the precise purpose of the increased HPA function during stress remains little understood.

The adrenal response to stress is mediated via the hypothalamus and anterior pituitary, but apparently the hypothalamic pathways controlling it are different from those controlling the circadian rhythm and feedback mechanisms. The response to stress will normally over-ride both of these, and the activity of the healthy HPA axis increase at any time during the 24 hr even in the presence of high circulating levels of corticosteroids or endogenous cortisol.

For a review of normal HPA function see James and Landon (1968).

From this consideration of the functioning of the HPA axis it is apparent that the source of the circadian rhythm of plasma cortisol secretion might arise at hypothalamic or pituitary level, or as a result of variation in adrenal sensitivity to ACTH. It is also possible that it could be due to a cyclic variation in the metabolic disposal of cortisol or in the concentration of the carrier protein to which it is bound in plasma. There is no evidence for either of the latter possibilities. Perkoff et al. (1959) infused cortisol in the morning, during the afternoon and at midnight and were unable to detect any difference in its rate of removal. Weitzman et al. (1971) studied the change in specific activity of the plasma following the intravenous administration of ^{14}C cortisol at different times, and showed that although there was some variability in the calculated plasma half time of cortisol this followed no clear circadian rhythm. Doe et al. (1964) were unable to detect any rhythmic change in the concentration of corticosteroid binding globulin.

On the other hand, there is a rhythmic variation in the sensitivity of the adrenal to ACTH. Perkoff et al. (1959) infused ACTH during the morning, during the afternoon and at midnight, and found that the plasma cortisol response to the infusion starting at midnight was lower than to the others. However, if the adrenal were submaximally stimulated by a low dose infusion of ACTH for several hours prior to the start of the maximally stimulating infusion at midnight, then the plasma cortisol response to the midnight infusion was equivalent to that produced by the infusions at other times of the day. The authors concluded that the lowered sensitivity of the adrenal at midnight was due to a diminished secretion of ACTH during the late daytime hours. Consequently their opinion was that the circadian rhythm of plasma cortisol was itself but a reflection of the circadian rhythm of plasma ACTH. This is now the generally held view, but it was some time before direct confirmation became possible, owing to the extreme difficulty of measuring plasma ACTH, particularly at the concentrations (< 20 pg/ml) found at the lower end of the normal range. However, with the development of sensitive radioimmunoassay systems and of new highly sensitive bioassays and radio receptor assays these difficulties are being overcome. Berson and Yalow (1968), using their radioimmunoassay, found a rhythm of plasma ACTH which closely paralleled that of corticosteroids, and Daly et al. (1973) using a new in vitro bioassay (Chayen et al., 1972; Daly et al., 1972) found plasma ACTH to be higher at 0800 (mean 69.8

pg/ml) than at 2000 (mean 23 pg/ml) with only one overlapping value in the 14 subjects studied. Krieger *et al.* (1971) using the Berson and Yalow radio-immunoassay measured plasma ACTH on samples withdrawn from four healthy subjects every 30 min for 24 hr. They found good correspondence between the times of peaks of plasma corticosteroid levels and those of ACTH levels. The major corticosteroid peaks were always accompanied by ACTH peaks; however they found no correlation in any given subject between a specific plasma cortisol level and a simultaneously obtained ACTH level (Fig. 6). Graber *et al.* (1965)

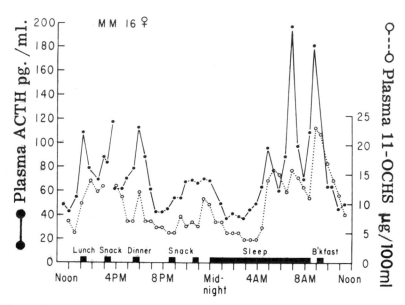

Fig. 6. The circadian rhythm of plasma corticosteroids and ACTH in a single healthy female demonstrated by very frequent sampling. The episodic nature of the secretion is apparent, as is the close phase relationship of the levels of ACTH and corticosteroids. Copied, with permission, from Krieger *et al.* (1971).

using one of the earlier bioassay systems (Lipscomb and Nelson, 1962) found the circadian rhythm of ACTH persisted in the presence of adrenal hypo-function.

Williams *et al.* (1972) thought the circadian rhythm of aldosterone followed that of plasma renin activity rather than that of ACTH, because they found that under some experimental conditions the aldosterone and cortisol rhythms could be dissociated.

Direct evidence that the circadian rhythm in ACTH secretion is accompanied in its turn by a circadian rhythm in hypothalamic CRF activity has been obtained from animal experiments. David-Nelson and Brodish (1969) showed a circadian rhythm in the CRF activity of the hypothalamus in the rat, and Seiden and Brodish (1972) showed this to persist in adrenalectomized and hypophysectomized animals. Similar results were obtained by Hiroshige and Sakakura (1971) who found a close resemblance between the fluctuation of CRF activity in the median eminence of the rat and the plasma concentration of corticosterone, although the two rhythms were slightly out of phase, the changes in the CRF activity always preceding those of the plasma corticosterone level (Fig. 7). Takebe *et al.* (1972) found the rhythm of CRF activity persisted in the

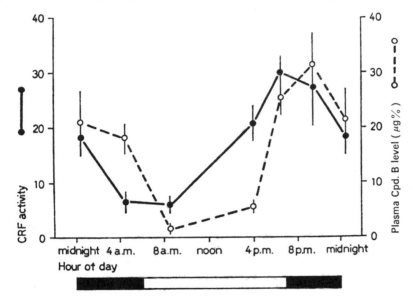

Fig. 7. The patterns of plasma corticosteroid level and of hypothalamic CRF activity in the rat. The corticosteroid level follows that of CRF activity. Note that in the rat, a nocturnal animal, the circadian rhythm of the HPA axis is almost exactly 12 hr out of phase with that of man. Copied, with permission, from Hiroshige and Sakakura (1971).

hypophysectomized or adrenalectomized rat as well as in the hypophysectomized-adrenalectomized animal, although the phase and amplitude of the rhythm were slightly altered by these procedures. It may be concluded, therefore, that the diurnal rhythm of hypothalamic CRF activity is an inherent property of the nervous system, and is not due to the feedback of peripheral hormones, although it may be influenced by this.

It is generally believed that the secretion of ACTH is dependent upon stimulation of the anterior pituitary by CRF. For evidence of this the reader is referred to reviews by Guillemin (1967), McCann *et al.* (1968), Mess and Martini (1968) and Yates *et al.* (1971). This being so, it seems reasonable to conclude that the circadian rhythm detected in hypothalamic CRF activity is the cause of the circadian rhythm in ACTH and hence corticosteroid secretion. This conclusion is supported by experiments in which drugs acting upon the central nervous system (CNS) or anatomical lesions produced at specific sites within it have been shown to modify the circadian rhythm of adrenal function in several species. Slusher (1964) found that lesions in the anterior hypothalamus of the rat, which bilaterally destroyed the periventricular zone and arcuate nuclei, abolished the circadian rise in plasma corticosterone. The response to noise or ether stress was not abolished by these lesions, although the response to noise, but not the circadian rise or response to ether stress, was prevented by lesions in the posterior tuber cinereum. She concluded that the integrity of anterior hypothalamic areas appeared essential for the normal circadian rise in plasma corticosterone, whilst more posterior areas were involved in mediation of the pituitary-adrenal response to the acute stress of sound. Krieger et al. (1968b) demonstrated that both atropine (an anti-cholinergic agent) and a short-acting barbiturate could prevent the normal circadian rise in plasma corticosteroids in the cat. They showed that these agents did not interfere with pituitary-adrenal responsiveness, hence the site of their blocking action was thought to be in the CNS. A notable feature of Krieger's data was that the administration of these drugs had to be timed very precisely in order to produce their effect, and this led the authors to speculate that the ACTH release responsible for the circadian peak occurred only during a relatively brief period of the 24 hr, and that the secretion throughout the rest of the day was basal, and regulated only by feedback or stress responses. This observation compares interestingly with the suggestion of Ceresa et al. (1969, 1970), that in man there is a once-a-day burst of ACTH activity corresponding to the circadian rise in adrenal secretion in the early morning hours, and that this is superimposed on basal activity of the HPA axis which persists throughout the remainder of the 24 hr. They found that this once-a-day impulsive activity was very sensitive to inhibition by exogenously administered corticosteroids, but that the basal secretion was very insensitive to feedback.

Krieger and Rizzo (1969) showed that drugs which affected the level of serotonin (5-hydroxytryptamine) in the CNS, or antagonized its action, could also prevent the normal circadian rise in plasma corticosteroids in the cat, and they again demonstrated that the pathways mediating the circadian rhythm in the CNS differed from those involved in the HPA response to stress. As a result of their series of experiments they concluded that the CNS regulates the circadian periodicity of corticosteroid secretion, and that cholinergic and serotonin-dependent pathways are involved in this regulation. These experiments, together with other evidence of the CNS control of the circadian rhythm of the pituitary-adrenal system, have recently been reviewed by Krieger (1970).

Little direct experimental evidence of the CNS control of the adrenal rhythm in man has been obtained, but there have been some studies performed in patients with chronic electrode implants in the brain. Electrical stimulation of the amygdala has been reported to cause a rise in plasma corticosteroids whilst stimulation of the hippocampus produced a fall (Mandell *et al.*, 1963; Rubin *et al.*, 1966). Evidence from pathological lesions in the CNS also suggests that the mechanism of the regulation of the rhythm may be similar to that in other mammalian species. However, as will be discussed in a later section, the adrenal circadian rhythm may be disturbed in a wide variety of pathological states, not all of which appear to involve the CNS, hence any conclusions concerning control which are drawn from observations on patients with CNS lesions should be tentative. Perkoff *et al.* (1959) showed that patients with altered states of consciousness or disturbed sleep patterns lost their adrenal circadian rhythm, in contrast to a wide variety of other pathological states in which the rhythm remained essentially normal. These findings were similar to those of Eik-Nes and Clark (1958) who studied four patients with severe CNS disorders and a profound degree of impairment of consciousness. All had loss of the normal circadian rhythm, with higher than normal mean levels of plasma corticosteroids. It was not clear from the study whether the abnormality was due to unawareness of environmental change, or due to a lesion in the neural pathways which might be responsible for regulation of the rhythm. Krieger (1961) studied two patients with lesions in the pretectal area, and two with lesions in the left temporal lobe. Each showed marked disturbance of both amplitude and phase of the plasma cortisol rhythm. Three patients with respectively a sphenoidal ridge meningioma, left occipital lobe cyst and cerebellar tumour showed no such disturbance. None of the patients had any alteration in consciousness, involvement of the pituitary or increased intracranial pressure, so the author concluded that her data supported the view that the pretectal area and temporal lobe are important in the regulation of ACTH release, and hence the circadian pattern of plasma corticosteroids which reflects it. A normal circadian rhythm was found in a number of patients with CNS disease, including temporal lobe lesions, by Oppenheimer *et al.* (1961), although one case of temporal lobe epilepsy had lost the rhythm. It is interesting to note that a normal rhythm was sometimes accompanied by abnormal responses to other endocrine tests such as metyrapone and dexamethasone suppression. This gave support to the view which had been derived from animal experiments that the mechanism leading to normal circadian rhythm was mediated via different pathways from the feedback and stress response mechanisms. Krieger and Krieger (1966) again showed that patients with CNS disease outside the hypothalamic-limbic system had a corticosteroid rhythm which did not differ significantly from the normal. On the other hand, of 27 patients with focal disease in the pretectum, temporal lobe or hypothalamus, 17 had an abnormal rhythm according to a strict definition of abnormality which the authors describe. In these patients, as in those of Oppenheimer *et al.* (1961), there was no correlation between the occurrence of an abnormal circadian pattern and an abnormal metyrapone response, and the rhythm abnormality could occur in alert, conscious patients with normal sleep patterns. In another study of 14 patients with circumscribed hypothalamic disease, Krieger and her group (Krieger et al., 1968) found 7 with abnormal circadian rhythm, and this was the parameter of endocrine function most frequently found to be abnormal.

Further indirect evidence of CNS control of the adrenal rhythm in man has been adduced from the variability at different times of day in the response of the HPA axis to the various function tests that have been devised for its clinical evaluation. These have been designed mainly to investigate stress and feedback responsiveness. Martin and Hellman (1964) reported that infusion of metyrapone between 0600 and 1200 hr was followed by a prompt rise in urinary 11-desoxycortisol, indicating a brisk ACTH response. Infusion of a similar dose during the afternoon produced a delayed response of lesser magnitude, although inhibition of 11β hydroxylation was shown to be adequate. Hence the response to metyrapone, i.e. to the feedback stimulus of a lowered plasma cortisol (Liddle et al., 1959), was greatest at the time of day when adrenocortical activity was maximal, and least when it was minimal. There is a similar diurnal variability in the feedback response to increased levels of circulating corticosteroids. Dexamethasone in a dose of 0.5 mg orally at 0800 or 1600 hr caused only temporary suppression of cortisol secretion, whereas the same dose given at midnight produced marked suppression of cortisol production for 24 hr (Nichols et al., 1965). Ceresa et al. (1969, 1970) studied the diurnal variation in feedback suppressibility of corticosteroid secretion by infusing 6-methylprednisolone at different times of day in doses that were not maximally suppressive. Suppression was obtained only from infusion during the nocturnal early morning hours, and not during the period 0800 to midnight. They postulate two phases of ACTH secretion, only one of which, the impulsive early morning peak, is sensitive to the feedback effect of submaximal doses of corticoids. This peak they suggest is due to "once a day" neural stimulation. The basal ACTH activity which forms the other phase might be due to autonomous CRF secretion by the hypothalamus, or to extrahypothalamic nervous stimuli which differ from those responsible for the circadian peak.

A diurnal rhythm of response to a synthetic vasopressin analogue which showed a phase opposite to the rhythmic variation of the metyrapone response was discovered by Clayton et al. (1963). There was a greater rise in the plasma corticosteroid level following vasopressin administration at midnight and at 1700 hr than at 0800; in other words the response varied inversely with the plasma corticosteroid level. A similarly phased rhythm of variation in response to hypoglycaemia has also been reported in man. The response of the plasma cortisol to insulin-induced hypoglycaemia at midnight was significantly greater than at 1000 hr, in contrast to the simultaneously measured growth hormone response which was greater at 1000 hr (Takebe *et al.*, 1969). This finding was confirmed for the plasma cortisol response by Ichikawa *et al.*, 1972, who found a greater increment at 2100 than at 0900 hr. Somewhat confusingly, however, they found the increment in the plasma ACTH was the same at both times. It is interesting that these observations of the variation in the human adrenal response to the stress of hypoglycaemia at different times are the inverse of those found by Gibbs (1970) in the response of the rat to ether stress. He reported that the plasma corticosterone response to ether is greater at the time of the circadian peak in this species than at the trough, although Hodges (1970) found the increment in plasma corticosterone to be the same in the morning and afternoon.

If it be correct that the site of feedback control of HPA function is in the hypothalamus then results of these tests add evidence, albeit indirect, in support of the view that the CNS controls the adrenal circadian rhythm in man. The exact location of the feedback site remains controversial however, and it seems most probable there are multiple sites of which the pituitary itself may be one (Yates *et al.*, 1971). Hence the precise significance of the diurnal variability in the HPA response to these clinical tests has not yet been defined.

C. SYNCHRONIZERS OF THE HPA CIRCADIAN RHYTHM

A large number of studies has been undertaken in an attempt to define the environmental change which forms the major synchronizer of the HPA rhythm. These have included investigation of the circadian rhythms of night workers, isolation of experimental subjects in caves, studies of the effect of continuous light and continuous darkness, alteration or reversal of sleeping patterns, observations of air travellers rapidly transported across time zones, and studies on blind individuals. Certainly the rhythm of sleep and wakefulness has an important synchronizing effect, but so, it appears, has the change from darkness to light, and Mills (1966) has suggested that contact with other people living a normal diurnal/nocturnal existence may be more important as a synchronizer than the habits of the subject himself.

Experiments designed to isolate the circadian synchronizer are extremely complex, as they necessitate removal of every rhythmic variable except the one being tested. In practice this is very difficult, and may involve, for example, separating periods of light from periods of wakefulness, and periods of darkness from periods of sleep, a procedure which is likely to be stressful to the experimental subject. It will be remembered that the circadian rhythm is only one of the determinants of cortisol secretion. There is also 'stress', a state provoked by many environmental stimuli, as well as such emotions as excitement, anger and fear, any of which may lead to a rise of plasma cortisol which can override the circadian mechanism. Experiments based on 'real life' situations, such as intercontinental air-travel, rather than on artificial laboratory situations, are also subject to such problems plus the added difficulties of precisely timed sample collection outside the laboratory environment.

It is thus understandable that the identity of the main HPA synchronizer has not been fully resolved despite the many experiments carried out, only a proportion of which can be reviewed here.

Migeon *et al.* (1956), studied plasma corticosteroid levels in night workers who had been on their shift for at least 6 months, and found that their rhythm was essentially similar to that of normal controls. However, it was pointed out that the night workers did not have an absolutely regular schedule, but worked 5 nights on and 2 off each week, and it could be that this break resulted in the failure of their rhythm to re-synchronize completely to the sleep/wake reversal of their nights on duty. This seems likely in view of the findings of Conroy *et al.* (1970) who used a fluorimetric technique for plasma corticosteroids (Spencer-Peet *et al.*, 1965) to study 3 groups of workers: day workers who worked from 0730 to 1630 hr, workers on monthly rotation of shifts with a night shift from 2200 to 0700 hr, and workers on permanent night work, from 2000 to 0800 hr. Not all the day workers were normal—4 out of 20 showed no consistent pattern, the reason for this was unexplained. The rotating-shift night workers were inconsistent, 10 out of 23 showed no discernible rhythm. Of the remainder some showed a maximum concentration around midnight and minimum at 0600, whilst others had a normal daytime type of rhythm. The workers on permanent night work showed a consistent rhythm with a maximum steroid concentration around 1400 hr, when they were arising from sleep, and minimal values in the early morning. The authors concluded that the adrenal cortical rhythm can be adapted to night work in a community in which this is universal, accepted and lifelong, but that such adjustment is unusual in men on night shift work for limited periods, and whose associates are mainly following a usual nycthemeral existence.

Experimental alteration of the sleeping pattern of normal subjects has been studied by a number of workers. Perkoff *et al.* (1959) subjected 4 healthy adult males and 4 healthy adult females to sleep reversal, the experiment lasting 5 days before reversal and 10 days after it. The subjects were confined to a hospital ward from which daylight was excluded. They slept from 0800 to 1600 hr and were active from 1600 to 0800 hr, taking meals at 0500, 0000 and 0700 hr. The relationship of meals to sleep/activity cycles seems rather unusual (e.g. dinner in the hour before retiring). The authors also do not state whether 'lights on' and 'lights off' were abrupt, or coincided exactly with the times of retirement and arousal. By the end of the reversal period, the diurnal pattern of plasma 17 OHCS level showed distinct inversion. It was noted that the amplitude of the reversed rhythm was less than that prior to reversal.

Sharp *et al.* (1961) studied the excretion of urinary corticosteroids during a sleep reversal experiment carried out at Spitzbergen during the continuous daylight of the Arctic summer. Four healthy adult males were investigated, and slept with light blindfolds. Three-hourly urine samples were collected between 0700 hr and 2200 hr, then a 9 hr nocturnal sample from 2200-0700. After sleep reversal (exact 12 hr shift) 3 hr sampling was from 1900-1000 and a 'night' sample from 1000-1900. 17 oxogenic steroids were measured on the 2nd, 4th, 6th and 8th days after reversal. During period 1 (control) 92.9% of daily total 17 oxogenic was excreted between 0700 and 2200 hr, 61.1% between 0700 and 1900 hr. In general there was a high morning output, a mid afternoon drop and a slightly higher evening output followed by a fall at night. After two days sleep reversal the rhythm of excretion was disrupted, but had reversed to a completely normal inverted pattern by the 8th day. There was a similar delay in adaptation of steroid excretion on reversing sleep back again to normal.

A very detailed experiment in which normal subjects in a metabolic ward were investigated on various sleep-wake schedules was performed by Orth et al. (1967). A 'normal' schedule and 3 experimental schedules of 12, 19 and 33 hr length were employed. A third of each cycle was spent in sleep. The rooms were darkened during the hours of sleep and well lighted during the hours of wakefulness. Sampling of blood was performed without awakening the subjects. Plasma corticosteroids were measured by the Porter-Silber method. With the 12 hr sleep-wake cycle all three subjects developed two cycles of plasma corticosteroid per 24 hr following 12 days of equilibration, but adaptation was not complete after shorter periods. The 12 hr adrenal cycle showed a normal shape, with lowest levels during the first hour or two of sleep, followed by a rapid rise and maximal values about the time of awakening. Two complete cycles occurred in the 24 hr period. With a 19 hr sleep-wake period the cycle became bimodal with 2 crests and 2 troughs; nevertheless there was definite phase synchronization with the sleep-wake schedule. On a 33 hr period, the curves were irregular, but the dominant rhythm again synchronized with the sleep-wake schedule. The authors concluded that the reason the 17 OHCS rhythm has a period of about 24 hr is because that is the duration of the habitual sleep-wake cycle which most people follow. If the sleep-wake cycle be altered the 17 OHCS rhythm gradually adapts to the new sleep-wake schedule. The fact that this adaptation is not immediate shows that the sleep-wake related determinants of pituitary-adrenal function are more subtle than the obvious clinical manifestations of sleep. These results differ from those found in animals, in which if the external synchronizer is altered beyond certain limits, usually to outside the range of 20 to 28 hours, then the signal no longer acts as a synchronizer and the rhythm becomes "free-running".

Later, the same group attempted to determine with greater precision the effect of light (Orth and Island, 1969). Normal subjects were studied in light-proof rooms and each slept from 2200 to 0600 hr. Three variations of the light-dark cycle were superimposed on the sleep-wake cycle. In the first, the 8 hr period of total darkness was from 1000 to 1800 hr, 12 hours out of phase with the sleep period, the subjects sleeping in well-lighted rooms. In the second, the darkness was in phase with sleep, but prolonged beyond waking, i.e. from 2200 to 1000 hr. In the third, subjects were in total darkness except for a single hour, 1800-1900 hr. Each schedule was maintained for 10-14 days prior to blood sampling. Blood samples were taken without waking the subjects. During the control phase—sleep in darkness—typical circadian rhythms were obtained, with the corticosteroid nadir during the first hour or two of sleep, levels which then rose rapidly towards mid-sleep, and a maximum at about the time of awakening and exposure to light. After 13 days on the schedule in which darkness was 12 hours out of phase with sleep, the dominant peak still occurred at about the time of wakening in the three subjects tested, but additional peaks occurred when the lights were turned on. In the period during which darkness persisted for 4 hr beyond awakening, i.e. till 1000 hr, the 3 subjects tested after 14 days on this regime showed the peak plasma cortisol at the time of the change from darkness to light. Three subjects who remained in darkness for 23 hr/day showed no rise in plasma cortisol during sleep, but only following sleep. A second significant peak occurred when the lights were turned on at 1800 hr.

The authors concluded that the plasma 17 OHCS cycle in man can be altered by modification of the dark-light cycle alone, and that the change from darkness to light is the important synchronizing stimulus.

Another attempt to separate the variables of darkness-light from sleep-wake as the determinant of the circadian rhythm of plasma cortisol was made by Krieger *et al.* (1969). After baseline studies on a normal schedule (sleep in darkness, midnight-0800) there followed 21 days of constant light, with a normal sleep-wake schedule, and finally 13 days of constant light with a reversed sleep-wake schedule. One healthy male and one healthy female were studied. Constant light with a normal sleep schedule produced a normal circadian rhythm. EEG monitoring of sleep showed normal percentage and time of occurrence of REM sleep. Reversal of the sleep-wake patterns resulted in phase reversal of the circadian rhythm of cortisol, despite persistent light. The authors concluded that the circadian rhythm of cortisol is not related to the presence of darkness, but is related to processes occurring in the course of sleep. No conclusion could be drawn as to the role of the presence of light.

A study of the circadian rhythm of urinary 17 OHCS excretion during continuous darkness has been made by Aschoff *et al.* (1971). Experimental subjects were enclosed in groups of two in an underground sound-proof room. There was a rigid time schedule, rest in bed being from 2330 to 0730 hr. For the first 4 days there was an artificial light-dark cycle, with the periods of darkness and light corresponding exactly with those of sleep and wakefulness. For a subsequent 4 days total darkness was maintained. Throughout both periods the timing of meals, sleep and the performance of various psycho-motor tests was strictly maintained. Urine was collected 3 hourly, and analysed for corticosteroids, catechol amines and sodium. No change in the circadian rhythm of excretion of any of these substances was observed between the light/dark and the total darkness periods. The authors considered their results showed that a light/dark cycle was unnecessary to entrain human circadian rhythms, at least for 4 days, but that the rhythm was entrained by social clues from the environment. However, it seems that as the subjects' sleeping time was maintained constant throughout the experiment this could have been the major synchronizer.

Studies of the adrenal rhythm in blind subjects, which might be expected to have made a contribution towards the resolution of the difficulty in deciding whether the light/dark cycle or the sleep/wake cycle is a primary synchronizer, have also yielded ambiguous results. Migeon et al. (1956) found normal circadian rhythms of plasma corticosteroids in 6 blind subjects. Three blind patients were investigated by Orth and Island (1969). Each had a circadian rhythm, one of which was normal in phase, i.e. with a peak level at about the time of waking, a second was abnormal in phase, with a peak prior to sleep rather than following it, and the third appeared to have a 'free-running', i.e. unsynchronized, rhythm with a period of about 24 hr 23 min.

Krieger and Rizzo (1971) studied a number of patients with partial light perception as well as some with total blindness. Of 7 subjects with partial light perception 5 had abnormal circadian patterns of plasma 11 OHCS, as defined by the authors, i.e. the level should be less than 75% of the 0800 level at any time after 0800 except noon. However, all showed a rise toward the end of sleep, though not necessarily to the peak, which may have occurred later, or earlier (e.g. 0400). Twelve subjects were totally blind, and of these 9 had abnormal circadian rhythms. All but 2, however, showed a rise toward the end of sleep, although the peak was not necessarily at 0800 hr. The abnormality did not correlate with age, sex or duration of blindness (which was always due to a peripheral cause). The authors concluded that the occurrence of a rise in plasma steroid levels with sleep-wake transition in all but 2 of the blind subjects indicated that sleep-wake rather than dark-light transition was the primary synchronizer. The abnormality throughout the rest of the day might have been due to the absence of light, which may normally modulate HPA function.

A further demonstration of the importance of sleep itself as a regulator of the adrenal rhythm was made by Simpson (1965). He sought to determine whether a population with a very precise routine of life such as that led by a tribe of equatorial American Indians might have a more marked rhythm than Europeans of more irregular habits. Comparing the 17 OHCS excretion of the Indians with that of Glasgow medical students he found the phase of the rhythm when referred to midnight differed between the Indians and the Scots, the peaks of excretion in the former occurring earlier, in keeping with their earlier time of retiring and rising. However, when this data was reanalysed, taking a time midway between retiring and rising instead of midnight as the reference point, the discrepancy between the phase of the circadian rhythm for the two population groups disappeared (Halberg and Simpson, 1967). This work showed the value of using an internal reference point within the biological system under study, rather than some external reference such as clock-time, particularly when comparing one rhythm with another.

Development of sleep-monitoring techniques such as those described in Section II. B above have enabled the circadian increase in adrenal secretion to be related not simply to sleep, but to definite sleep stages. Mandell and Mandell (1965, 1969) and Mandell *et al.* (1966b) measured corticosteroid excretion during EEG monitored sleep, employing continuous urine collections via a urethral catheter. They found an increase in urinary corticosteroids towards the end of, or immediately following, a REM period, and suggested that REM sleep might be a concomitant of a periodic discharge of the neuro-endocrine apparatus triggered by low circulating required metabolites, perhaps glucose or fatty acids, and that the gluconeogenic influence of periodic glucocorticoid discharge might be a rhythmic energy feeding mechanism to maintain the organism through the long fast of sleep.

Similar results to those of the Mandells and their colleagues were obtained by Weitzman *et al.* (1966) who sampled blood at 30 min intervals during EEG monitored sleep in 6 subjects and found peak elevations associated with REM periods. Weitzman's group confirmed this relationship in subsequent studies (Hellman *et al.*, 1970a; Weitzman *et al.*, 1971), and found that nearly half the total cortisol produced in the 24 hr was secreted during this REM sleep associated phase. Yet they point out that there is no simple one-to-one ratio between a REM and a secretory period. It is clear from the sleep reversal experiments cited earlier in this section, that REM sleep and corticosteroid secretion can be separated, at least temporarily, and Weitzman *et al.* (1968) themselves showed such dissociation during a sleep reversal experiment. Other studies have also shown the persistence of the corticosteroid rhythm in the complete absence of sleep (Halberg *et al.*, 1961, Frank *et al.*, 1966), but Rubin *et al.* (1969) showed that when sleep deprivation was prolonged to between 120 and 205 hours some disruption of the rhythm began to appear.

Anders *et al.* (1970) could detect no rise in plasma cortisol associated with REM sleep in 4 normal infants from 1-15 weeks old, although there was a rise during crying.

A variant of the sleep reversal experiment is provided by East-West intercontinental air travel which involves rapid alteration of both sleep-wake and light-dark cycles. As long ago as 1959 Flink and Doe showed that it took 11 days for the circadian pattern of urinary corticosteroid excretion to become fully adapted to the new societal time following a flight from Minneapolis to

Korea (time shift 9 hr), whilst on the first day after arrival the rhythm remained appropriate to the previous time zone. A number of similar studies have been made and their results and significance reviewed by Siegel et al. (1969). In a recent experiment of this type volunteers were studied for 7 days in England, then flown to San Francisco, where testing was continued for 10 days, and finally studied for a further 7 days after return to England (Evans et al., 1972). The changes in plasma corticosteroids were reported by Daly (1970). Blood was sampled 4 hourly on several days during each phase of the experiment, and plasma corticosteroids determined fluorimetrically (Spencer-Peet et al., 1965). The East to West journey produced immediate disruption of the rhythm, with apparently random peaks and considerable variation between individuals, but with a nadir persisting at about midnight British time (mid afternoon Pacific Coast time). On the fourth day the rhythm had completely re-phased to Pacific Coast time, but the amplitude of the oscillation was less than during the control period. On the tenth day the rhythm was normal in both phase and amplitude. After return to England the rhythm was again completely disrupted and showed no sign of recovery at the conclusion of the experiment. It was uncertain whether this meant it was harder to adapt to West to East travel than to East to West, or whether the circadian control mechanisms were rendered less adaptable owing to their having had to make another considerable adjustment only a short time before.

Although all these studies have not enabled us to characterize with certainty and precision the sole synchronizer of the HPA circadian rhythm it seems that the major one is somehow related to the mechanism of sleep, for although the circadian peak can be uncoupled from sleep, 'the ultimate resynchronization of the sleep cycle with the steroid release cycle following geographic and laboratory phase shifts, nevertheless indicates the importance of the sleep period as one of the determinants in the timing of ACTH release' (Hellman et al., 1970a).

D. ALTERATIONS OF THE HPA CIRCADIAN RHYTHM IN DISEASE

Disturbances of the HPA axis which occur in organic CNS disease have been discussed in the previous section, but abnormalities have also been described in affective disease, as well as in some pathological states in which there is no obvious organic or functional disorder of the nervous system. Acute illness, particularly when accompanied by pain or fever, as well as surgery and trauma, cause stress activation of the HPA axis, and this may over-ride the circadian rhythm. Loss of rhythm has been described in congestive heart failure by Connolly and Wills (1967) and Knapp et al. (1967), using the fluorimetric method of Mattingly (1962) for plasma corticosteroids, but the reason for this is unclear.

Sholiton et al. (1961) investigated the circadian rhythm of plasma and urinary corticosteroids using the methods of Nelson and Samuels (1952) and

Glenn and Nelson (1953) respectively, methods based on the Porter-Silber reaction. Their patients fell into three main groups: (1) chronically ill patients who were alert and rational. These were subdivided into three subgroups—miscellaneous, cirrhotic and uraemic. Each subgroup showed similar and normal plasma and urinary circadian rhythms. (2) Patients with bronchial carcinoma, who were subdivided into ambulatory and advanced. These showed a significant difference between the two subgroups. A circadian rhythm was present in the ambulatory patients but was lost in the advanced subgroup, who also showed greatly raised levels of plasma corticosteroids. This might have been due to the stress of terminal illness or to the inclusion in the group of some cases of ectopic ACTH syndrome, which had not been clearly defined at the time Sholiton and his colleagues published their work. (3) Patients acutely ill with fever, half of whom were mentally confused, formed the final group. Those acutely ill, but normally conscious, showed a normal circadian rhythm of corticosteroids. Those who were confused, however, had a completely disrupted rhythm with raised corticosteroid levels.

Alteration in cortisol metabolism may be expected to cause disturbances of adrenal rhythm in liver disease, but Tucci et al. (1966) did not think that this alone accounted for the abnormalities observed in plasma and urinary corticosteroids in their patients. Metabolic abnormalities leading to circadian disturbances might also be expected in thyroid disease, and this was confirmed by Martin et al. (1965) who found raised urinary corticosteroids with an increased amplitude of the circadian rhythm in thyrotoxicosis, and reduced excretion with loss of rhythm in myxoedema. Gallagher et al. (1972) found that in thyrotoxicosis the number of adrenal secretory eposides during the 24 hr was increased from 7-9 in controls to 12-16 in 4 thyrotoxic patients they studied in detail. There was thus a substantially increased cortisol secretion rate in thyrotoxicosis, but the plasma half-time of cortisol was correspondingly reduced by the increased metabolic rate, and hence the average quantity perfusing the tissues was no greater than normal. The very low secretion characteristic of mid-sleep occurred normally in the thyrotoxic patients.

Cushing's Syndrome is the best known of all pathological states causing loss of the circadian rhythm of the HPA axis, and this is so no matter whether the cause of the syndrome be sustained hypothalamopituitary over-drive leading to adrenal hyperplasia, tumour of the adrenal leading to autonomous cortisol secretion, or ectopic ACTH syndrome. This loss of the rhythm in Cushing's Syndrome has been described by, among others, Doe et al. (1960), Ekman et al. (1961) and Knapp et al. (1967). Hellman et al. (1970b) studied one patient with Cushing's Syndrome in detail, and found the secretion of cortisol was episodic, as it is in normal subjects, but the general level of secretion was much higher than normal. There is a sleep disturbance in Cushing's Syndrome associated with adrenal hyperplasia, with a decrease in the amount of time spent in REM sleep as well as in stages 3 and 4 (Krieger and Glick, 1972). This may perhaps indicate a CNS abnormality responsible both for the sleep disturbance and the loss of circadian rhythm and also perhaps for the psychiatric disturbance which is a feature of Cushing's Syndrome. However, psychiatric disorder has been reported in patients with Cushing's Syndrome due to adrenocortical adenoma (Regestein *et al.*, 1972), as well as during prolonged high dosage corticosteroid therapy. Hence the raised level of corticosteroid in itself may be responsible. Gillin *et al.* (1972) have shown that exogenously administered glucocorticoid can markedly reduce the percentage of REM sleep.

There have been many studies of adrenocortical activity in psychiatric disease (see Rubin and Mandell, 1966, and Mason, 1968 for reviews). The magnitude of the disturbance both of sleep and of adrenocortical activity correlates with the degree of psychic turmoil, and this may well be a non-specific stress response (Curtis *et al.*, 1966). However, despite somewhat conflicting evidence, there appears to be a more or less specific disturbance of the HPA circadian rhythm in depression. The general level of secretion is high (McClure, 1966; Bridges and Jones, 1966) and the phasing may be different from normal, with both nadir and the morning rise occurring earlier (Knapp *et al.* 1967; Conroy *et al.*, 1968; Fullerton *et al.*, 1968), or completely disrupted (Butler and Besser, 1968). Roffwarg *et al.* (1970) in a study of 8 depressives sampled blood every 20 min throughout the night with EEG monitoring of sleep, and found that although the general shape of the plasma cortisol rhythm and the number of secretory episodes was similar to normal, the low basal levels which healthy subjects show early in the night were raised in the depressed patients and the later peaks were very high.

In contrast, Knapp *et al.* (1967) have found a normal HPA circadian rhythm in schizophrenia. It is possible that the circadian abnormality in depression is related to the early wakening and profound disturbance of both orthodox and REM sleep which occur in this disease (Snyder, 1969), whilst the normal circadian pattern in schizophrenia may be associated with the unchanged REM intensities and somewhat reduced percentage of REM (Kupfer *et al.*, 1970). However, the evidence concerning the sleep disturbances found in psychotic illness is unfortunately still very conflicting, and many of the early studies neglected the effects of prolonged medication. This problem has been discussed by St. Laurent (1971) and Mendels and Hawkins (1971).

IV. SECRETION OF GROWTH HORMONE (GH)

A. RELATION OF GH SECRETION TO SLEEP

The secretion of GH from the anterior pituitary, like that of ACTH, appears to be dependent on a releasing factor from the hypothalamus. Secretion occurs in response to a wide range of stimuli, including exercise, stress, fasting, hypoglycaemia, amino acid infusion, and a decrease in plasma fatty acids. There is evidence that certain of these stimuli in the wakeful state may be mediated via alpha-adrenergic receptors in the CNS (Blackard and Heidingsfelder, 1968). Despite the wide range of potential stimulants of secretion the circulating level of GH is normally very low during the day (< 2.0 ng/ml). The general physiology of GH release has been reviewed by Glick et al. (1965) and Tanner (1972).

Because of the low levels of circulating GH and the variety of exogenous stimuli which may affect it, recognition of a circadian rhythm has been difficult, and Goldsmith and Glick (1970) found periodic increases which appeared unrelated to any previously described stimulus of GH release. It was noted by several investigators that GH levels tended to be particularly high during the night (Quabbe et al., 1966; Hunter et al., 1966; Hunter and Rigal, 1966), and later work by many groups has shown a clear relationship of secretion to certain well-defined sleep stages, in which GH shows an interesting contrast to the nocturnal pattern of HPA activity.

Takahashi et al. (1968) and Honda et al. (1969) independently discovered an almost invariable association between GH secretion and early sleep. They studied healthy young subjects, sampling plasma every 20 or 30 min throughout the night with full EEG monitoring of sleep. A rise in GH was noted some 20-40 min after sleep onset with the peak occurring 39-165 min (mean 70) after onset. Takahashi's group reported peak values of 13-72 ng/ml (mean 34), whilst Honda's group found peak values of 3.7-40 ng/ml. The former group employed a double antibody radioimmunoassay technique (Schalch and Parker, 1964), and the latter a radioimmunoassay using electrophoretic separation of bound and free hormone (Glick et al., 1963). Differences in technique and in antibody and standard used make direct comparisons of levels obtained in different centres difficult to interpret. However, both groups of workers noted the peak to be of a magnitude similar to that obtained with previously described stimulants of GH release such as insulin-hypoglycaemia or arginine infusion. Both also noted an association with stage 3 and 4 sleep, and Honda et al. considered there was inhibition of GH release coincident with the onset of a REM phase.

These observations of the occurrence of GH secretion with great regularity early in sleep have now been repeatedly confirmed, and the very close relationship between its secretion and some component of sleep itself has also been demonstrated (Fig. 8). Parker et al. (1969) showed that the association between stage 3 and 4 sleep and GH release was not simply due to the coincidence of these shortly after sleep onset, but that secretion was directly related to the sleep stage. Smaller rises in GH occurred fairly frequently throughout sleep after the initial major peak, and the majority of these later peaks were also associated with slow wave (stage 3 and 4) sleep. The authors considered that since slow wave sleep is a cortical event and initiation of GH secretion is probably hypothalamic, there may be activity in a common subcortical centre which is basic to both events.

Numerous experiments have been carried out in an attempt to dissociate slow wave sleep from GH release by means of delaying, interrupting, reversing and preventing sleep. In their original report Takahashi *et al.* (1968) also described their results with some experiments of this type. Sleep was delayed in some of their subjects by 3-3½ hr. The expected rise in GH did not occur at the usual clock time, the subjects being still awake, but occurred some 30-90 min after sleep was permitted, and during an episode of slow wave sleep. Honda *et al.* (1969) obtained similar results whether sleep was delayed or brought forward in

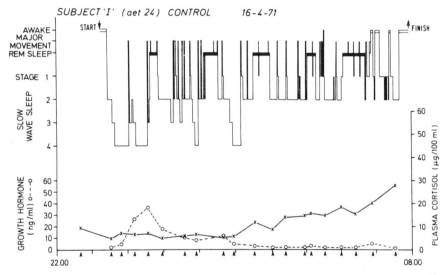

Fig. 8. Correlation between the sleep histogram and the plasma levels of corticosteroids (X———X) and GH (o ____ o) in a normal man.

time. In either event the GH peak moved with sleep, and was not related to clock time. Likewise both Takahashi *et al.* and Honda *et al.* found that prolonged interruption of sleep after the initial GH peak had occurred produced a second peak shortly after resumption of sleep was permitted. When sleep was reversed from night-time to daytime sleep GH secretion also reversed immediately, and the peak occurred early in the first sleep period after reversal and was associated with a slow wave cycle (Sassin *et al.*, 1969a). During the 24 hr of wakefulness that had to be maintained to accomplish the reversal there was no period of GH secretion corresponding in clock time to sleep on the control nights. These workers found no evidence of an endogenous rhythm of GH secretion independent of sleep.

Deprivation of slow wave sleep has been achieved by inflicting electrical stimulation to the dorsum of the foot every time the EEG trace showed signs of entry into stage 3 (Sassin *et al.*, 1969b). Shocks were repeated until a change in the EEG was noted. Total sleep time was not diminished by this procedure, and although as many as 300 shocks might have been administered during the two nights of slow-wave-deprived sleep, only three or four were remembered. Deprivation of slow-wave sleep resulted in delay in GH secretion in three subjects of the five tested, with lower peaks in two of these, and complete absence of the peak in the remaining two subjects. Othmer *et al.* (1969) conducted a study in which the subjects were deprived of REM sleep, and found such deprivation significantly increased GH levels.

Finkelstein *et al.* (1971) studied GH secretion in infants and found consistently low plasma levels (< 5 ng/ml) during quiet wakefulness, and no rise during arousal or distress, although the plasma cortisol showed a distinct rise during distressed crying as early as the first week of life. They also found no significant increase of GH level in association with any sleep stage, but point out that the typical EEG changes of stage 3 and 4 sleep are not seen in infants of the age group studied (15 weeks). In another study these authors (Shaywitz *et al.*, 1971) studied newborn infants and found that at two days old GH levels were very high (75-150 ng/ml), but had fallen considerably by the fourth day. They were unable to demonstrate any relationship between GH secretion and quiet sleep, which is considered to be the ontogenic precursor of the slow wave sleep of adults. A statistically significant difference between GH levels during sleep and wakefulness is apparent in infants older than 3 months (Vigneri *et al.*, 1971). Children between 5 and 14 show a clear relationship between slow wave sleep and GH release, with peak levels comparable to those achieved during hypoglycaemia (Underwood *et al.*, 1971).

Vigneri *et al.* (1971) also noted that nocturnal GH peaks were diminished in the elderly (60-90 years) in whom it is known, as pointed out in Section II above, that there is less slow wave sleep than in younger age groups.

These experiments have revealed a marked contrast between the relationship of sleep to GH secretion on the one hand, and ACTH secretion on the other. GH secretion occurs maximally during the first two hours of sleep; ACTH secretion is at its lowest level during this time. GH secretion is related to slow-wave sleep; insofar as there is any relationship with ACTH, slow-wave sleep would appear to inhibit its secretion. ACTH secretion rises during late sleep, possibly in association with REM periods; GH secretion appears to be inhibited during this phase (Fig. 8). During sleep deprivation the GH peak fails to appear; ACTH secretion appears at the same clock-time that would normally have coincided with late sleep. During sleep reversal there is immediate association between GH secretion and the new time of sleep onset; ACTH secretion takes between 4 and 10 days to become adjusted to the new sleep/wake rhythm.

B. METABOLIC CORRELATES OF SLEEP-ASSOCIATED GH RELEASE

GH causes a rise in plasma free fatty acids, and its secretion is provoked by hypoglycaemia, hence it has been suggested that it may be a minute-to-minute regulator of substrate availability. The metabolic significance of its nocturnal release is thus of great interest.

Hyperglycaemia inhibits GH release during the wakeful state in normal subjects, but Quabbe *et al.* (1971) found no correlation during sleep between the level of plasma GH and that of glucose, free fatty acids and immunoreactive insulin.

VanderLaan *et al.* (1970) and Parker and Rossman (1971a) infused glucose during sleep and produced blood glucose levels of between 132 and 332 mg/100 ml. They collected blood samples every 20-30 min during EEG monitored sleep and found no significant difference in the peak GH level between the glucose infusion and the control nights. These findings were confirmed by Lucke and Glick (1971a), who found, however, that in three of their subjects whose plasma glucose reached between 350 and 480 mg/100 ml some suppression of GH did occur. There was no suppression in seven studies in which the glucose reached from 180-320 mg/100 ml. Schnure *et al.* (1971) also found glucose infusion did not alter nocturnal GH secretion in their subjects. They then studied the effect of the nocturnal GH peak on glucose tolerance. Intravenous glucose tolerance tests (GTT) were performed at 0800 hr after a normal night's sleep, and on a subsequent morning after a night during which slow-wave sleep had been prevented. On a third occasion the GTT was performed after slow-wave sleep had been delayed until 0400 hr and then permitted. Levels of GH remained basal during the slow wave deprived night, and the subsequent GTT was similar to the control. Following the night of delayed slow-wave sleep, which resulted in the appearance of a GH peak at around 0400 hr, there was significant impairment in the morning GTT. In another study a GTT was performed at 0100 hr during maintained wakefulness, so that no GH peak occurred, and on a subsequent night during sleep at about 90 min after the GH peak. There was significant impairment of glucose tolerance in the sleep GTT, whilst that performed at about the same time, but with the subject awake, was normal. These results were confirmed using oral GTT. Hence the nocturnal GH peak, whenever it occurs, causes significant impairment of glucose tolerance as measured both by intravenous and oral GTT, although no difference was demonstrated in the levels of immunoreactive insulin. Nakagawa (1971) found the GH response to hypoglycaemia was diminished during sleep if it followed the sleep-related GH peak, but there was no impairment of the night-time response if sleep was not permitted.

Parker *et al.* (1972) studied sleep-related GH release during an 80 hr fast, and also during 6 days of a 600 g carbohydrate, 4,000 calorie diet. Normal sleep and

GH patterns were exhibited throughout both situations, although the GH peak was higher during fasting, but the timing and frequency of peaks were unchanged. This was depite the changes in plasma glucose and non-esterified fatty acids which were provoked by the experimental conditions.

Lipman et al. (1972) recently reported they had succeeded in suppressing GH release during sleep in 4 young men by elevating their plasma-free fatty acid levels with an orally administered lipid preparation.

There is a circadian rhythm in the level of plasma amino acids in man, a feature of which is a decline during early sleep, between the hours of 2200 and 0200. As it is known that GH lowers plasma amino acids it was considered the circadian decline in these at night might be secondary to the sleep-associated GH peak. This was investigated by Zir et al. (1972) who measured plasma tyrosine and GH during sleep. They confirmed that the decline in plasma tyrosine and the rise in GH occurred concurrently, but a sleep delay experiment shifted the GH peak but not the decline in tyrosine, which occurred at the customary clock-time. Likewise subjects without a GH peak, including 3 with pan-hypopituitarism, showed the usual decline in plasma tyrosine.

Exercise is a recognized stimulator of GH release. However, exercise of what Zir et al. (1971) describe as 'moderate intensity', but which produced fatigue in all the fit young Naval personnel who formed the experimental subjects, did not alter the pattern of sleep-related GH secretion. Two of the 10 subjects tested did have rather higher peaks following exercise.

These experiments collectively show that although nocturnal GH release does have measurable metabolic effects, its control seems remarkably immune to those metabolic stimuli which normally modify GH secretion. It appears that sleep release of GH is regulated by a rhythm in the CNS which is scarcely altered by substrate availability, and may be mediated via different pathways from those of the mechanism of daytime GH release. The rhythmic release of GH during sleep presumably enhances the rate of amino acid incorporation into protein, hence it may serve an important anabolic function. It thus provides evidence of a possible role of slow-wave sleep in tissue growth and repair.

C. EFFECT OF STEROIDS AND DRUGS ON NOCTURNAL GH RELEASE

Not only is the sleep-related release of GH resistant to the usual influences on day time GH secretion, but it is also uninfluenced by a number of drugs which might have been expected to affect it.

Takahashi et al. (1968) tested a variety of drugs known to have an effect on the CNS. They found no inhibition of the sleep-related GH peak by chlorpromazine, phenobarbitone, diphenylhdantoin, isocarboxazid or chlordiazepoxide, although the first two of these did cause some variation in the secretory pattern throughout the night in some, but not all, of the subjects studied. Two out of four subjects treated with imipramine, however, showed suppression of the GH peak.

Blockers of α-adrenergic receptors, such as phentolamine, have been reported to block GH secretion during insulin-hypoglycaemia or arginine infusion, and β-adrenergic blockers, such as propranalol, to enhance it. Lucke and Glick (1971a) therefore studied the effect of these drugs on sleep-related GH release. Neither phentolamine infusion, nor propranalol infusion, significantly altered the GH peaks from those which occurred on control nights when saline was infused.

Certain steroids may inhibit the nocturnal GH peak under appropriate circumstances. Medroxyprogesterone acetate (6-methyl-17α-hydroxypro-gesterone acetate) suppresses the GH response to insulin-hypoglycaemia and arginine infusion (Simon et al., 1967), and its effect on the sleep-induced GH peak was studied by Lucke and Glick (1971b). They found that 10 mg/day for four days was followed by partial suppression of the nocturnal GH peak in 5 normal males.

Krieger et al. (1971) failed to suppress the nocturnal GH peak with an injection of cortisol one hour prior to sleep, or with a cortisol infusion throughout sleep. Eastman et al. (1971), on the other hand, found that chronic steroid administration could lead to suppression of the nocturnal GH peak. In a group of 10 asthmatic children with corticosteroid-induced growth retardation 2 failed to show the nocturnal peak, and in another 3 the values were subnormal. The remaining 5 children had normal peaks.

It appears, however, that administration of steroids may not need to be prolonged for suppression of nocturnal GH release to occur, because administration of prednisolone in divided doses for 36 hours has been observed to suppress the peak in some normal individuals (Glass et al., 1973). Likewise administration of 1 mg of α^{1-24} corticotrophin-zinc (Depot Synacthen-Ciba) at 0800 hr, which produced a sustained rise of plasma corticosteroid throughout the next 24 hr, resulted in suppression of the nocturnal GH peak in 6 healthy young males (Fig. 9), without altering slow-wave sleep itself (Evans et al., 1973). The effect of corticosteroids is interesting as Krieger and Glick (1972) showed the nocturnal secretion of GH to be absent in Cushing's Syndrome, and Stiel et al. (1970) previously noted absence of GH peaks in this disease throughout both the day and night. Krieger and Glick (1972) and James et al. (1968) considered the failure of GH secretion in Cushing's Syndrome might be a primary defect in this disease. In the 4 patients studied by Krieger and Glick (1972) there was a marked reduction in slow-wave sleep, and this is probably important in the lack of a GH peak. Corticosteroids have been reported to decrease REM sleep but not slow-wave sleep (Gillin et al., 1972), hence it seems unlikely that the reduction of slow-wave sleep in Cushing's Syndrome is secondary to the high circulating corticosteroids. The effect of corticosteroids on GH release has been the subject of conflicting reports. Stiel *et al.* (1970) found no inhibition of random GH peaks occurring throughout the 24 hr following 15 mg of prednisolone given in a single daily dose at 0800 hr for a week. Frantz and Rabkin (1964) and Hartog *et al.* (1964) found the GH response to hypoglycaemia to be impaired in corticosteroid treated subjects, as did Stempfel *et al.* (1968), whilst Morris *et al.* (1968) did not. Daly and Glass (1971) found impaired GH response to hypoglycaemia in 10 patients on long-term ACTH therapy. The precise relationship between raised corticosteroids and GH release remains confused and further study is needed. It seems differences in the timing

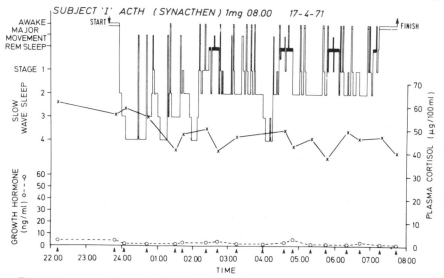

Fig. 9. The same subject as in Fig. 8 on the night following an injection of 1 mg of α^{1-24} corticotrophin Zn at 0800 hr. There is a sustained rise in the corticosteroid level (X——X) with complete suppression of GH (O— — —O). For details of the experimental data of this and Fig. 8, see Evans *et al.* (1973).

and frequency of administration as well as the dose and duration of corticosteroid therapy may be factors causing the apparently contradictory observations of different groups.

The experiments with drugs show that although GH release during sleep shows considerable resistance to pharmacological interference, some drugs (only imipramine, medroxyprogesterone acetate and corticosteroids so far having been reported as effective) may suppress the GH peak without altering slow-wave sleep. Thus, although the connection between slow-wave sleep and GH release is clearly a very close one, there are circumstances in which they may become dissociated. Failure to influence the GH peak with α- and β-receptor blockers suggests the sleep related pathways of GH release are not adrenergic, in contrast to those which mediate the response to hypoglycaemia and arginine infusion.

D. SLEEP-RELATED GH RELEASE IN CERTAIN PATHOLOGICAL STATES

As might be anticipated, hypopituitarism is associated with loss of the normal sleep-induced GH release (Underwood *et al.*, 1971; Eastman *et al.*, 1971) and GH secretion in acromegaly shows spontaneous fluctuations which are randomly distributed throughout sleep, irrespective of the stage of sleep revealed by the EEG (Eastman *et al.*, 1971) and levels which change very little during the day or night (Cryer and Daughaday, 1969).

VanderLaan *et al.* (1970) suggested there might be impairment of secretion in obesity, and this was confirmed by Quabbe *et al.* (1971), but the latter group found normal peaks in two non-obese children with heights at or above the 97th percentile, although a third had reduced peaks. Children with constitutional dwarfism also appeared to have normal peaks, as did four children with retarded growth associated with long-standing renal disease.

Blindness, somewhat surprisingly, was found by Krieger and Glick (1971) to be associated with failure to demonstrate a normal nocturnal GH peak in five subjects. However, the amount of time spent in slow-wave sleep was decreased in all the subjects compared with normally sighted controls, and two of them showed no slow-wave sleep at all.

Rosenbloom *et al.* (1970) found both the sleep characteristics and GH release to be normal in progeria.

The abnormality of nocturnal GH release in Cushing's Syndrome has been discussed in the previous section.

Hansen and Johansen (1970) found the average level of GH was higher throughout the 24 hr in 5 untreated male patients with juvenile diabetes. There were several peaks during the night, to values considerably higher than in the healthy controls, but a major peak was present in all during the first 2 hr of sleep. The EEG stage of sleep was not monitored in this study. Parker and Rossman (1971b) studied the sleep-related GH peak in 5 treated juvenile diabetics. Despite blood glucose levels of up to 382 mg/100 ml the GH peaks were normal and related to slow-wave sleep. During a night in which spontaneous hypoglycaemia occurred in one subject the sleep peak of GH was greater in duration and magnitude than on the other nights, although it remained related to slow-wave sleep.

Recently, in one 45 years old male patient suffering from juvenile diabetes, we have found an apparent effect of plasma glucose level on GH release in sleep. On nights when the plasma glucose was consistently elevated or within the normal range, no GH peaks occurred (Fig. 10); however, on nights during which hypoglycaemia occurred spontaneously there were several GH peaks related to Stage 3 and 4 sleep. The latter observation is in agreement with the findings of Parker and Rossman (1971b) but the absence of GH peaks on nights without hypoglycaemia is surprising, and will obviously require further study. Occur-

J. R. DALY AND J. I. EVANS

rence of slow wave sleep was normal (see Table 1). This illustrates the fact that as yet our picture of the variables which control nocturnal GH peaks may be incomplete.

Table 1. *Amount of stages 3 and 4 sleep in diabetic subject (see Fig. 10)*

Date	Total sleep time (min)	Stage 3 and 4 sleep (min)	Percent. stage 3 and 4
12.4.72	420	86	20.4
19.4.72		Recording defective	
26.4.72	426	84	19.7
10.5.72	435	151	35.8

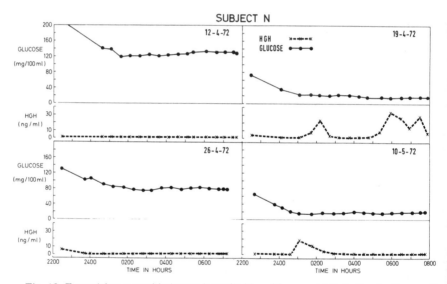

Fig. 10. Four nights at weekly intervals studied in a 45 years old diabetic who frequently suffered from attacks of hypoglycaemia despite much effort to regulate his insulin intake and diet. GH peaks occur only on hypoglycaemic nights. For sleep data on this subject see Table 1.

Further illustration of the association of GH peaks with slow-wave sleep occurs in patients suffering from the Pickwickian Syndrome (Burwell *et al.*, 1956). These obese patients suffer from somnolence and show signs of hypercapnia, hypoxia, cyanosis, compensatory polycythaemia and right sided cardiac failure. During sleep they show a unique pattern of severe disruption of orthodox sleep (Jung and Kuhlo, 1965). When drowsy the patient develops hypoventilation and at times apnoea; PCO_2 levels rise and hypoxia increases (Drachman and Gumnit 1962). Hypoxia is a potent arousal stimulus and the patient wakes often with a tremendous snort and body twitch. Stages 3 and 4 sleep are therefore rare and short lived, but REM sleep periods continue, only slightly disrupted by the snorting respiration. In our studies of this syndrome we

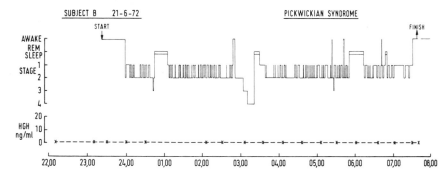

Fig. 11. Pickwickian Syndrome. The severe disruption of orthodox sleep due to the respiratory abnormality of this patient prevents the appearance of stage 3 and 4 slow wave sleep, apart from one brief period near mid-sleep. GH levels are consistently less than 1 ng/ml.

have found (Fig. 11) that usually no GH peaks occur in sleep. However on one occasion a minor peak appeared slightly in advance of the only period of Stage 3 and 4 sleep that night.

V. THE HYPOTHALAMO-PITUITARY-GONADAL (HPG) AXIS

A. GENERAL OBSERVATIONS ON SLEEP RELATIONSHIPS OF HPG SECRETION

The characteristics of the secretion of the hormones of the HPG axis have been less fully worked out than those of the HPA axis. This is both due to the greater complexity of the relationships between the hormones of the HPG axis and to the fact that whereas satisfactory methods have been available for the determination of plasma corticosteroids for nearly twenty years, methods for the measurement of hormones of HPG axis in plasma have been developed only relatively recently.

There have been conflicting reports as to whether there is any circadian rhythm in plasma testosterone, but the consensus now appears to be that it shows a rhythm very similar in phase to that of cortisol, but of lower amplitude (Faiman and Winter, 1971). In this study dexamethasone caused no suppression of the testosterone level, hence it was thought the rhythm was not dependent on the ACTH rhythm, which would have been inhibited by dexamethasone (Fig. 12).

Evans *et al.* (1971a and b), sampled blood every 30 min throughout EEG monitored sleep in 6 healthy young subjects and found peaks of testosterone occurred in conjunction with or adjacent to periods of REM sleep, although the rise was often noted to precede the REM period. Sleep reversal in one subject resulted in reversal of the circadian rhythm of plasma testosterone, peaks

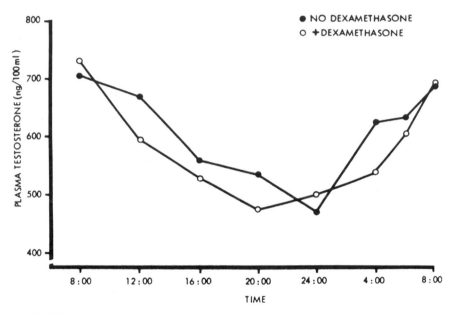

Fig. 12. Circadian rhythm of plasma testosterone. The failure of dexamethasone to alter the pattern indicates that the rhythm, although of similar phase to that of the HPA axis, is not controlled by ACTH. Copied, with permission, from Faiman and Winter, (1971).

occurring in association with REM periods during the daytime sleep. The authors point out that the testosterone association with REM sleep is interesting in view of the penile tumescence with which this phase of sleep is commonly associated.

Luteinizing hormone (LH) is regarded as the trophic hormone for testosterone secretion, but no circadian rhythm was found by Krieger *et al.* (1972) in 4 healthy men who had normal cortisol and GH rhythms. Sixteen healthy young men were studied by Rubin *et al.* (1972), and were found to have episodic but unrelated peaks of both LH and follicle stimulating hormone (FSH). The patterns differed both between subjects and from night to night in the same subject. It was found, however, that LH secretion was slightly higher during REM than during other stages of sleep. FSH was not increased during REM sleep. The authors note that the increase of LH in REM fits the data of Evans et al. (1971) cited above, concerning testosterone.

Okamoto et al. (1971) found no significant differences at different times of day in the plasma LH, although they found plasma testosterone to be high in the morning. They did not make a specific examination of nocturnal or sleeping levels. Faiman and Winter (1971) found no circadian rhythm of LH, but unlike Krieger et al. (1972) they did find a rhythm of FSH, which showed a parallelism to the testosterone cycle. The authors speculated as to whether FSH and testosterone secretion may be linked rather than LH and testosterone as generally held. Faiman and Winter did not study sleep relationships. Boyar et al. (1972b) sampled blood every 20 min in 5 normal adult males throughout the 24 hr, with EEG monitoring of sleep. They found that LH was secreted in a series of irregularly occurring episodes throughout the day and night. From 9 to 14 such episodes occurred during the 24 hr. The typical incremental change in such episodes varied from 3.0 mIU/ml to 14.0 mIU/ml above basal levels, (i.e. 36-311%). There was no evidence of there being more episodes of secretion during sleep, nor of such episodes being associated with any particular phase of sleep. These findings in adults contrast most interestingly with the findings of the same group (Boyar et al., 1972a) in males and females during puberty. In this situation there was a very clear association between LH secretion and sleep. LH levels rose soon after sleep onset to values about four times above daytime levels. Sleep delay resulted in delay of LH secretion, hence the phenomenon appeared to be sleep-related and not merely a function of clock-time. REM periods seemed to exert an inhibitory effect on secretion. The authors stress that this sleep-related LH secretion is a feature of puberty, and was not seen either in pre-pubescent children or in adults. As they point out, their study underlines the importance of considering hormone secretion as a dynamic 24 hr process with periods of episodic secretion causing widely fluctuating plasma levels.

Runnebaum et al. (1972) found no diurnal variation in plasma progesterone during the luteal phase of the menstrual cycle or in early pregnancy. During the latter half of pregnancy, however, a circadian rhythm appeared, with a rise from 0800 hr to a peak between 1600 and 2000 hr, followed by a fall to the following 0800.

VI. CONCLUSION

It will be seen from the foregoing necessarily selective account that there has been an enormous amount of research into hormonal rhythms during the past 20 years or so, but that a great deal remains to be explained. The development of sleep-monitoring techniques, together with methods of plasma sampling that enable very frequent specimens to be taken without disturbing the subject or arousing him from sleep, offers tremendous scope for further investigations, and is already giving new and profound insight into the relationships between endocrine systems and the CNS. The work of Dr. E. D. Weitzman and his colleagues in New York has challenged many ideas of hormonal regulation that had become "received doctrine". The finding of the episodic nature of cortisol secretion, and the timing of the episodes, has necessitated rethinking the notion of feedback control of the HPA system, and the recognition of augmented LH secretion during sleep in adolescence invites speculation as to what other hitherto unsuspected physiological events may be revealed by the study of sleep-related endocrinology.

The importance of these findings for the clinician as well as the experimental endocrinologist is obvious. It has been recognized for several years that demonstration of loss of the HPA circadian rhythm is an important diagnostic point in the recognition of Cushing's Syndrome, but as Dr. D. T. Krieger and her group have shown, it may also be the earliest endocrinological abnormality to be found in hypothalamic disease. The discovery of sleep-related GH release has added an important new investigation to the well-established insulin hypoglycaemia and arginine infusion tests. A GH level of more than 5 ng/ml during early sleep makes hypopituitarism most unlikely (Daughaday, 1969). This test is simple and disturbs the patient very little, yet a normal result may relieve him of the necessity of undergoing one of the more complex provocative tests of GH release. So regular is the sleep-related GH peak in normal subjects that a sample 60-90 min after behaviourally observed sleep onset may be adequate, without need of elaborate sleep monitoring. An abnormal result from this simple procedure is not, of course, diagnostic of pituitary disorder, but an indication of the need for more extensive investigation. The usefulness of sleep-related GH release in diagnosis in both adults and children has been discussed by Mace *et al.* (1970, 1972). Underwood *et al.* (1971) consider that the best time for sampling in children is 60 min after sleep onset, and that this will detect a raised GH in 70% of normal subjects.

An interesting field for investigation is provided by comparison of the data of Hellman *et al.* (1970a, 1970b) on the episodic secretion of cortisol and that of Ceresa *et al.* (1969, 1970), showing there to be two apparent phases of cortisol secretion, basal and impulsive, only one of which—the "impulsive" early morning peak, is sensitive to corticosteroid inhibition. The effect of exogenous steroids on the different secretory episodes occurring throughout the day needs to be studied. Meanwhile, as Ceresa points out, it may be of value in corticosteroid therapy to limit administration of the drug to a time of day when it will cause minimal HPA suppression. A study by Myles *et al.* (1972) suggests this may have practical therapeutic significance.

The possible anabolic role of nocturnal GH secretion has been discussed, but the function of the circadian rise in corticosteroids is less clear. It has been suggested that it may have an arousal function. However, patients on corticosteroid or ACTH therapy, or having replacement therapy for Addison's Disease or adrenogenital syndrome, have profoundly disturbed circadian rhythm of the HPA axis, but none of the symptons of these conditions has been demonstrated to be specifically due to the rhythmic upset. Likewise the symptoms allegedly produced by rapid travel across time zones have not been proved to be circadian, still less to be directly related to the undoubted disruption of the HPA rhythm (see Siegel *et al.*, 1969 for review), but with the increase in rapid air travel, and the development of space flight, the significance of circadian disruption will no doubt be recognized, together with the need for further research (Chemin, 1970).

Despite the work already done the need for further study into the endocrinology of sleep is apparent; because of it, techniques are now available for new and major advances in neuroendocrinology.

REFERENCES

Anders, T. F., Sachar, E. J., Kream, J., Roffwarg, H. P. and Hellman, L. (1970). *Pediatrics* **46**, 532-537.

Aschoff, J. (1965). *Science, N.Y.* **148**, 1427-1432.

Aschoff, J., Fatranska, M., Giedke, H., Doerr, P., Stamm, D. and Wisser, H. (1971). *Science, N.Y.* **171**, 213-215.

Aserinsky, E. and Kleitman, N. (1953). *Science, N.Y.* **118**, 273-274.

Aserinsky, E. and Kleitman, N. (1955). *J. appl. Physiol.* **8**, 11-18.

Asfeldt, V. H. (1971). *Scand. J. clin. Lab. Invest.* **28**, 61-70.

Bartter, F. C., Delea, C. S. and Halberg, F. (1962). *Am. N.Y. Acad. Sci.* **78**, 969-983.

Berger, H. (1929-1930). *J. Physiol. Neurol.* **40**, 160-179.

Berger, R. (1961). *Science, N.Y.* **134**, 840.

Berson, S. A. and Yalow, R. S. (1968). *J. clin. Invest.* **47**, 2727-2751.

Blackard, W. G. and Heidingsfelder, S. A. (1968). *J. clin. Invest.* **47**, 1407-1414.

Blake, H., Gerard, R. W. (1937). *Amer. J. Physiol.* **119**, 692-703.

Blake, H., Gerard, R. W. and Kleitman, N. (1939). *J. Neurophysiol.* **2**, 48-60.

Bliss, E. L., Sandberg, A. A., Nelson, D. H. and Eik-Nes, K. (1953). *J. clin. Invest.* **32**, 818-823.

Boyar, R., Finkelstein, J., Roffwarg, H., Kapen, S., Weitzman, E. D. and Hellman, L. (1972a). *New Eng. J. Med.* **287**, 582-586.

Boyar, R., Perlow, M., Hellman, L., Kapen, S. and Weitzman, E. (1972b). *J. clin. Endocr.* **35**, 73-81.

Braunsberg, H. and James, V. H. T. (1960). *J. Endocr.* **21**, 327-340.

Bridges, P. K. and Jones, M. T. (1966). *Brit. J. Psychiat.* **112**, 1257-1261.

Brooks, C. Mc. C., Hoffman, B. F., Suckling, E. E., Kleyntjens, F., Koenig, E. H., Coleman, K. S. and Treumann, II. J. (1956). *J. appl. Physiol.* **9**, 97-104.

Burwell, C. S., Robin, E. D., Whaley, R. D. and Bickelmann, A. G. (1956). *Amer. J. Med.* **21**, 811-818.

Butler, P. W. P. and Besser, G. M. (1968). *Lancet* i, 1234-1236.

Carli, G., Armengol, V., Zanchetti, A. (1965). *Arch. ital. Biol.* **103**, 725–788.

Ceresa, F., Angeli, A., Boccuzzi, G. and Molino, G. (1969). *J. clin. Endocr.* **29**, 1074-1082.

Ceresa, F., Angeli, A., Boccuzzi, G. and Perotti, L. (1970). *J. clin. Endocr.* **31**, 491-501.

Chayen, J., Loveridge, N. and Daly, J. R. (1972). *Clin. Endocrinol.* **1**, 219-233.

Chemin, P. (1970). *Presse Méd.* **78**, 81-84.

Clayton, G. W., Librik, L., Gardner, R. L. and Guillemin R. (1963). *J. clin. Endocr.* **23**, 975-980.

Connolly, C. K. and Wills, M. R. (1967). *Brit. med. J.* **2**, 25-27.

Conroy, R. T. W. L., Hughes, B. D. and Mills, J. N. (1968). *Brit. med. J.* **3**, 405-407.

Conroy, R. T. W. L., Elliott, A. L. and Mills, J. N. (1970). *Brit. J. industr. Med.* **27**, 170-174.

Critchlow, V., Liebelt, R. A., Bar-Sela, M., Mountcastle, W. and Lipscomb, H. S. (1963). *Amer. J. Physiol.* **205**, 807-815.

Cryer, P. E. and Daughaday, W. H. (1969). *J. clin. Endocr.* **29**, 386-393.

Curtis, G. C., Fogel, M. C., McEvoy, D. and Zarate, C. (1966). *Psychosom. Med.* **28**, 696-713.

Daly, J. R. (1970). *Clin. Trials Journal* **32**, 179-185.

Daly, J. R. and Glass, D. (1971). *Lancet* i, 476-477.

Daly, J. R. and Elstein, M. (1972). *J. Obstet. Gynaec. Brit. Cmnwlth.* **79**, 544-549.

Daly, J. R., Loveridge, N., Bitensky, L. and Chayen, J. (1972). *Ann. clin. Biochem.* **9**, 81-84.

Daly, J. R., Fleischer, M. R., Scott, J. T. and Chayen, J. (1973). *J. Endocr.* **58**, ix.

Daughaday, W. H. (1969). *Postgrad. Med.* **46**, 84-91.

David-Nelson, M. A. and Brodish, A. (1969). *Endocrinology* **85**, 861-866.

Dement, W. and Kleitman, N. (1957). *Electroenceph. clin. Neurophysiol.* **9**, 673-690.

Denisova, M. D. and Figurin, N. L. (1926). *Novoe u Refleksologii i Fiziologii Rerunci Sistemy* **2**, 338-345.

Doe, R. P., Flink, E. B. and Goodsell, M. G. (1956). *J. clin. Endocr.* **16**, 196-205.

Doe, R. P., Vennes, J. A. and Flink, E. B. (1960). *J. clin. Endocr.* **20**, 253-264.

Doe, R. P., Fernandez, R. and Seal, U.S. (1964). *J. clin. Endocr.* **24**, 1029-1039.

Drachman, D. B. and Gumnit, R. J. (1962). *Arch. Neurol.* **6**, 471-477.

Eastman, C. J., Mitchell, R. P. and Lazarus, L. (1971). *Proc. Endocrin. Soc. Australia* **36**.

Eik-Nes, K. and Clark, L. D. (1958). *J. clin. Endocr.* **18**, 764-768.

Ekman, H., Håkansson, B., McCarthy, J. D., Lehmann, J. and Sjögren, B. (1961). *J. clin. Endocr.* **21**, 684-694.

Evans, J. I., Lewis, S. A., Gibbs, I. A. M. and Cheetham, M. (1968). *Brit. med. J.* **4**, 291-293.

Evans, J. I., Maclean, A. M., Ismail, A. A. A. and Love, D. (1971a). *Nature, Lond.* **229**, 261-262.

Evans, J. I., Maclean, A. M., Ismail, A. A. A. and Love, D. (1971b). *Proc. roy. Soc. Med.* **64**, 841-842.

Evans, J. I., Christie, G. A., Lewis, S. A., Daly, J. R. and Moore-Robinson, M. (1972). *Arch. Neurol.* **26**, 36-48.

Evans, J. I., Glass, D., Daly, J. R. and Maclean, A. M. (1973). *J. clin. Endocr.* **36**, 36 41.

Faiman, C. and Winter, J. S. D. (1971). *J. clin. Endocr.* **33**, 186 192.

Finkelstein, J. W., Anders, T. F. Sachar, E. J., Roffwarg, H. P. and Hellman, L. D. (1971). *J. clin. Endocr.* **32**, 368-371.

Flink, E. B. and Doe, R. P. (1959). *Proc. Soc. exp. Biol. N.Y.* **100**, 498-501.

Fontana, F. (1765). Ricerche de motu del iride, Giusta, Lucca.

Frank, G., Halberg, F., Harner, R., Matthews, J., Johnson, E., Gravem, H. and Andrus, V. (1966). *J. psychiat. Res.* **4**, 73-86.

Franks, R. C. (1967). *J. clin. Endocr.* **27**, 75-78.

Frantz, A. G. and Rabkin, T. (1964). *New Eng. J. Med.* **271**, 1375-1381.

Fullerton, D. T., Wenzel, F. J., Lohrenz, F. N. and Fahs, H. (1968): *Arch. gen. Psychiat.* **19**, 674-681.

Gallagher, T. F., Hellman, L., Finkelstein, J., Yoshida, K., Weitzman, E. D., Roffwarg, H. D. and Fukushima, D. K. (1972). *J. clin. Endocr.* **34**, 919-927.

Gibbs, F. P. (1970). *Amer. J. Physiol.* **219**, 288-292.

Gillin, J. C., Jacobs, L. S., Fram, D. H. and Snyder, F. (1972). *Nature, Lond.* **237**, 398-399.

Glass, D., Motson, R., Daly, J. R. and Rudolf, N. de M. (1973) in preparation.

Glenn, E. M. and Nelson, D. H. (1953). *J. clin. Endocr.* **13**, 911-921.

Glick, S. M., Roth, J., Yalow, R. and Berson, S. A. (1963). *Nature, Lond.* **199**, 784-787.

Glick, S. M., Roth, J., Yalow, R. S. and Berson, S. A. (1965). *Recent Progr. Hormone Res.* **21**, 241-283.

Goldsmith, S. J. and Glick, S. M. (1970): *Mt. Sinai J. Med.* **37**, 501-509.

Gordon, R. D., Spinks, J., Dulmanis, A., Hudson, B., Halberg, F. and Bartter, F. C. (1968). *Clin. Sci.* **35**, 307-324.

Graber, A. L., Givens, J. R., Nicholson, W. E., Island, D. P. and Liddle, G. W. (1965). *J. clin. Endocr.* **25**, 804-807.

Grant, S. D., Pavlates, F. C. and Forsham, P. H. (1965). *J. clin. Endocr.* **25**, 1057-1066.

Guillemin, R. (1967). *Ann. Rev. Physiol.* **29**, 313-348.

Halberg, F. (1959). *Z. Vitamin. Hormon. u. Fermentforsch.* **10**, 225-296.

Halberg, F. (1969). *Ann. Rev. Physiol.* **31**, 675-725.

Halberg, F. and Haus, E. (1960). *Amer. J. Physiol.* **199**, 859-862.

Halberg, F. and Simpson, H. (1967). *Hum. Biol.* **39**, 405-413.

Halberg, F., Frank, G., Harner, R., Matthews, J., Aaker, H., Gravem, H. and Melby, J. (1961). *Experientia* **17**, 282-284.

Hansen, A. P. and Johansen, K. (1970). *Diabetologia* **6**, 27-33.

Hartmann, E. (1967). 'The Biology of Dreaming', Chas. C. Thomas, Springfield, Ill.

Hartog, M., Gaafar, M. A. and Fraser, R. (1964). *Lancet* ii, 376-378.

Hastings, J. W. (1970). *New Eng. J. Med.* **282**, 435-441.

Hellman, L., Nakada, F., Curti, J., Weitzman, E. D., Kream, J., Roffwarg, H., Ellman, S., Fukushima, D. K. and Gallagher, T. F. (1970a): *J. clin. Endocr.* **30**, 411-422.

Hellman, L., Weitzman, E. D., Roffwarg, H., Fukushima, D. K., Yoshida, K. and Gallagher, T. F. (1970b). *J. clin. Endocr.* **30**, 686-689.

Hess, W. R. (1933). *Klin. Wschr.* **12**, 129-134.

Hinton, J. M. and Marley, E. (1959). *J. Neurol. Neurosurg. Psychiat.* **22**, 137-140.

Hiroshige, T. and Sakakura, M. (1971). *Neuroendocrinology* 7, 25-36.

Hodges, J. R. (1970). *Progr. Brain Res.* 32, 12-20.

Honda, Y., Takahashi, K., Takahashi, S., Azumi, K., Irie, M., Sakuma, M., Tsushima, T. and Shizume, K. (1969). *J. clin. Endocr.* 29, 20-29.

Howell, W. H. (1897). *J. exper. Med.* 2, 313-345.

Hunter, W. M. and Rigal, W. M. (1966). *J. Endocr.* 34, 147-153.

Hunter, W. M., Friend, J. A. R. and Strong, J. A. (1966). *J. Endocr.* 34, 139-146.

Ichikawa, Y., Nishikai, M., Kawagoe, M., Yoshida, K. and Homma, M. (1972). *J. clin. Endocr.* 34, 895-898.

Jacobson, A., Kales, A., Lehman, D., Hoedemacher, F. (1964). *Exp. Neurol.* 10, 418-424.

James, V. H. T. and Landon, J. (1968). *In* 'Recent Advances in Endocrinology' (V. H. T. James, ed.), Churchill, London.

James, V. H. T., Landon, J., Wynn, V., Greenwood, F. C. (1968). *J. Endocr.* 40, 15-28.

Jouvet, M. (1961): *In* Ciba Foundation Symposium 'Nature of Sleep' (G. Wolstenholm and M. O'Connor, eds.), pp. 188-208, Churchill, London.

Jouvet, M. (1965). *Progr. Brain Res.* 18, 20-57.

Jouvet, M. (1969). *In* 'Sleep, Physiology and Pathology' (A. Kales, ed.), pp. 89-100, Lipincott, Philadelphia.

Jung, R. and Kuhlo, W. (1965). *Progr. Brain Res.* 18, 140-159.

Karacan, I., Goodenough, D. R., Shapiro, A. and Starker, S. (1966). *Arch. gen. Psychiat.* 15, 183-189.

Karacan, I., Hursch, C. J., Williams, R. L. and Thornby, J. I. (1972). *Arch. gen. Psychiat.* 26, 351-356.

Knapp, M. S., Keane, P. M. and Wright, J. G. (1967). *Brit. med. J.* 2, 27-30.

Kohlschutter, E. (1862). *Z. ration. Med.* 17, 209-253.

Kream, J., Fishman, R., Gallagher, T. F. and Hellman, H. (1970). *Psychophysiology* 7, 323.

Krieger, D. T. (1961). *J. clin. Endocr.* 21, 695-698.

Krieger, D. T. (1970). *Trans. N.Y. Acad. Sci.* 32, 316-329.

Krieger, D. T. and Krieger, H. P. (1966). *J. clin. Endocr.* 26, 929-940.

Krieger, D. T. and Rizzo, F. (1969). *Amer. J. Physiol.* 217, 1703-1707.

Krieger, D. T. and Glick, S. (1971). *J. clin. Endocr.* 33, 847-850.

Krieger, D. T. and Rizzo, F. (1971). *Neuroendocrinology* 8, 165-179.

Krieger, D. T. and Glick, S. M. (1972). *Amer. J. Med.* 52, 25-40.

Krieger, D. T., Glick, S., Silverberg, A. and Krieger, H. P. (1968a). *J. clin. Endocr.* 28, 1589-1598.

Krieger, D. T., Silverberg, A. I., Rizzo, F. and Krieger, H. P. (1968b). *Amer. J. Physiol.* 215, 959-967.

Krieger, D. T., Kreuzer, J. and Rizzo, F. A. (1969). *J. clin. Endocr.* 29, 1634-1638.

Krieger, D. T., Albin, J., Paget, S. and Glick, S. (1971a). Abstr. of the 53rd Meeting American Endocrine Soc., 215.

Krieger, D. T., Allen, W., Rizzo, F. and Krieger, H. P. (1971b). *J. clin. Endocr.* 32, 266-284.

Krieger, D. T., Ossowski, R., Fogel, M. and Allen, W. (1972). *J. clin. Endocr.* 35, 619-623.

Kupfer, D. J., Wyatt, R. J., Scott, J. and Snyder, F. (1970). *Amer. J. Psychiat.* 126, 1213-1223.

Laidlaw, J. C., Jenkins, D., Reddy, W. J. and Jakobson, T. (1954). *J. clin. Invest.* **33**, 950.

Liddle, G. W., Estep, H. L., Kendall, J. W. Jnr., Williams, W. C. Jnr. and Townes, A. W. (1959). *J. clin. Endocr.* **19**, 857-894.

Lipman, R. L., Taylor, A. L., Schenk, A. and Mintz, D. H. (1972). *J. clin. Endocr.* **35**, 592-594.

Lipscomb, H. S. and Nelson, D. H. (1962). *Endocrinology* **71**, 13-23.

Loomis, A. L., Harvey, E. N. and Hobart, G. A. (1935). *Science, N.Y.* **81**, 597-598.

Loomis, A. L., Harvey, E. N. and Hobart, G. A. (1937). *J. exp. Psychol.* **21**, 127-144.

Lucke, C. and Glick, S. M. (1971a). *J. clin. Endocr.* **32**, 729-736.

Lucke, C. and Glick, S. M. (1971b). *J. clin. Endocr.* **33**, 851-853.

McCann, S. M., Dhariwal, A. P. S. and Porter, J. C. (1968). *Ann. Rev. Physiol.* **30**, 589-640.

McClure, D. J. (1966). *J. Psychosom. Res.* **10**, 189-195.

Mace, J. W., Gotlin, R. W., Sassin, L. F., Parker, D. C. and Rossman, L. G. (1970). *J. clin. Endocr.* **31**, 225-226.

Mace, J. W., Gotlin, R. W. and Beck, P. (1972). *J. clin. Endocr.* **34**, 339-341.

MacWilliam, J. A. (1923). *Brit. med. J.* **2**, 1196-1200.

Magnes, J., Moruzzi, G. and Pompeiano, O. (1961). *Arch. ital. Biol.* **99**, 33-67.

Magnussen, G. (1944): 'Studies of Respiration during Sleep.' Lewis, London.

Mandell, A. J. and Mandell, M. P. (1965). *Amer. J. Psychiat.* **122**, 391-401.

Mandell, A. J. and Mandell, M. P. (1969). *Exp. Med. Surg.* **27**, 224-236.

Mandell, A. J., Chapman, L. F., Rand, R. W. and Walter, R. D. (1963). *Science, N.Y.* **139**, 1212.

Mandell, M. P., Mandell, A. J., Rubin, R. T., Brill, P., Rodnick, J., Sheff, R. and Chaffey, B. (1966a). *Life Sci.* **5**, 583-587.

Mandell, A. J., Chaffey, B., Brill, P., Mandell, M. P., Rodnick, J., Rubin, R. T. and Sheff, R. (1966b). *Science, N.Y.* **151**, 1558-1560.

Martin, M. M. and Hellman, D. C. (1964). *J. clin. Endocr.* **24**, 253-260.

Martin, M. M., Mintz, D. H. and Tanagaki, H. (1965). *J. clin. Endocr.* **23**, 242-243.

Mason, J. W. (1968). *Psychosom. Med.* **30**, 576-607.

Mattingly, D. (1962). *J. clin. Pathol.* **15**, 374-379.

Mendels, J. and Hawkins, D. R. (1971). *J. Nerv. Ment. Dis.* **153**, 274-277.

Mess, B. and Martini, L. (1968): *In* 'Recent Advances in Endocrinology' (V. H. T. James, ed.), Churchill, London.

Migeon, C., Tyler, F. H., Mahoney, J. P., Florentin, A. A., Castle, H., Bliss, E. L. and Samuels, L. T. (1956). *J. clin. Endocr.* **16**, 622-633.

Mills, J. N. (1966). *Physiol. Revs.* **46**, 128-171.

Morris, H. G., Jorgensen, J. R. and Jenkins, S. A. (1968). *J. clin. Invest.* **47**, 427-435.

Moruzzi, G. and Magoun, H. (1949). *Electroenceph. clin. Neurophysiol.* **1**, 455-460.

Murphy, B. P., Engelberg, W. and Patee, C. J. (1963). *J. clin. Endocr.* **23**, 313-348.

Myles, A. B., Bacon, P. A. and Daly, J. R. (1971). *Ann. rheum. Dis.* **30**, 149-153.

Nakagawa, K. (1971). *J. clin. Endocr.* **33**, 854-856.

Nelson, D. H. and Samuels, L. T. (1952). *J. clin. Endocr.* **12**, 519-526.

Nichols, T., Nugent, C. A. and Tyler, F. H. (1965). *J. clin. Endocr.* **25**, 343-349.

Nichols, C. T. and Tyler, F. H. (1967). *Ann. Rev. Med.* **18**, 313-324.

Ohlmeyer, P., Brilmayer, H., Hillstrung, H. (1944). *Pflugers. Arch. ges. Physiol.* **248**, 559-560.

Okamoto, M., Setaishi, C., Nakagawa, K., Horiuchi, Y., Moriya, K. and Itoh, S. (1971). *J. clin. Endocr.* **32**, 846-851.

Oppenheimer, J. H., Fisher, L. V. and Jailer, J. W. (1961). *J. clin. Endocr.* **21**, 1023-1036.

Orth, D. N. and Island, D. P. (1969). *J. clin. Endocr.* **29**, 479-486.

Orth, D. N., Island, D. P. and Liddle, G. W. (1967). *J. clin. Endocr.* **27**, 549-555.

Oswald, I. (1962). *Proc. roy. Soc. Med.* **55**, 910-912.

Oswald, I. (1969). *Nature, Lond.* **223**, 893-897.

Oswald, I. (1970). *New Scientist* **46**, 170-172.

Othmer, E., Daughaday, V. and Guze, S. (1969). *Electroenceph. clin. Neurophysiol.* **27**, 685.

Parker, D. C. and Rossman, L. G. (1971a). *J. clin. Endocr.* **32**, 65-69.

Parker, D. C. and Rossman, L. G. (1971b). *Diabetes* **20**, 691-695.

Parker, D. C., Rossman, L. G. and VanderLaan, E. F. (1972). *Metabolism* **21**, 241-251.

Parker, D. C., Sassin, J. F., Mace, J. W., Gotlin, R. W. and Rossman, L. G. (1969). *J. clin. Endocr.* **29**, 871-874.

Parmeggiani, P. and Zanocco, G. (1963). *Arch. ital. Biol.* **101**, 385-412.

Perkoff, G. T., Eik-Nes, K., Nugent, C. A., Fred, H. L., Nimer, R. A., Rush, L., Samuels, L. T. and Tyler, F. H. (1959). *J. clin. Endocr.* **19**, 432-443.

Peterson, R. E. (1957). *J. clin. Endocr.* **17**, 1150-1157.

Pincus, G. (1943). *J. clin. Endocr.* **3**, 195-199.

Pompeiano, O. (1967). *Res. Publ. Ass. nerv. ment. Dis.* **45**, 351-423.

Pompeiano, O. and Morrison, A. (1965). *Arch. ital. Biol.* **103**, 569-595.

Quabbe, H.-J., Schilling, E. and Helge, H. (1966). *J. clin. Endocr.* **26**, 1173-1177.

Quabbe, H.-J., Helge, H. and Kubicki, S. (1971). *Acta endocr. (Kbh.)* **67**, 767-783.

Regestein, Q. R., Rose, L. I. and Williams, G. H. (1972). *Arch. intern. Med.* **130**, 114-117.

Robin, E. D., Whaley, R. D., Crump, C. H. and Travis, D. M. (1958). *J. clin. Invest.* **372**, 981-989.

Roffwarg, H., Muzio, J. and Dement, W. (1966): *Science, N.Y.* **152**, 604-619.

Roffwarg, H. P., Sachar, E., Finkelstein, J., Curti, J., Ellman, S., Kream, J., Fishman, R., Gallagher, F. T. and Hellman, H. (1970). *Psychophysiology* **1**, 323.

Rosenbloom, A. L., Karacan, I. J. and DeBusk, F. L. (1970). *J. Pediat.* **77**, 692-695.

Rubin, R. T. and Mandell, A. J. (1966). *Amer. J. Psychiat.* **123**, 387-400.

Rubin, R. T., Mandell, A. J. and Crandall, P. H. (1966). *Science, N.Y.* **153**, 767-768.

Rubin, R. T., Kollar, E. J., Slater, G. G. and Clark, B. R. (1969). *Psychosom. Med.* **31**, 68-79.

Rubin, R. T., Kales, A., Adler, R., Fagan, T. and Odell, W. (1972). *Science, N.Y.* **175**, 196-198.

Runnebaum, B., Rieben, W., Bierwirth-v. Munstermann, A.-M. and Zander, J. (1972). *Acta endocr. (Kbh.)* **69**, 731-738.

St. Laurent, J. (1971). *Canad. psychiat. Ass. J.* **16**, 327-336.

Samuel, J. G. (1964). *Brit. J. Psychiat.* **110**, 711-719.

Sassin, J. F., Parker, D. C., Johnson, L. C., Rossman, L. G., Mace, J. W. and Gotlin, R. W. (1969a). *Life Sci.* **8**, 1299-1307.

Sassin, J. F., Parker, D. C., Mace, J. W., Gotlin, R. W., Johnson, L. C. and Rossman, L. G. (1969b). *Science, N.Y.* **165**, 513-515.

Schalch, D. S. and Parker, M. L. (1964). *Nature, Lond.* **203**, 1141-1142.

Schnure, J. J., Raskin, P. and Lipman, R. L. (1971). *J. clin. Endocr.* **33**, 234-241.

Seiden, G. and Brodish, A. (1972). *Endocrinology* **90**, 1401-1403.

Sharp, G. W. G., Slorach, S. A. and Vipond, H. J. (1961). *J. Endocr.* **22**, 377-385.

Shaywitz, B. A., Finkelstein, J., Hellman, L. and Weitzman, E. D. (1971). *Pediatrics* **48**, 103-109.

Sholiton, L. J., Werk, E. E. and Marnell, R. T. (1961). *Metabolism* **10**, 632-646.

Siegel, P. V., Gerathewohl, S. J. and Mohler, S. R. (1969). *Science, N.Y.* **164**, 1249-1255.

Silber, R. H. and Porter, C. L. (1954). *J. biol. Chem.* **210**, 923-932.

Silverberg, A., Rizzo, F. and Krieger, D. T. (1968). *J. clin. Endocr.* **25**, 1661-1663.

Simon, S., Glick, S. M., Schiffer, M. and Schwartz, E. (1967). *J. clin. Endocr.* **27**, 1633-1636.

Simpson, H. (1965). *J. Endocr.* **32**, 179-185.

Slusher, M. A. (1964). *Amer. J. Physiol.* **206**, 1161-1164.

Smyth, H. S., Sleight, P. and Pickering, G. W. (1969). *Circulat. Res.* **24**, 109-121.

Snyder, F. (1967). *Res. Publ. ass. nerv. ment. Dis.* **45**, 469-487.

Snyder, F. (1969). *Biol. Psychiat.* **1**, 119-130.

Snyder, F. (1971). *Clin. Neurosurg.* **18**, 503-536.

Sollberger, A. (1969). *Exp. Med. Surg.* **27**, 80-104.

Spencer-Peet, J., Daly, J. R. and Smith, V. (1965). *J. Endocr.* **31**, 235-244.

Stempfel, R. S., Sheikholislam, B. M., Lebowitz, H. E., Allen, E. and Franks, R. C. (1968). *J. Pediat.* **73**, 767-773.

Stiel, J. N., Island, D. P. and Liddle, G. W. (1970). *Metabolism* **19**, 158-164.

Takahashi, Y., Kipnis, D. M. and Daughaday, W. H. (1968). *J. clin. Invest.* **47**, 2079-2090.

Takebe, K., Kunita, H., Sawano, S., Horiuchi, Y. and Mashimo, K. (1969). *J. clin. Endocr.* **29**, 1630-1633.

Takebe, K., Sakakura, M. and Mashimo, K. (1972). *Endocrinology* **90**, 1515-1520.

Tanner, J. M. (1972). *Nature, Lond.* **237**, 433-439.

Tarchanoff, J. (1894). *Arch. ital. Biol.* **21**, 318-321.

Tucci, J. R., Albacete, R. A. and Martin, M. M. (1966). *Gastroenterology* **50**, 637-644.

Tyler, F. H. Migeon, C., Florentin, A. A. and Samuels, L. T. (1954). *J. clin. Endocr.* **14**, 774.

Underwood, L. E., Azumi, K., Voina, S. J. and Van Wyk, J. J. (1971). *Pediatrics* **48**, 946-954.

VanderLaan, W. P., Parker, D. C., Rossman, L. G. and VanderLaan, E. F. (1970). *Metabolism* **19**, 891-897.

Vankirk, K. and Sassin, J. F. (1969). *Amer. J. EEG. Technol.* **9**, 143-146.

Vigneri, R., D'Agata, R. and Polosa, P. (1971). *Il Progresso Medico* **27**, 366-372.

Weitzman, E. D., Schaumberg, H. and Fishbein, W. (1966). *J. clin. Endocr.* **26**, 121-127.

Weitzman, E. D., Goldmacher, D., Kripke, D., MacGregor, P., Kream, J. and Hellman, L. (1968). *Trans. Amer. Neurol. Assoc.* **93**, 153-157.

Weitzman, E. D., Fukushima, D., Nogeire, C., Roffwarg, H., Gallagher, T. F. and Hellman, L. (1971). *J. clin. Endocr.* **33**, 14-22.

Williams, G. H., Cain, J. P., Dluhy, R. F. and Underwood, R. H. (1972). *J. clin. Invest.* **51**, 1731-1742.

Williams, H. L. (1971). *J. Psychiat. Res.* **8**, 445-478.

Yates, F. E., Russell, S. M. and Maran, J. W. (1971). *Ann. Rev. Physiol.* **33**, 393-444.

Zir, L. M., Smith, R. A. and Parker, D. C. (1971). *J. clin. Endocr.* **32**, 662-665.

Zir, L. M., Parker, D. C., Smith, R. A. and Rossman, L. G. (1972). *J. clin. Endocr.* **34**, 1-6.

CHEMISTRY AND BIOLOGICAL ACTIVITY OF VITAMIN D, ITS METABOLITES AND ANALOGS

M. F. HOLICK AND H. F. DeLUCA

Department of Biochemistry,
College of Agricultural and Life Sciences,
University of Wisconsin-Madison, Madison, Wisconsin, U.S.A.

I. INTRODUCTION

The history of vitamin D investigation can be separated into five distinct phases. The first phase, which might be considered as the recognition of an antirachitic factor, began with the experimental demonstration of the disease rickets by Sir Edward Mellanby and its cure and prevention by the administration of cod liver oil (Mellanby, 1919a,b). Huldshinsky (1919) at the same time demonstrated that this disease could be cured by sunlight or artifically produced ultraviolet light. McCollum *et al.* (1922) established that the antirachitic activity of cod liver oil is due to a new vitamin which they designated as vitamin D. Steenbock and his coworkers (1924) and almost immediately thereafter Hess and his group (1925) demonstrated that ultraviolet light induces vitamin D activity in the sterol fraction of biological material. This discovery ushered in the second phase, i.e. the isolation and identification of the D vitamins. Thus in 1931 vitamin D_2 derived from ergosterol was isolated and identified (Askew *et al.*, 1931). In 1935 and 1936 Windaus and his collaborators (Windaus *et al.*, 1935, 1936) established the structure of vitamin D_3 derived from 7-dehydrocholesterol.

The third phase, i.e. the delineation of physiologic functions of vitamin D, began with the conclusive demonstration of its central role in stimulating intestinal calcium absorption in 1937 by Nicolaysen and coworkers (Nicolaysen and Eeg-Larsen, 1953). Carlsson and coworkers (Carlsson, 1952; Bauer *et al.*, 1955) established the role of vitamin D in the mobilization of calcium from bone while the possible role of vitamin D in renal tubular reabsorption of ions, in intestinal absorption of phosphate and in calcification remains to be established.

The fourth phase, i.e. the functional metabolism of vitamin D to its active form(s), began with the demonstration of highly biologically active metabolites of vitamin D in 1966 (Lund and DeLuca, 1966). In 1968 the first such metabolite, i.e. 25-hydroxyvitamin D_3 (25-OH-D_3) was isolated and identified (Blunt *et al.,* 1968) and synthesized (Blunt and DeLuca, 1969). The most potent metabolite, i.e. 1,25-dihydroxyvitamin D_3 (1,25-$(OH)_2D_3$) has recently been isolated, identified (Holick *et al.*, 1971a,b; Lawson *et al.*, 1971) and synthesized (Semmler *et al.*, 1972). In addition, other metabolites have been identified, the enzyme systems involved in some of the conversions have been studied, and their feed-back regulation established.

The fifth phase, i.e. the molecular or cellular mechanism whereby vitamin D carries out its physiological functions, is still in its infancy. Although some progress has been made in this area, it will not be discussed in this review inasmuch as it has recently been reviewed and no new information is available (Wasserman and Taylor, 1972; Omdahl and DeLuca, 1973; DeLuca, 1972).

In this review, major emphasis will be placed on the chemistry and biochemistry of vitamin D, its metabolites and their analogs. This will be discussed with special focus on new information available on the structure-functional relationship especially in regard to the separate physiologic functions of the vitamin, i.e. calcium absorption, bone calcium mobilization and calcification of bone.

No attempt will be made to review all aspects of vitamin D in which progress has been made. Readers interested in other aspects or emphases are directed to a large number of recent reviews (Norman, 1968; DeLuca, 1967; Sebrell and Harris, 1954, 1971; DeLuca and Suttie, 1970; Wasserman, 1963).

II. HISTORY OF THE EXPERIMENTS CONDUCTED ON THE METABOLISM OF VITAMIN D_3

A. 25-HYDROXYVITAMIN D_3 (25-OH-D_3)

In 1966 the concept that vitamin D must be metabolically activated before it can function was introduced. Equipped with tritiated vitamin D_3 of high specific activity, Lund and DeLuca (1966) demonstrated the existence of a polar metabolite(s) of vitamin D, which possessed a high degree of biological activity. Not only was it effective in the cure of rickets in rats, but it also acted more rapidly than vitamin D_3 in initiating intestinal calcium transport (Lund et al., 1967). This metabolite was isolated in pure form from porcine plasma and identified as the 25-hydroxy derivative of the parent vitamin (Fig. 1) (Blunt et al., 1968). The 25-hydroxylation was subsequently shown to take place in the liver (Horsting and DeLuca, 1969; Ponchon et al., 1969; Ponchon and DeLuca, 1969) and to be regulated in some unknown manner (Bhattacharyya and DeLuca, 1973). Suda et al. (1969) also isolated in pure form from hog plasma a metabolite derived from vitamin D_2 and identified its structure as 25-hydroxy-vitamin D_2 (25-OH-D_2).

B. BIOLOGICALLY ACTIVE METABOLITES MORE POLAR THAN 25-OH-D_3

The successful synthesis of $[26,27-^3H]$-25-OH-D_3 (Suda et al., 1971) made possible the studies on the further metabolism of 25-OH-D_3. Of major interest was a more polar metabolite of vitamin D_3 and 25-OH-D_3, which appeared in the target tissues, namely in the intestine and bone (Cousins et al., 1970a,b; Haussler et al., 1968; Lawson et al., 1969a). Haussler et al. (1968) were the first to demonstrate that this metabolite obtained from intestine of chicks given $[1,2^{-3}H]$-vitamin D_3 possesses marked biological activity in the stimulation of intestinal calcium transport. This metabolite acts more rapidly than 25-OH-D_3 in the initiation of intestinal calcium transport (Haussler *et al.*, 1971; Omdahl *et al.*, 1971; Myrtle and Norman, 1971). It also acts more rapidly and to a greater extent than 25-OH-D_3 in the mobilization of calcium from bone (Tanaka and DeLuca, 1971). Lawson and coworkers (1969a) studied the metabolism of $[1\alpha^{-3}H]$-vitamin D_3, but were unable to demonstrate the presence of this new polar metabolite in chicken intestine as reported by Haussler *et al.* (1968). They quickly realized that $[1\alpha^{-3}H]$-vitamin D_3 lost greater than 85% of its tritium during conversion to the intestinal metabolite. They, therefore, concluded that the loss of tritium must result from the insertion of a hydroxyl on C-1 or on a vicinal carbon atom. They also noted that a level of 1 nanogram/gram of tissue of this metabolite could not be exceeded in intestine by increasing the dose of vitamin D_3 or 25-OH-D_3 given to the animals.

C. ISOLATION AND IDENTIFICATION OF PLASMA METABOLITES

During this same period of time Suda *et al.* (1970b,c) reported the isolation and identification of 21,25-dihydroxyvitamin D_3 (21,25-(OH)$_2$D$_3$) and 25,26-dihydroxyvitamin D_3 (25,26-(OH)$_2$D$_3$) (Fig. 1) from porcine plasma.

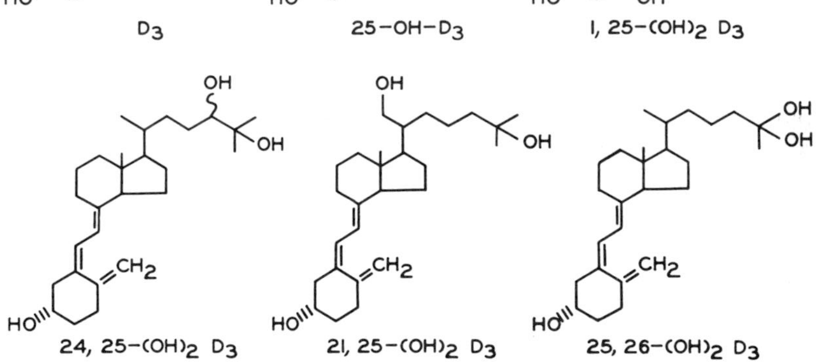

Fig. 1. Structures of vitamin D_3 and its metabolites. Abbreviations: D_3, vitamin D_3; 25-OH-D_3, 25-hydroxycholecalciferol; 1,25-(OH)$_2$D$_3$, 1,25-dihydroxycholecalciferol; 24,25-(OH)$_2$D$_3$, 24,25-dihydroxycholecalciferol; 21,25-(OH)$_2$D$_3$, 21,25-dihydroxycholecalciferol; 25,26-(OH)$_2$D$_3$, 25,26-dihydroxycholecalciferol.

Although $21,25\text{-}(OH)_2D_3$ had preferential activity in mobilizing calcium from the bone, while $25,26\text{-}(OH)_2D_3$ appeared to have its greatest effect in stimulating intestinal calcium transport, it was clear that neither of these metabolites was the tritium-deficient intestinal metabolite.

D. ROLE OF KIDNEY IN VITAMIN D METABOLISM

In 1970 Fraser and Kodicek made the important observation that the tritium deficient metabolite was made solely by the kidney and demonstrated that this metabolite could be generated *in vitro* from $25\text{-}OH\text{-}D_3$ with chicken kidney homogenates (Fraser and Kodicek, 1970). This was quickly confirmed by Gray *et al.* (1971) and Norman *et al.* (1971a).

E. ISOLATION AND IDENTIFICATION OF 1,25-DIHYDROXYVITAMIN D_3 (1,25-$(OH)_2D_3$)

In 1971, two years after it was first observed that the intestinal polar metabolite was biologically active, two laboratories simultaneously reported the structural identification of the intestinally active metabolite. Starting with 1500 chickens dosed with 2.5 μg of ^{3}H-vitamin D_3, Holick *et al.* (1971a,b) isolated 10 μg of the metabolite in 22 g of lipid extract. After several chromatographic procedures the metabolite (2 μg) was isolated in pure form as the mono-trimethylsilyl ether derivative. The ultraviolet absorption spectrum of the isolated metabolite showed a λ_{max} 265 nm and a λ_{min} 228 nm leaving little doubt that the 5,6-cis-triene system for the D vitamins was still intact. A mass spectrum of the metabolite and its tritrimethylsilyl ether derivative (TMS) (Fig. 2) showed molecular ion peaks m/e 416 and 632 respectively, demonstrating the presence of three hydroxyl functions in the molecule. The intense fragment m/e 131 in the mass spectrum of the TMS derivative established one of the hydroxyls on C-25. It was further assumed that the 3β-hydroxyl of vitamin D_3 was still intact leaving one hydroxyl unaccounted for. Fragments at m/e 287, 269 (287-H_2O) and 251 (287-2 H_2O) in the mass spectrum of the metabolite were accounted for by the loss of the entire side chain, that is, bond cleavage at C-17, C-20, thus suggesting that the additional hydroxyl was not on the side chain. The mass spectrum showed prominent fragments at m/e 152 and 134 (152-H_2O) which can only result from an additional oxygen function on ring A, since the ultraviolet absorption spectrum ruled out C_6, C_7 and C_{19} as possible positions. Therefore, the additional hydroxyl function had to be on C-1, 2 or 4. Since positions on C-1 and C-4 were allylic to the triene system it was possible to demonstrate by catalytic reduction with PtO_2 and hydrogen that the extra hydroxyl in the A ring was on either C-1 or C-4, since the hydroxyl group in the A ring was eliminated by the reduction to yield hexahydro-25-OH-D_3.

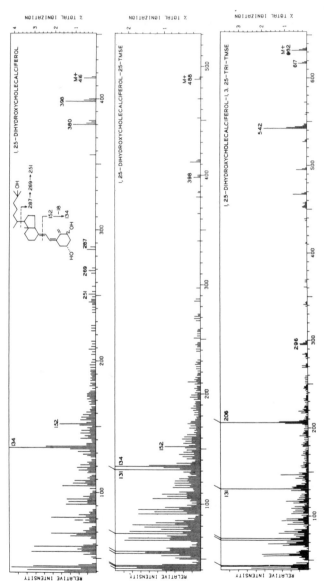

Fig. 2. Mass spectrum of 1,25-(OH)$_2$D$_3$, 1,25-(OH)$_2$D$_3$-25-monotrimethylsilyl ether and 1,25-(OH)$_2$D$_3$-1,3,25-tri-trimethylsilyl ether.

Treatment of the metabolite with sodium metaperiodate for 24 hours at room temperature showed no reaction while many vicinal hydroxyl steroids showed the expected cleavage within 4 hours, thus eliminating both C-2 and C-1 as positions for the new hydroxyl. These data made it clear that the additional oxygen function must be on C-1. Therefore, the structure of the intestinal metabolite is $1,25\text{-}(OH)_2D_3$ (Fig. 1). Simultaneously, Lawson *et al.* (1971) isolated the metabolite from kidney homogenates and reported that the metabolite had a λ_{max} 269 nm and λ_{min} 232 nm. The mass spectrum of the metabolite showed a molecular ion at m/e 416 and fragment peaks at m/e 287, 269, 251, 152 and 134. Furthermore they reported that greater than 95% of the tritium which was located in the 1α position was lost in its biosynthesis from $[1\alpha\text{-}^3H, 4\text{-}^{14}C]\text{-}25\text{-}OH\text{-}D_3$. These results led them to conclude that their tritium deficient metabolite was also $1,25\text{-}(OH)_2D_3$. Recently confirmatory mass spectral data have been provided for the metabolite from kidney homogenates (Norman *et al.*, 1971b).

F. ISOLATION AND IDENTIFICATION OF 24,25-DIHYDROXYVITAMIN D_3 $(24,25\text{-}(OH)_2D_3)$

Boyle *et al.* (1971) were the first to demonstrate that the further hydroxylation of $25\text{-}OH\text{-}D_3$ is closely controlled in the kidney by a direct or indirect action of serum calcium concentration. When the animals are hypocalcemic, the need for calcium is interpreted in some way by the kidney resulting in the production of $1,25\text{-}(OH)_2D_3$. On the other hand normal or hypercalcemia results in the production of another metabolite designated as peak Va. This metabolite was first demonstrated in both hogs and chickens that had received excess amounts of vitamin D_3 (Suda *et al.*, 1970b). Similarly, Holick and DeLuca (1971) noted that intestinal lipid extracts from chickens that had received 2.5 µg of vitamin D_3 24 hours before sacrifice contained three metabolites more polar than $25\text{-}OH\text{-}D_3$, one of which was peak Va (Fig. 3). However, when chickens received only $\frac{1}{10}$ this amount of vitamin D_3, only $1,25\text{-}(OH)_2D_3$ (peak V) was observed as the more polar metabolite. Recently Boyle *et al.* (1972b), Omdahl and DeLuca (1971, 1972) and Omdahl *et al.* (1972) have shown that peak Va is made in the kidney from animals maintained on either a high calcium diet or a diet in which strontium replaced calcium.

The peak Va metabolite was generated from $25\text{-}OH\text{-}D_3$ with kidney homogenates from chickens maintained on the high calcium diet supplemented with 0.25 µg of vitamin D_3 orally each day. Approximately 20 µg of the metabolite was recovered in 1 g of lipid residue. Its application to a number of chromatographic systems similar to those used in the isolation and identification of $1,25\text{-}(OH)_2D_3$ (Holick *et al.*, 1971b) resulted in the isolation of 11 µg of the metabolite in pure form. The ultraviolet absorption spectrum for the metabolite showed a λ_{max} 265 nm and λ_{min} 228 nm, demonstrating the presence of the 5,6-cis triene chromophore characteristic for vitamin D. The

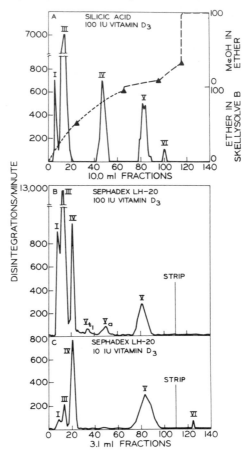

Fig. 3. Comparison of the chromatography of intestinal lipid extracts from groups of 3 chicks that received [1,2-³H]-vitamin D_3. (A) Silicic acid chromatography of an intestinal lipid extract from chicks that received 2.5 μg of ³H-vitamin D_3; (B) Sephadex LH-20 (CHCl₃:Skellysolve B 65:35) chromatography of intestinal lipid extract from chicks that received 2.5 μg ³H-vitamin D_3; and (C) Sephadex LH-20 chromatography of intestinal lipid extract from chicks that received 0.25 μg ³H-vitamin D_3. (Reproduced with the kind permission of the publisher, Holick and DeLuca, 1970.)

mass spectrum of the metabolite (Fig. 4) showed a molecular ion at m/e 416, suggesting the incorporation of an additional oxygen function in the parent 25-OH-D_3. Furthermore the peaks at m/e ratio 271 and 253 (271-H_2O) as well as fragments at m/e 136 and 118 (136-H_2O) mimic those for both vitamin D_3

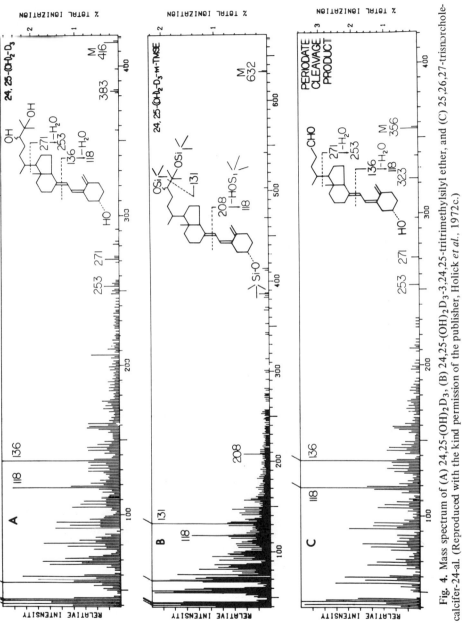

Fig. 4. Mass spectrum of (A) 24,25-(OH)₂D₃, (B) 24,25-(OH)₂D₃-3,24,25-tritrimethylsilyl ether, and (C) 25,26,27-trisnorcholecalcifer-24-al. (Reproduced with the kind permission of the publisher, Holick *et al.*, 1972c.)

and 25-OH-D$_3$, thus requiring that the additional oxygen function be on the side chain. The tritrimethylsilyl ether derivative of the metabolite (Fig. 4) displayed a molecular ion at m/e 632, demonstrating the presence of 3 hydroxyl functions in the molecule, while the strong peak at m/e 131 firmly established the presence of a C-25 hydroxyl function.

Upon treatment with periodate, 95% of the tritium in the metabolite on C-26 and C-27 could not be accounted for. The mass spectrum of this product showed a molecular ion at m/e 356 which could only result from the cleavage of the C-24, C-25 bond to yield the corresponding aldehyde (Fig. 4) Thus the data could only be interpreted in one way: this metabolite (peak Va) is the 24-hydroxy derivative of 25-OH-D$_3$ (Holick et al., 1972c) (Fig. 1). Because it had been reported that the peak Va metabolite generated in vivo from hogs was 21,25-(OH)$_2$D$_3$, it was of interest to reexamine that metabolite in light of the results obtained for the structure of the in vitro peak Va metabolite. Peak Va metabolite, isolated from porcine plasma according to the procedure of Suda et al. (1970b), was obtained in pure form. The ultraviolet absorption spectrum and mass spectrum corresponded in identical fashion with those reported for 24,25-(OH)$_2$D$_3$. The porcine peak Va was also sensitive to periodate treatment and the mass spectrum of the resulting product was identical to that obtained for the in vitro generated 24,25-(OH)$_2$D$_3$, thus demonstrating that this metabolite is also 24,25-(OH)$_2$D$_3$ and not the 21-hydroxy derivative of 25-OH-D$_3$ (Holick et al., 1972c).

G. METABOLISM OF 1,25-(OH)$_2$D$_3$

Although 1,25-(OH)$_2$D$_3$ can stimulate intestinal calcium transport in anephric (Boyle et al., 1972a) and actinomycin D-poisoned rats (Tanaka et al., 1971), it was still possible that 1,25-(OH)$_2$D$_3$ might require further metabolic alteration before it can act in stimulating intestinal calcium transport. Frolik and DeLuca (1971) biosynthesized [^{3}H]-1,25-(OH)$_2$D$_3$ from either [26,27-^{3}H]-25-OH-D$_3$ or [2-^{3}H]-25-OH-D$_3$ with chicken kidney homogenates and dosed what they considered a physiological amount of [^{3}H]-1,25-(OH)$_2$D$_3$ (62.5 pmoles) to vitamin D-deficient chickens. Twelve hours later the blood and the intestines were collected, extracted, and the extracts chromatographed on a Sephadex LH-20 chromatographic system using 75:23:2 chloroform : Skellysolve B : methanol. The results demonstrated that at a time when the intestine was maximally transporting calcium in response to this meta-bolite, greater than 80% of the radioactivity remained as 1,25-(OH)$_2$D$_3$, while the remaining radioactivity was dispersed throughout the chromatogram with no other definite metabolite appearing (Fig. 5). This work was repeated in the rat with similar results (Frolik and DeLuca, 1972). As late as 24 hours after a dose of 60 pmoles [26,27-^{3}H]-1,25-(OH)$_2$D$_3$, greater than 80% was recovered as 1,25-(OH)$_2$D$_3$. They also noted that at 6 and 12 hours after dosing, when bone calcium mobilization was maximally stimulated, the major metabolite in the bone was unaltered 1,25-(OH)$_2$D$_3$. As the bone calcium mobilization response began to decrease at 24 hours, there was a corresponding increase in the percent of bone radioactivity in the regions of the chromatogram both less and more polar than 1,25-(OH)$_2$D$_3$. However, since these metabolites appear to the greatest

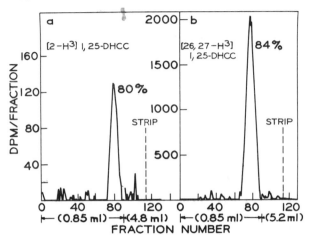

Fig. 5. Sephadex LH-20 chromatographic (chloroform : Skellysolve B : methanol 75 : 23 : 2) profile of intestinal mucosa extract from chicks dosed intravenously with (A) 62 pmoles [2-³H]-1,25-(OH)$_2$D$_3$ and (B) 62.5 pmoles [26,27-³H]-1,25-(OH)$_2$D$_3$ 12 hours earlier. (Reproduced with the kind permission of the publisher, Frolik and DeLuca, 1971.)

extent at a time when bone calcium mobilization response was beginning to decline, it would appear that these metabolites are not responsible for the early bone mobilization response.

H. THE DISCRIMINATION OF BIRDS AND NEW WORLD MONKEYS BETWEEN VITAMIN D$_2$ AND VITAMIN D$_3$

Steenbock and his colleagues were the first to recognize that the vitamin D derived from ergosterol was not as effective as fish liver oils in the prevention of rickets in chicks (Steenbock *et al.*, 1932). Waddell (1934) convincingly demonstrated that irradiated ergosterol was not as effective as irradiated impure cholesterol (7-dehydrocholesterol) in preventing vitamin D deficiency symptoms in chicks while both preparations were equally effective in the rat. He correctly concluded that the pro-vitamin in cholesterol was not identical to ergosterol and that the chick discriminated between the two irradiation products. After a careful study, Chen and Bosman (1964) concluded that vitamin D$_2$ is about $\frac{1}{10}$ as active as vitamin D$_3$ in curing rickets in chicks.

This discrimination has also been observed in other fowl such as turkeys (Boucher, 1949) and in new-world monkeys (Hunt et al., 1967). In contrast to this, rats, man and most other mammals appear to respond equally as well to vitamin D_2 and vitamin D_3.

Rachitic chicks injected with 0.25 μg of randomly labeled ^{14}C vitamin D_2 (Imrie et al., 1967) show a rapid disappearance of ^{14}C from the blood and a concomitant increase of radioactivity in the feces and the bile as compared to the disappearance of ^{3}H from the blood of chicks that had received the the same amount of tritiated vitamin D_3. This suggested that vitamin D_2 or a metabolite thereof is excreted in the bile at a more rapid rate and is thus turned over more quickly than vitamin D_3. Drescher et al. (1969) continued the work on the metabolism of vitamin D_2 and confirmed the previous results of Imrie et al. (1967) which suggested that vitamin D_2 or a metabolite is rapidly excreted, thereby reducing its effective life time. In the course of his studies, he demonstrated that vitamin D_2 is metabolized to a more polar metabolite (peak IV) (Drescher et al., 1969). However, chicks do not respond to the 25-OH-D_2 while showing a marked response to 25-OH-D_3. The discrimination is therefore somewhere beyond the 25-hydroxylation stage. This interesting problem will undoubtedly come under close examination in the next few years with the recent synthesis of [3H]-vitamin D_2 of high specific activity (Pelc and Kodicek, 1971).

III. FEED-BACK REGULATION OF 25-OH-D_3 METABOLISM TO 1,25-(OH)$_2$D$_3$ OR 24,25-(OH)$_2$D$_3$

A. ROLE OF DIETARY AND SERUM CALCIUM

Rottensten (1938), Fairbanks and Mitchell (1935) and Nicolaysen et al. (1953b) demonstrated that animals and man possess a marked ability to adapt to low dietary calcium intakes. When fed diets low in calcium, they adapt by markedly increasing their efficiency of absorption while they show poor calcium absorption ability when fed high calcium diets. This ability to adapt requires the presence of vitamin D. In addition, Nicolaysen et al. (1953b) noted that man deprived of calcium for a long period of time and then shifted to normal calcium diets retains the high efficiency of absorption until the skeleton is completely recalcified. They postulated the existence of an endogenous factor secreted by the skeleton which would inform the intestine of the skeletal needs for calcium. This 'factor' has remained unidentified until recently.

With the demonstration that 1,25-(OH)$_2$D$_3$ is likely the metabolically active form of vitamin D_3 in the initiation of intestinal calcium transport it occurred to Boyle et al. (1971) that if dietary calcium could in some manner regulate the biosynthesis of 1,25-(OH)$_2$D$_3$, then the 1,25-(OH)$_2$D$_3$ could represent at least in part the 'endogenous factor' of Nicolaysen in the adaptation of animals to low calcium diets. An examination of this question resulted in the demonstration

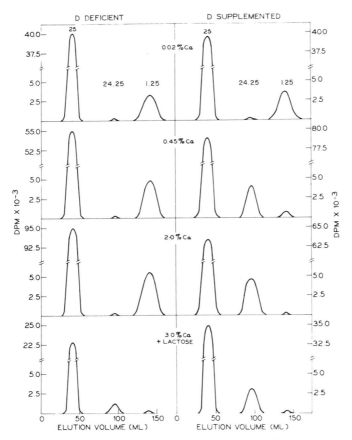

Fig. 6. Influence of dietary calcium on metabolism of ^{3}H 25-OH-D$_3$ to either 1,25-(OH)$_2$D$_3$ or 24,25-(OH)$_2$D$_3$. Rats were fed diets containing 0.3% phosphorus and the various levels of calcium indicated with and without 0.025 μg vitamin D$_3$ each day. After 2–3 weeks each rat was injected with 325 pmoles ^{3}H-25-OH-D$_3$ and 12 hours later their plasma was extracted and chromatographed. (Reproduced with the kind permission of the publisher, Boyle *et al.*, 1971.)

that rats on low calcium diets produce large amounts of 1,25-(OH)$_2$D$_3$ while those on higher dietary calcium intake have reduced 1,25-(OH)$_2$D$_3$ production until at high calcium levels little or no 1,25-(OH)$_2$D$_3$ is made (Fig. 6). As the production of 1,25-(OH)$_2$D$_3$ is shut down by dietary calcium, another metabolite, i.e. 24,25-(OH)$_2$D$_3$ is produced in increasing amounts in an almost reciprocal manner. Since the function of this metabolite is not yet known, its regulation will not be discussed further here. Thus the $1,25\text{-}(OH)_2D_3$ would represent the 'endogenous factor' which is responsible for the adaptation phenomenon. Confirmation of this belief was obtained by the demonstration that chicks maintained on $1,25\text{-}(OH)_2D_3$ as their source of vitamin D show high calcium absorption rates independent of dietary calcium while animals maintained on $25\text{-}OH\text{-}D_3$ clearly show the adaptation phenomenon (Omdahl and DeLuca, unpublished results). These experiments demonstrate that $1,25\text{-}(OH)_2D_3$ serves as the messenger for stimulation of intestinal calcium absorption under circumstances of low dietary calcium.

The feeding of strontium in place of calcium to animals given vitamin D causes rickets and reduced calcium absorption (Omdahl and DeLuca, 1971, 1972). Strontium feeding has also been shown to reduce to low levels both *in vivo* and *in vitro* production of $1,25\text{-}(OH)_2D_3$ (Omdahl and DeLuca, 1971, 1972). Furthermore the administration of $1,25\text{-}(OH)_2D_3$ to strontium fed chicks restores their calcium absorption to normal levels illustrating that a major lesion of strontium is the inhibition of $1,25\text{-}(OH)_2D_3$ production which then results in markedly inhibited calcium absorption (Omdahl and DeLuca, 1971, 1972).

B. ROLE OF PARATHYROID HORMONE, CALCITONIN AND CYCLIC AMP

Although it seems clear that the $1,25\text{-}(OH)_2D_3$ is regulated by dietary calcium, there remains the question of what actually triggers the synthesis of $1,25\text{-}(OH)_2D_3$ in the kidney. The production of $1,25\text{-}(OH)_2D_3$ in intact rats is related to the serum calcium concentration (Fig. 7) (Boyle *et al.*, 1972). Hypocalcemia is associated with marked production of $1,25\text{-}(OH)_2D_3$ while normal and hypercalcemia results in a turn-off of $1,25\text{-}(OH)_2D_3$ synthesis and a stimulation of $24,25\text{-}(OH)_2D_3$ production. It is therefore apparent that the need for calcium is translated into hypocalcemia which in some fashion stimulates $1,25\text{-}(OH)_2D_3$ production, a hormone in turn responsible for the mobilization of calcium from intestine and bone.

It has now become clear that the parathyroid glands play an important role in the regulation of $1,25\text{-}(OH)_2D_3$ synthesis (Fig. 8) (Garabedian *et al.*, 1972). Thyroparathyroidectomy of rats on low calcium diets results in an elimination of $1,25\text{-}(OH)_2D_3$ production and an increase in $24,25\text{-}(OH)_2D_3$ production. Parathyroid hormone (10 units/6 hours) restores the ability to produce $1,25\text{-}(OH)_2D_3$ and reduces $24,25\text{-}(OH)_2D_3$ synthesis to preoperation levels. Rasmussen and his colleagues have shown that parathyroid hormone or cyclic AMP added to isolated chick renal tubules stimulates $1,25\text{-}(OH)_2D_3$ production (Rasmussen *et al.*, 1972). Galente *et al.* (1972a,b) have reported that large doses

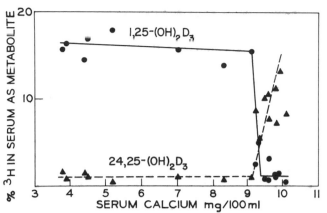

Fig. 7. The relationship of serum calcium concentration to the ability of rats to produce 1,25-$(OH)_2D_3$ from 25-OH-D_3. Animals were fed diets containing various amounts of calcium and phosphorus with and without vitamin D_3 for three weeks. At that time all animals received an intravenous injection of ^{3}H-25-OH-D_3. Twelve hours later blood was taken from each animal, extracted and chromatographed to reveal the metabolites formed. All animals, regardless of treatment were used in this plot. Note the sharp switch-over point at 9.5 mg % calcium. The 24,25-$(OH)_2D_3$ represents another metabolite of vitamin D whose function is not yet known. (Reproduced with the kind permission of the publisher, Boyle *et al.*, 1972a.)

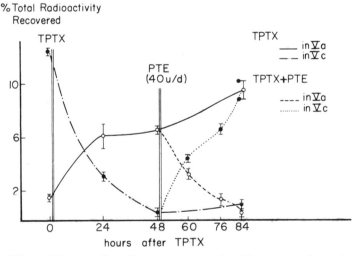

Fig. 8. Effect of thyroparathyroidectomy and parathyroid extract on the production of two polar metabolites of 25-OH-D_3. Va (24,25-$(OH)_2D_3$) and Vc (1,25-$(OH)_2D_3$) in the blood are shown as percent of total radioactivity recovered from the column of Sephadex LH-20 (chloroform : Skellysolve B 65 : 35). The rats received 325 pmoles of ^{3}H-25-OH-D_3 intrajugularly 12 hours before death. Half of the rats received 10 units of parathyroid extract (second vertical bars) 48 hours after the operation (first vertical bars) and 10 units every 6 hours thereafter. Each point is the mean ± standard deviation of the mean of 5 rats. ^{3}H in Va with (- - -) or without (——) parathyroid extract; ^{3}H in Vc with (····) or without (— · —) parathyroid extract. (Reproduced with the kind permission of the publisher, Garabedian *et al.*, 1972.)

of parathyroid hormone to rats on high calcium high phosphorus diets actually reduces while calcitonin stimulates $1,25\text{-}(OH)_2D_3$ production. Unfortunately their experiments were carried out with intact animals. It is possible that a large pulse of parathyroid hormone produced a compensatory release of endogenous calcitonin which may actually be responsible for the reduced $1,25\text{-}(OH)_2D_3$ production. Their experiments must be repeated using thyroparathyroid-ectomized animals before firm conclusions can be drawn.

C. ROLE OF INORGANIC PHOSPHATE

Rats on low phosphorus diets produce large amounts of $1,25\text{-}(OH)_2D_3$ in spite of hypercalcemia or thyroparathyroidectomy (Tanaka and DeLuca, 1973). Thus hypophosphatemia can also trigger $1,25\text{-}(OH)_2D_3$ synthesis (Tanaka and DeLuca, 1973). If rats on low calcium diet are TPTXed they produce no $1,25\text{-}(OH)_2D_3$ (Garabedian et al., 1972). If they are given instead of parathyroid hormone, calcium gluconate and glucose in their drinking water, the serum phosphorus falls and they begin to produce $1,25\text{-}(OH)_2D_3$. In fact after three days of such treatment their $1,25\text{-}(OH)_2D_3$ production is completely restored. A plot of serum phosphorus versus production of $1,25\text{-}(OH)_2D_3$ or $24,25\text{-}(OH)_2D_3$ in thyroparathyroidectomized rats reveals that at phosphorus levels below 7–8 mg/100 ml (Fig. 9) $1,25\text{-}(OH)_2D_3$ is produced while at high values, $24,25\text{-}(OH)_2D_3$ is produced. Because parathyroid hormone inhibits tubular phosphate reabsorption while calcitonin increases cellular phosphate (Kennedy and Talmage, 1972; Talmage et al., 1972) it seems that the renal cell inorganic phosphorus level may be the mechanism underlying the regulation of $1,25\text{-}(OH)_2D_3$ production by parathyroid hormone, calcitonin and hypophos-phatemia. In fact there is a very good correlation between renal cortex inorganic phosphorus level and production of $1,25\text{-}(OH)_2D_3$. When cortex inorganic phosphorus falls below 400 μg/g tissue, $1,25\text{-}(OH)_2D_3$ is made while values above that figure correlate with $24,25\text{-}(OH)_2D_3$ production. Thus the basic regulation of metabolism of $25\text{-}OH\text{-}D_3$ to either $1,25\text{-}(OH)_2D_3$ or $24,25\text{-}(OH)_2D_3$ may be the renal cell level of inorganic phosphate.

In the intact animal undoubtedly the parathyroid mechanism operates to regulate $1,25\text{-}(OH)_2D_3$ synthesis except under abnormal hypophosphatemic conditions. Clearly the renal system responsible for $1,25\text{-}(OH)_2D_3$ production must now be recognized as an important calcium homeostatic system. It is possible that much of the calcium regulation previously attributed to the parathyroid hormone may be through its regulation of the renal system responsible for the conversion of $25\text{-}OH\text{-}D_3$ to $1,25\text{-}(OH)_2D_3$.

Clinically, it seems likely that hypoparathyroid patients are probably unable to produce $1,25\text{-}(OH)_2D_3$. Thus the compound of choice in their management is probably $1,25\text{-}(OH)_2D_3$ or one of its analogs.

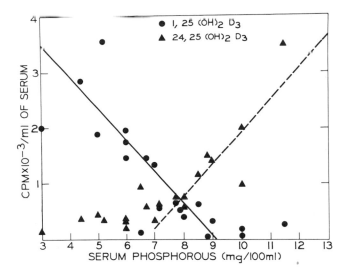

Fig. 9. Relationship of serum inorganic phosphorus to *in vivo* synthesis of 24,25-$(OH)_2D_3$ or 1,25-$(OH)_2D_3$. For this plot thyroparathyroidectomized rats were prepared in the following diverse manners. (1) They were fed a high calcium, low phosphorus diet for 2 weeks and then given 325 pmoles 25-OH-D_3 orally 24 hours prior to thyroparathyroidectomy. (2) They were fed a high calcium, adequate phosphorus diet for 2 weeks and were given 325 pmoles 25-OH-D_3 orally every day for 5 days prior to thyroparathyroidectomy. The rats from these two groups were shifted to various diets. Some of the latter rats were given calcium gluconate-glucose solutions. Three days after each shift in diet rats were injected intravenously with 325 pmoles ^{3}H-25-OH-D_3 and 12 hours later their serum was taken for serum calcium, serum phosphorus and chromatographic analysis of ^{3}H labeled vitamin D metabolites. The serum phosphorus is plotted versus production of 24,25-$(OH)_2D_3$ or 1,25-$(OH)_2D_3$ for all rats regardless of treatment. No correlation is found between metabolite levels and serum calcium concentration. (Reproduced with the kind permission of the publisher, Tanaka and DeLuca, 1973.)

IV. CHEMICAL SYNTHESIS OF VITAMIN D$_3$, ANALOGS AND METABOLITES

A. COMPLETE SYNTHESIS OF VITAMIN D$_3$ AND PREVITAMIN D$_3$

The discovery of Steenbock and associates that vitamin D is produced by irradiation of plant and animal sterol fractions led to the synthesis of vitamin D$_2$ and vitamin D$_3$ by the irradiation of ergosterol and 7-dehydrocholesterol. This work was pioneered by the brilliant efforts of Windaus and coworkers (Windaus *et al.*, 1932, 1935; Schenck, 1937) and Askew and coworkers (Askew *et al.*, 1931). After many years of working with various isomers of vitamin D$_3$, Inhoffen (1960) reported the total synthesis of vitamin D$_3$. In order to understand the intrinsic nature of the vitamin D structure, Inhoffen and coworkers chose to decompose

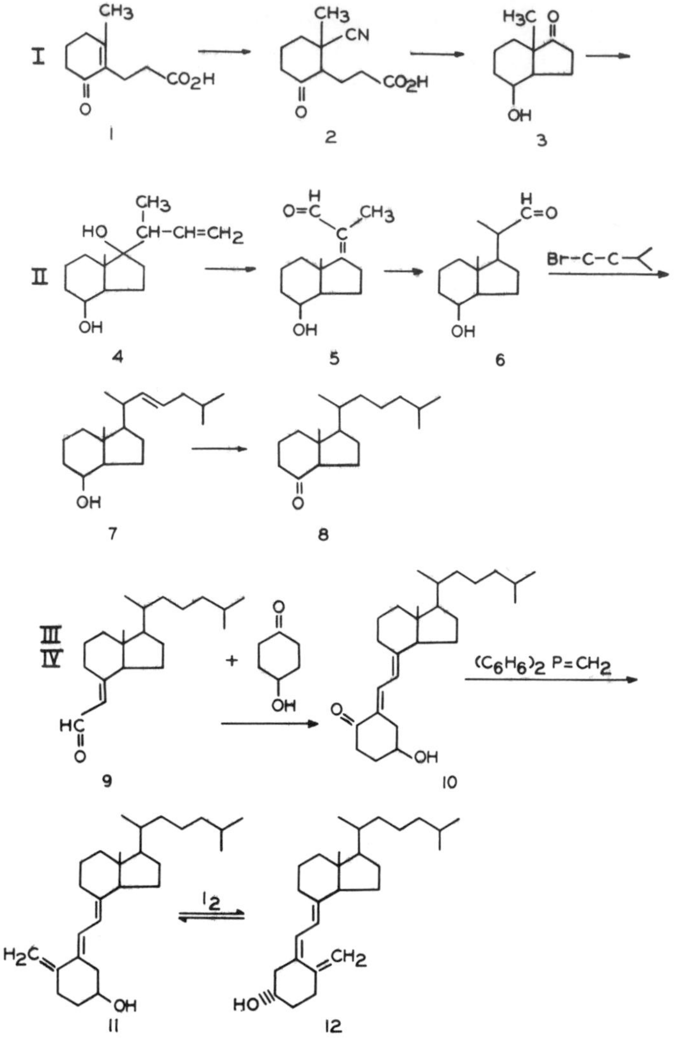

Fig. 10. Synthesis of vitamin D_3 by a non-photochemical method.

the vitamin with a number of oxidation procedures. They isolated the products, identified them, and then undertook the task of synthesizing the decomposition products. Finally these were put back together as if assembling a puzzle.

The vitamin was built in four basic steps as outlined in abbreviated form in Fig. 10. In the first series of reactions (I) the C and D ring system was made. The next major undertaking as shown in Step II, was the addition of the iso-octyl

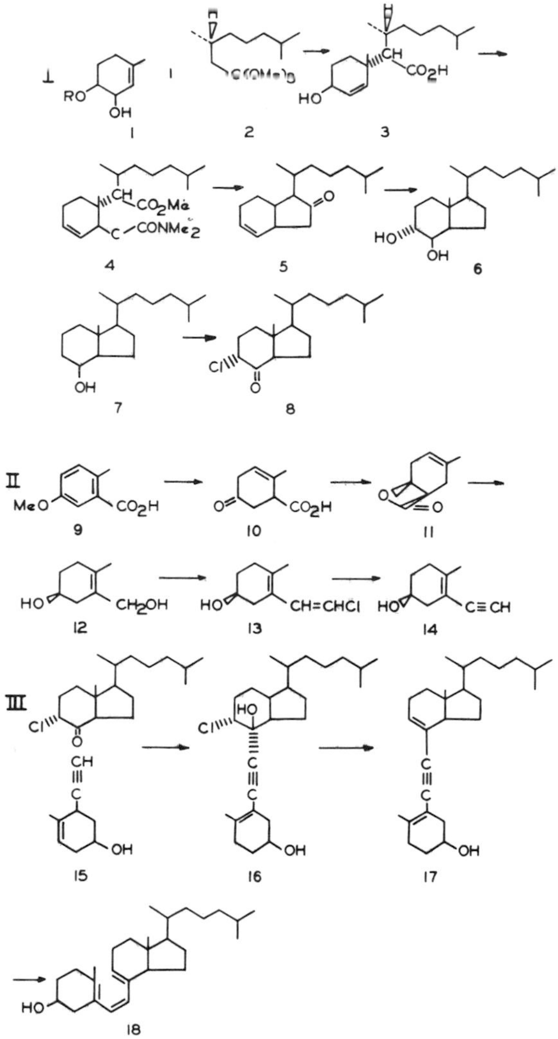

Fig. 11. Synthesis of previtamin D$_3$ by a non-photochemical method.

side chain. In step III the bridge carbons were put into place, using a Wittig reaction, and then altered in preparation for step IV, the addition of ring A. An aldol condensation of 9 with *p*-hydroxycyclohexanone yielded the hydroxy ketone, 10. The 3β isomer was then isolated and the C-19 methylene was introduced by a Wittig reaction to yield the 5,6-trans isomer of vitamin D$_3$. After many years of experience with isomers of vitamin D$_3$, these brilliant workers had

had no difficulty in isomerizing their product to the desired 5,6-cis triene, thus completing the first total synthesis of vitamin D_3.

Ten years later, Lithgoe and colleagues reported the total synthesis of precholecalciferol by a non-photochemical method as outlined in abbreviated form in Fig. 11. With similar brilliance and after numerous steps, this group synthesized the C and D ring system with the vitamin D_3 side chain attached to it (Bolton et al., 1970). The A ring was then synthesized from the methoxy acid 9 (Dawson et al., 1970) to 14 (Bruck et al., 1967; Harrison and Lithgoe, 1970) and then attached to the rest of the molecule 8, by the acetylene link of the en-yn-ene to give 17. Semi-hydrogenation of 17 yielded the precholecalciferol 18.

B. SYNTHESIS OF 25-OH-D_3

The importance of metabolically active forms of vitamin D_3 came as a direct result of the synthesis of $[1,2-^3H]$-vitamin D_3 of high specific activity. This was prepared by the heterogeneous catalytic reduction of cholesta-1,4-diene-3-one with $^3H_2$ to yield the $[1,2-^3H]$-cholesterol which was used in the synthesis (Neville and DeLuca, 1966). In a similar fashion the synthesis of $[1\alpha-^3H]$-vitamin D_3 was achieved by palladium-charcoal catalytic reduction of cholesta-1-en-3-one with tritium to $[1-^3H]$-cholestanone, which was subsequently converted to the 5,7-diene for irradiation to the precholecalciferol (Callow et al., 1966).

The use of high specific activity $[1,2-^3H]$-vitamin D_3 in metabolism studies led DeLuca and coworkers to isolate and identify a biologically active metabolite of

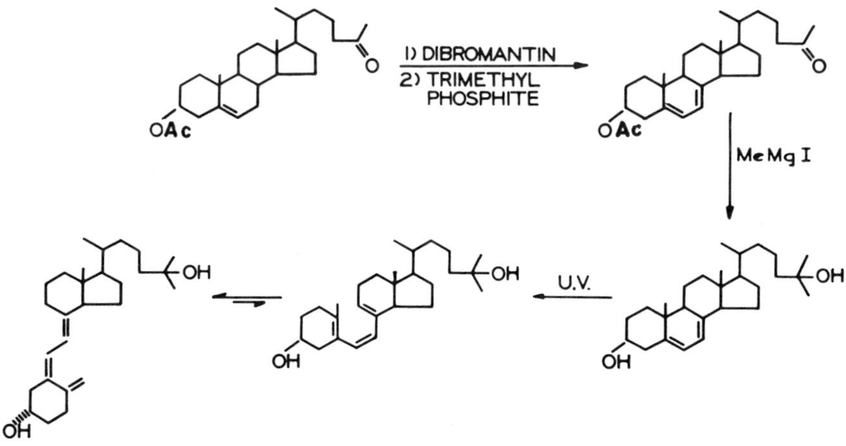

Fig. 12. Synthesis of 25-hydroxycholecalciferol.

vitamin D_3, 25-OH-D_3. Soon after its identification Blunt and DeLuca (1969) reported two routes for the synthesis of 25-OH-D_3. Starting with either 26-nor-cholesta-5-en-25-on-3βyl acetate (Fig. 12) or 25 hydroxycholesteryl acetate they reported the synthesis of 25-OH-D_3 in overall yields of 3.6 and 3.2%, respectively. A similar synthesis was reported by Halkes and Vam Vliet (1969). A short time later Campbell and coworkers (Campbell *et al.*, 1969) demonstrated the feasibility of synthesizing the same metabolite from 3β-hydroxy-chol-5-enic acid.

C. CHEMICAL SYNTHESIS OF 1α,25-(OH)$_2$D$_3$ AND 1α-OH-D$_3$

Using the synthetic method of Blunt and DeLuca (1969), Suda *et al.* (1971) prepared [26,27-^{3}H]-25-OH-D_3 of high specific activity. With this tool, the existence of more polar biologically active metabolites was demonstrated (Cousins *et al.*, 1970a,b). This led to the isolation and identification of an even more active metabolite of vitamin D_3 (1,25-(OH)$_2$D$_3$). Although biological data on the loss of ^{3}H during the conversion of [1α-^{3}H]-vitamin D_3 to 1,25-(OH)$_2$D$_3$ suggested the configuration of 1-OH to be alpha (Lawson *et al.*, 1969a, 1971), sufficient evidence for such a conclusion was unavailable. Recently Semmler *et al.* (1972) have reported a 21-step synthesis for 1α-25-(OH)$_2$D$_3$ (Fig. 13), starting with *i*-homocholanic acid methyl ester 1. The major steps were to protect the Δ^5 by conversion to a 5-ketone which could be protected as a ketal before introducing the Δ^1 by a series of reactions. This was accomplished by oxidation at the 3 position to 6, allylic bromination to 8 and elimination to the Δ^1 9. Epoxidation of 9 to 1α,2α-epoxide 10 and subsequent reduction with LiAlH$_4$, provided the 1,3-diol, 11. Unfortunately only the 3α isomer was recovered so that it was necessary to invert the 3α-hydroxyl by selective oxidation of 11 to 12. A subsequent sodium borohydride reduction yielded 1α,3β,25-trihydroxy-6,6'-dioxyethylene cholesterol 13. This compound was then acetylated and the ketal was removed by acid hydrolysis to yield 15. Selective reduction of 15 to 16 with NaBH$_4$ an isopropanol and subsequent dehydration with POCl$_3$ in pyridine yielded 1α,3β,25-triacetoxycholesterol 17. Allylic bromination and dehydrohalogenation yielded the corresponding 5,7-diene 20. The 5,7-diene triacetate was subjected to ultraviolet irradiation and the triacetoxy previtamin D_3 was recovered. Saponification of 20 yielded 1α,3β,25-dihydroxycholecalciferol. This product, and its 3α isomer, were used in co-chromatography studies with biosynthetic 1,25-(OH)$_2$D$_3$. The 1α,3β-25-(OH)$_2$D$_3$ comigrated with biosynthetic material, while the 3α isomer did not. The chemically synthesized products were tested for their biological activity and compared with the biosynthetic material as shown in Table 1. Clearly the 1α,3β-25-(OH)$_2$D$_3$ proved to be identical with biosynthetic 1,25-(OH)$_2$D$_3$ in endochondral calcification, intestinal calcium transport and bone calcium mobilization activity, while 1α,3α-25-(OH)$_2$D$_3$ has little if any effect in any of these systems. (It is interesting to note that Inhoffen (1960) reported that epivitamin D_3, i.e. 3α-vitamin D_3, is only about 15% as active as vitamin D_3. It now appears that the $1\alpha,3\alpha$-25-$(OH)_2D_3$ has approximately the same biological activity.)

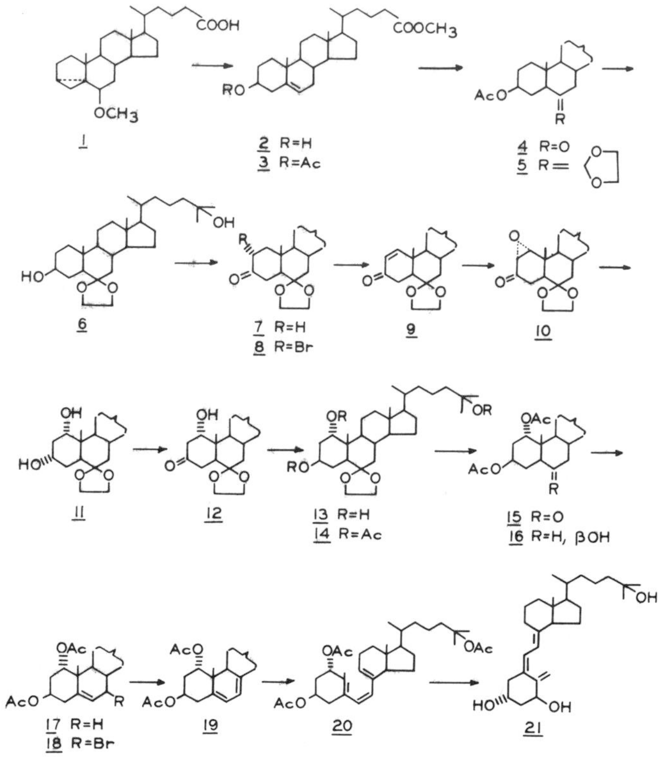

Fig. 13. Synthesis of $1\alpha,25$-dihydroxycholecalciferol. (Reproduced with the kind permission of the publisher, Semmler *et al.*, 1972.)

The ultraviolet absorption spectrum and mass spectrum of the chemically synthesized $1\alpha,3\beta$-25-$(OH)_2D_3$ were also identical with that of the biosynthetic material. Therefore, the chemical synthesis of $1\alpha25$-$(OH)_2D_3$ confirms the structure reported for the intestinal metabolite (Holick *et al.*, 1971a,b; Lawson *et al.*, 1971). Although there is no absolute proof that the 1-hydroxyl of the biosynthetic material is in the alpha rather than beta position, the identical biological and chemical properties it has in common with the chemically synthesized $1\alpha,3\beta,25$-$(OH)_2D_3$ provides strong evidence that it is in the alpha position.

The 1α-hydroxyvitamin D_3 (Holic et al., 1973a) was also synthesized as a direct result of the chemical synthesis of $1\alpha,3\beta$-25-$(OH)_2D_3$, and have reported that it is similar in biological activity to $1,25$-$(OH)_2D_3$ in inducing intestinal calcium transport, bone calcium mobilization and in healing rachitic lesions as shown in Table 1.

Table 1. *Biological activity of 1α-hydroxyvitamin D compounds*

Compound	Route of administration	^{45}Ca serosal/ ^{45}Ca mucosal	Milligrams Ca/100 ml serum	Antirachitic activity (I.U./µg)
Control	i.v. in 95% EtOH	1.5 ± 0.2	4.0 ± 0.1	
0.125 µg 1,25-$(OH)_2D_3$ (biosynthetic)	i.v. in 95% EtOH	3.5 ± 0.2	6.6 ± 0.2	
0.125 µg 1α,3β,25-$(OH)_2D_3$ (synthetic)	i.v. in 95% EtOH	3.7 ± 0.2	6.2 ± 0.1	
0.25 µg 1α,3α,25-$(OH)_2D_3$ (synthetic)	i.v. in 95% EtOH	1.9 ± 0.2	4.7 ± 0.1	
0.025 µg 1α-OHD_3	i.v. in 95% EtOH	2.8 ± 0.3	5.8 ± 0.1	
1α-OHD_3	orally in propylene glycol			80
1α-OHD_3	i.v. in 95% EtOH			200
1α,25-$(OH)_2D_3$ (biosynthetic)	orally in propylene glycol			80
1α,25-$(OH)_2D_3$ (biosynthetic)	i.v. in 95% EtOH			400
1α,3β,25-$(OH)_2D_3$ (synthetic)	i.v. in 95% EtOH			400
vitamin D_3	orally in oil			40

Determinations of biological activity were carried out by methods described in Omdahl et al. (1971) and Holic et al. (1972d).

V. BIOLOGICALLY ACTIVE ANALOGS OF VITAMIN D

A. METABOLISM AND BIOLOGICAL ACTIVITY OF DIHYDROTACHYSTEROL

Following the chemical work of Askew et al. (1931) and of Windaus (1935, 1936) on the elucidation of the structures of vitamins D_2 and D_3, many investigators have made analogs of vitamin D and tested them for their biological potency in the calcification of bone either by the 'line test' method or by increase in bone ash. One of the more interesting biologically active compounds was reported by von Werder (1939). He reduced tachysterol with sodium-propanol to yield dihydrotachysterol. Although this compound has very little antirachitic activity in comparison to vitamin D_3 (1/450), this group of analogs displayed preferential activity at large doses in the mobilization of calcium from the bone in thyroparathyroidectomized rats (Roborgh and DeMan, 1960; Harrison *et al.*, 1968). Recently Suda and coworkers postulated that the 25-hydroxy derivative would be more active than dihydrotachysterol (DHT). They synthesized 25-OH-DHT$_3$, and demonstrated that on a weight basis this hydroxylated form was more active than DHT$_3$, both as an antirachitic agent and as an agent for inducing intestinal calcium transport and bone calcium mobilization (Suda *et al.*, 1970).

Hallick and DeLuca (1971) synthesized $[1,2-^3H]$-DHT$_3$ and studied its metabolism in vitamin D-deficient rats. They demonstrated that $[1,2-^3H]$-DHT$_3$ is metabolized to more polar metabolites and that the major metabolite in the blood migrated on the chromatogram in a position similar to 25-OH-DHT$_3$. By co-chromatography studies with authentic 25-OH-DHT$_3$ in various chromatographic systems, they convincingly demonstrated that the major metabolite of DHT in the blood is the 25-OH derivative. Furthermore, they demonstrated that rat liver homogenates produce this metabolite from DHT$_3$ which is responsible for the mobilization of calcium from bone and probably intestinal calcium transport since at biologically active doses of $[1,2-^3H]$-DHT$_3$ virtually no metabolites more polar than 25-OH-DHT$_3$ were detected in those tissues (Hallick and DeLuca, 1972). Similarly Trummel *et al.* (1971) demonstrated in embryonic rat bone cultures that 25-OH-DHT$_3$ is at least 150 times more effective than DHT$_3$ in promoting the release of calcium from fetal bones.

B. ISOMERS OF VITAMIN D_3

During the 1950's and early 1960's much effort was directed to the synthesis and characterization of the various isomers of vitamin D_3. Verloop and coworkers (1955) reported the synthesis of the 5,6-*trans* isomer of vitamin D_3 by iodine catalysis and demonstrated its biological activity in chickens to be about $\frac{1}{30}$ that of vitamin D_3 (Verloop *et al.*, 1959). Although this isomer appeared to be of little use as a biologically active analog of vitamin D_3, the *cis–trans* equilibration in the presence of iodine proved to be a useful tool in the completion of the total synthesis of vitamin D_3.

Recently as a result of new concepts emanating from an understanding of the metabolism of both vitamin D_3 and DHT$_3$, Holick *et al.* (1972d) compared the structure of 5,6-*trans*-vitamin D_3 to DHT$_3$ and 1,25-(OH)$_2$D$_3$. Although the ring A is substantially different from either 1,25-(OH)$_2$D$_3$ or DHT, it does have an hydroxyl in the position occupied by the 1-hydroxyl of 1,25-(OH)$_2$D$_3$ or the 3-hydroxyl of DHT (Fig. 14). Unlike vitamin D_3 or 25-OH-D$_3$, 5,6-*trans*-vitamin

D_3 can stimulate both intestinal calcium transport and bone calcium mobilization in anephric rats as has been demonstrated for DHT_3 (Hallick and DeLuca,
1972; Harrison and Harrison, 1972), thus mimicing the action of $1,25$-$(OH)_2D_3$
(Holick et al., 1972a; Boyle et al., 1972a). In vitamin D-deficient animals, 25 μg
of this analog elicited an intestinal calcium transport response as early as 3 hours

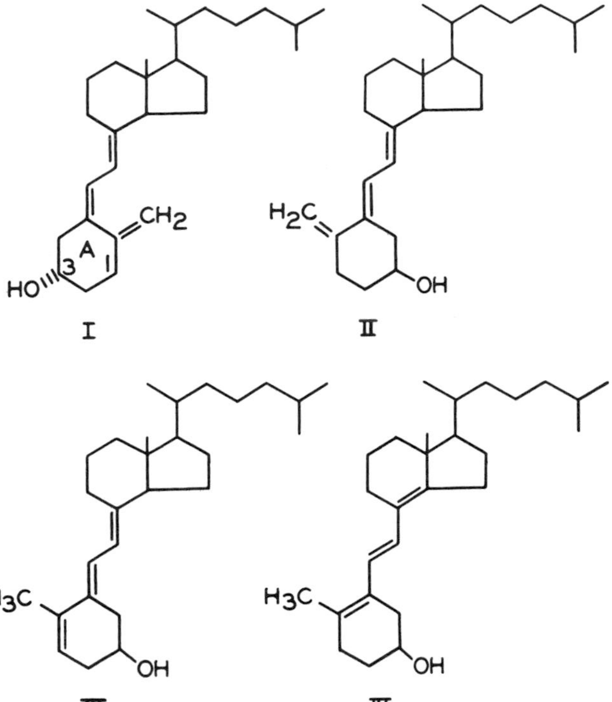

Fig. 14. Structures of (I) vitamin D_3; (II) 5,6-*trans*-vitamin D_3; (III) isovitamin D_3, and
(IV) isotachysterol$_3$.

after its administration and showed a maximum response at 6 hours (Fig. 15(a)).
Similarly this analog showed a small but significant bone calcium mobilization
response after 3 hours and a maximum response at 12 hours (Fig. 15(b)). As
little as 2.5 μg of 5,6-*trans*-vitamin D_3 will elicit a response in both the intestine
and the bone. Because it was demonstrated that the 25-OH derivatives of DHT_3,
vitamin D_2 and vitamin D_3 are biologically more active than their non-
hydroxylated analogs (Suda et al., 1970a,d; Blunt et al., 1969), it was of interest
to see if this might also be the case for 5,6-*trans*-vitamin D_3. Although on a
weight basis the 25-OH derivative of 5,6-*trans*-D_3 did not appear to be more

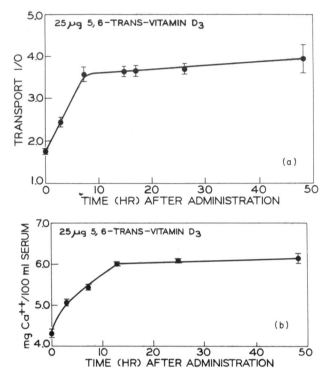

Fig. 15. Intestinal calcium transport and bone calcium mobilization response of vitamin D deficient rats on a low calcium diet to a 25 μg dose of 5,6-*trans*-D$_3$. The vertical bars represent the standard error of the mean for six animals. (Reproduced with the kind permission of the publisher, Holick *et al.*, 1972d.)

Table 2. *Intestinal calcium transport and bone calcium mobilization response to various analogs of vitamin D$_3$ in normal and anephric rats according to the procedure of Holick* et al. *(1972b)*

Dose	Condition of animal	^{45}Ca serosal/^{45}Ca mucosal	Milligrams Ca/100 ml serum
50 μl 95% ETOH	normal	1.8 ± 0.2	4.2 ± 0.1
25 μg 5,6-*trans*-D$_3$	normal	4.2 ± 0.2	6.2 ± 0.1
25 μg 5,6-*trans*-25-OH-D$_3$	normal	4.4 ± 0.3	4.8 ± 0.1
25 μg 25-OH-D$_3$	normal	4.5 ± 0.8	6.4 ± 0.1
5 μg isotachysterol	normal	3.5 ± 0.2	6.4 ± 0.1
5 μg isovitamin D$_3$	normal	3.2 ± 0.2	6.2 ± 0.1
50 μl 95% ETOH	anephric	1.5 ± 0.2	4.3 ± 0.1
25 μg 5,6-*trans*-D$_3$	anephric	3.3 ± 0.3	6.5 ± 0.1
25 μg 5,6-*trans*-25-OH-D$_3$	anephric	3.3 ± 0.3	4.9 ± 0.1
25 μg 25-OH-D$_3$	anephric	1.9 ± 0.3	4.4 ± 0.1

active than 5,6-*trans*-vitamin D_3 in inducing intestinal calcium transport in anephric rats, it was surprising that this derivative had little activity in the mobilization of calcium from the bone (Table 2) (Holick *et al.*, 1972d). These results suggest that at least in the bone the 5,6-*trans*-vitamin D_3 may act by itself without 25-hydroxylation.

C. ISOTACHYSTEROL AND ISO-VITAMIN D_3

In their initial efforts to achieve the partial synthesis of vitamin D_2, Inhoffen and coworkers accomplished the synthesis of two new triene isomers of vitamin D (Inhoffen *et al.*, 1954). They reported that vitamin D_3 in the presence of either borontrifluoride etherate or phosphoric acid/acetic anhydride isomerized to a new isomer which had λ_{max} at 302, 290 and 280 nm (ϵ_{290} = 40,800). They called this isomer isotachysterol (Fig. 14). In another attempt to synthesize cholecalciferol, they reported the synthesis of isovitamin D_3 (Fig. 14), which had an ultraviolet absorption spectrum similar to isotachysterol except that the entire ultraviolet absorption spectrum shifted 1–2 nm to give λ_{max} at 300, 288 and 278 nm (ϵ_{288} = 41,800).

Recently Murray *et al.* (1966) noted that after treatment with antimony trichloride, vitamin D_2 isomerizes to a compound with an ultraviolet absorption spectrum similar to that if isovitamin D_3 as reported by Inhoffen *et al.* (1954).

Because the A ring of both these isomers is rotated 180°, similar to both 5,6-*trans*-vitamin D_3 and dihydrotachysterol such that the 3β-hydroxyl is also in the pseudo 1-hydroxyl position, it was reasonable to assume that these analogs would also by biologically active, similar to the 5,6-*trans*-vitamin D_3 and DHT. Recently these analogs have been synthesized and shown to be active in inducing intestinal calcium transport and bone calcium mobilization in vitamin D-deficient rats (Table 2) (Holick *et al.*, 1972b). However, isovitamin D_3 is not biologically active in anephric rats which might suggest that the A ring is not rotated 180° as suggested for the structure of isovitamin D_3.

D. SIDE-CHAIN ANALOGS OF VITAMIN D

Windaus and coworkers (1935, 1936) were the first to attempt the synthesis of antirachitic compounds with the 5,6-*cis*-triene system of vitamin D_2 with differing side chain structures. They successfully synthesized an analog of ergosterol which had a cholesterol side chain and reported that one of its irradiation products possessed about the same antirachitic potency as vitamin D_2. However, when the side-chain is replaced by a hydroxyl group (Dimroth and Paland, 1939) or by a bile acid side chain (Haselwood, 1939), the compounds are devoid of vitamin D activity. Vitamin D_4 (22,23-dihydrovitamin D_2) has 75% the biological activity of vitamin D_3 in rats and 10% in the case of chicks

(McDonald, 1936; DeLuca *et al.*, 1968). Irradiation mixtures produced from the 5,7-diene of stigmasterol (Rosenberg, 1942) and sitosterol (Grab, 1936) gave approximately 5–10% of the antirachitic activity of vitamin D_3.

Because it is now possible to determine different biological activities for various side chain analogs and their 5,6-*trans*-isomers, the 24-nor,27-nor,26,27-bisnor derivatives of 25-OH-D_3 (Fig. 16) were assayed for their ability to stimulate intestinal calcium transport and bone calcium mobilization and for

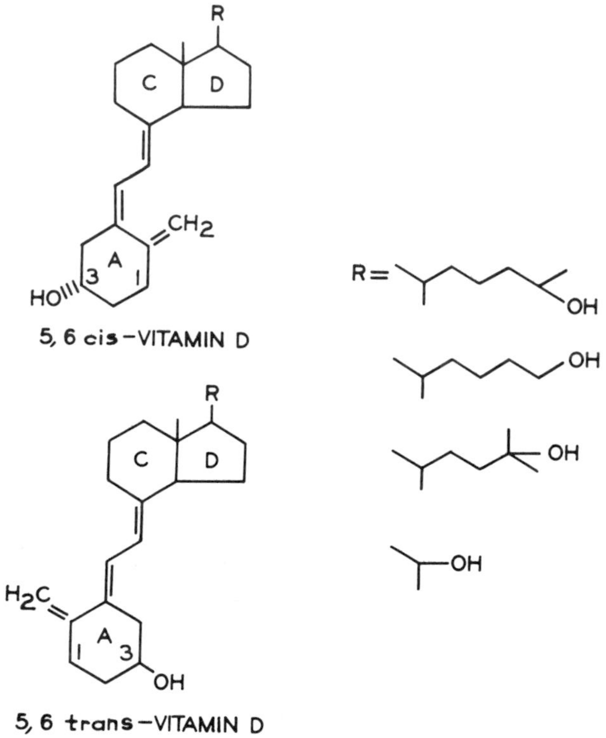

Fig. 16. Hydroxy side-chain analogs of vitamin D_3 and 5,6-*trans*-D_3.

their potency to heal rachitic lesions (Holick, Garabedian and DeLuca, unpublished results). It appears that each of these analogs is about 1–10% as active as 25-OH-D_3 in initiating intestinal calcium transport and mobilizing calcium from the bone. However, if 5 μg of each of these compounds is dosed orally to rachitic rats none of these compounds are able to heal rickets. Using pregnenolone as a starting material, an analog of vitamin D_3 devoid of a side chain but with a 20-hydroxyl function was prepared (Fig. 16). Twenty-five μg of this analog did not stimulate either intestinal calcium transport or bone calcium mobilization. Even when this analog was isomerized to the 5,6-*trans* isomer to provide a pseudo-1-hydroxyl function, it was not biologically active. Since the 24-nor-27-nor and 26,27-bisnor 25-OH-D_3 are somewhat biologically active in both the bone and the intestine, this suggests that at least part of the side chain is necessary for biological activity. However, because these analogs of 25-OH-D_3 are inactive in anephric rats while their 5,6-*trans* isomers restore activity, it appears that they must be hydroxylated on C-1 before they can function.

VI. TOOLS FOR ISOLATION AND IDENTIFICATION OF VITAMIN D METABOLITES

A. MASS SPECTROMETRY OF VITAMIN D AND ITS METABOLITES

The use of mass spectrometry as an important tool for the identification of various vitamin D metabolites was first demonstrated by Blunt et al. (1968). Vitamin D fragments in such a way that it is easy to distinguish whether an additional oxygen function is incorporated into the side chain, C-D ring system or in the A ring. There are two basic cleavages of the vitamin D molecule in an electron beam. Loss of the side chain representing the cleavage of the C-17, C-20 bond gives rise to the fragments m/e 271 and m/e 253 (271-H_2O). The most intense fragments, however, are at m/e 136 and m/e 118 (136-H_2O), accountable by the cleavage of the C-7, C-8 bond (Fig. 17).

The mass spectrum of the first hydroxylated metabolite of vitamin D was isolated from hog plasma and showed a molecular ion of 400, which suggested the incorporation of an additional oxygen function into the parent molecule (MW 384). The mass spectrum of the metabolite showed fragments at m/e 136, 118, 271 and 253, clearly indicating that the additional oxygen function was on the side chain and a fragment at m/e 59 suggesting a cleavage of the C-24,C-25 bond (Fig. 17) (Blunt et al., 1968). The mass spectrum of the ditrimethylsilyl ether derivative of 25-OH-D_3 exhibits an intense peak at 131 which could only arise from fragment $(CH_3)_2C=O-Si(CH_3)_3$ providing additional evidence that the oxygen function was on carbon 25. This intense fragment peak for the TMS derivative of vitamin D metabolites is usually diagnostic for the C-25 hydroxyl function (Suda et al., 1969; Holick et al., 1971a,b, 1972c). In a similar fashion Suda et al. (1969) isolated and identified the 25-hydroxy derivative of vitamin D_2 from hogs that had received large doses of vitamin D_2. The mass spectrum of 25-OH-D_2 displayed intense fragments at m/e 136 and 118 as well as fragment peaks at m/e 271 and 253, requiring that the additional oxygen function be on

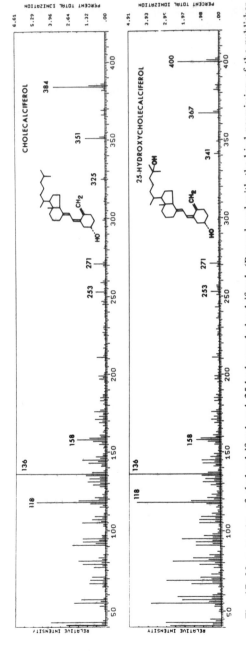

Fig. 17. Mass spectra of cholecalciferol and 25-hydroxycholecalciferol. (Reproduced with the kind permission of the publisher, Blunt *et al.*, 1968.)

the side chain. However, because of the Δ^{22} in the side chain and the additional methyl group at C-24, the fragmentation of the side chain for vitamin D_2 and 25-OH-D_2 is different from that for vitamin D_3 and its 25-OH derivative. A minor fragment at m/e 354 represents the bond cleavage of C-24,C-25.

In their quest to isolate metabolites of vitamin D more polar than 25-OH-D_3, Suda and coworkers (1970b,c) isolated two metabolites more polar than 25-OH-D_3 from porcine plasma. The mass spectrum of the first metabolite, peak Vc (25,26-dihydroxyvitamin D_3) has a molecular weight of 416 suggesting the incorporation of two additional oxygen functions into the vitamin D_3 molecule. Since the mass spectrum also showed fragments at m/e 271, 253, 136 and 118 it was clear that the additional oxygen functions were in the side chain. In addition to these peaks the mass spectrum for Vc showed a peak at M-18-31 or m/e 367, indicating the presence of CH_2OH group, suggesting a 20,21 or 25,26 dihydroxylated side chain (Fig. 18). The mass spectrum of the tritrimethylsilyl ether derivative of the metabolite supported the 25,26-dihydroxy structure. The relatively intense peak at m/e 529 corresponds to the loss of 103 mass units, $M-CH_2OSi(CH_3)_3$ and a peak at m/e 219 can result by cleavage of the C-24,C-25 bond. Further proof of a vicinal glycol grouping was provided by periodate cleavage of the metabolite which gave a compound of MW 384 as expected for the transformation of a 25,26-dihydroxy compound to the corresponding 25-keto derivative (Suda et al., 1970c). The peak Va metabolite also showed a molecular ion at 416 demonstrating that the metabolite was a dihydroxy-cholecalciferol (Suda et al., 1970b). Fragments at 118, 136, 253 and 271 clearly demonstrated that the additional oxygen functions were in the side chain while the mass spectrum of the tritrimethylsilyl ether derivative showed an intense peak at 131 demonstrating that one of the hydroxyl functions was on carbon 25. The sensitivity of this metabolite to periodate and the mass spectrum of the periodate cleavage product left little doubt that the structure for this metabolite was the 24,25-dihydroxy derivative of vitamin D_3 (Figs 1 and 4) (Holick et al., 1972c).

The only metabolite of vitamin D_3 isolated to date which has an oxygen function in a place other than the side chain is 1,25-dihydroxyvitamin D_3 (Holick et al., 1971a,b; Lawson et al., 1971). The mass spectrum of this metabolite clearly demonstrated the usefulness of mass spectrometry in identifying vitamin D_3 metabolites. The mass spectrum of this metabolite as shown in Fig. 2 showed intense fragments at 134 and 152 (oxygen analogs of 118 and 136) demonstrating that the additional oxygen function was either in the A ring or on carbon C-6, C-7 or C-19, while the tritrimethylsilyl ether derivative of this compound exhibited an intense fragment at 131 clearly identifying at least one of these hydroxyl functions to be on carbon 25. Using various chemical techniques it was established that the additional oxygen function was on carbon 1.

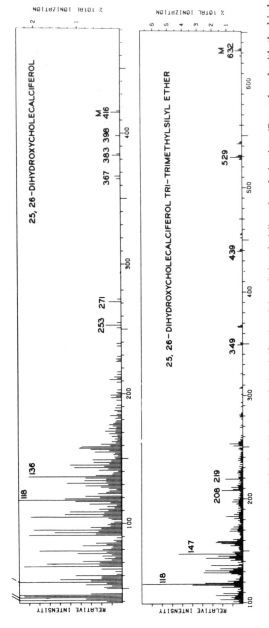

Fig. 18. Mass spectra of 25,26-dihydroxycholecalciferol and its tritrimethylsilyl ether derivative. (Reproduced with the kind permission of the publisher, Suda et al., 1970c.)

B. MASS SPECTROMETRY OF VARIOUS ISOMERS OF VITAMIN D_3

The mass spectrum of the 5,6-*trans* isomer of vitamin D_3 is very similar to the 5,6-*cis* vitamin D_3 mass spectrum as shown in Fig. 19. Characteristic fragments for the loss of the side chain (m/e 271, 253) as well as cleavage at C-7, C-8 are present in the mass spectrum for the 5,6-*trans* isomer. However, fragment m/e 259 in the spectrum for the 5,6-*trans* isomer is not found in the vitamin D mass spectrum (Figs 17 and 19). The mass spectra for both isovitamin D_3 and isotachysterol$_3$, however, are distinctly different from both vitamin D_3 and 5,6-*trans*-vitamin D_3.

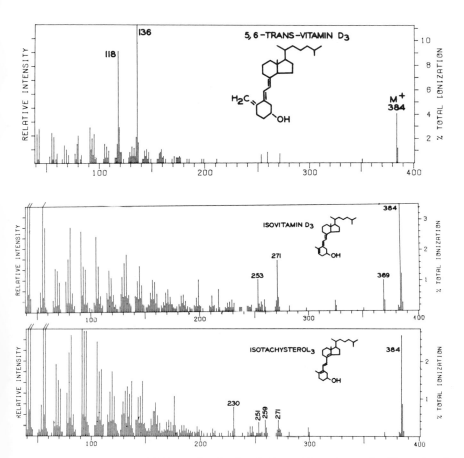

Fig. 19. Mass spectra of 5,6-*trans*-D_3; isovitamin D_3 and isotachysterol$_3$. (Reproduced with the kind permission of the publisher, Holick *et al.*, 1972d.)

Although the $\Delta^{5,7}$ part of the triene system for isovitamin D_3 is similar to both the 5,6-*cis* and *trans* vitamin D_3, the mass spectrum of this isomer does not show the C-7,C-8 bond cleavage (m/e 136 and 118). Instead it displays fragments 271 and 253 characteristic for the C-17,C-20 bond cleavage and a fragment M-15 (m/e 369) accountable by the loss of a CH_3^+ and little else. The mass spectrum for isotachysterol$_3$ exhibits fragments m/e 271 and 253 similar to the other isomers and fragments m/e 230, 259 and 299 which are not present in the mass spectra of vitamin D_3 and isovitamin D_3 (Holick *et al.*, 1973b).

The mass spectrum of dihydrotachysterol$_3$ displays a molecular ion m/e 386 and fragments at m/e 255 and 273 typical for the M—side chain—H_2O. This analog also exhibits a fragment at m/e 259, similar to 5,6-*trans*-vitamin D_3 and isotachysterol$_3$, possibly arising by the sequence of M→301→259 that is elimination of a 6 carbon fragment from the side chain to yield an ion of composition $C_{21}H_{33}O$ (MW 301) followed by loss of ketone involving the hydroxyl function of ring A. A less common fragment at m/e 247 accountable by the loss of ring A and carbons 6 and 7 is also present in the spectrum (Suda *et al.*, 1970d).

C. ULTRAVIOLET ABSORPTION SPECTROPHOTOMETRY FOR VITAMIN D AND ITS ISOMERS

Ultraviolet absorption spectrophotometry is another extremely useful tool for the structural identification of vitamin D metabolites. Based on this technique, it has been determined that each of the hydroxylated metabolites of vitamin D_3 have retained the 5,6-*cis* triene configuration of the parent structure, since only the 5,6-*cis* triene exhibits a λ_{max} 265 (ϵ = 18,200) and λ_{min} 228 (Fig. 20) (Blunt *et al.*, 1968; Suda *et al.*, 1969, 1970a,b; Holick *et al.*, 1971b, 1972c). Although the mass spectrum of the 5,6-*trans* isomer is very similar to the vitamin (especially bond cleavage C-7,C-8 (m/e 136, 118)), its ultraviolet absorption spectrum λ_{max} 273.5 (ϵ = 24,200) and λ_{min} 232 (Fig. 21) clearly distinguishes it from the 5,6-*cis* triene of the D metabolites (Verloop *et al.*, 1953; Nair *et al.*, 1968; Holick *et al.*, 1972d). Although the ultraviolet absorption spectra for isovitamin D_3 (λ_{max} 300, 288, 278) (Inhoffen *et al.*, 1954) and isotachysterol$_3$ (λ_{max} 302, 290, 280) (Inhoffen *et al.*, 1954) as shown in Fig. 22 are very similar, they could never be mistaken for the 5,6-*cis* triene of vitamin D_3.

Tachysterol, one of the irradiation products of 7-dehydrocholesterol, also exhibits an untraviolet spectrum much different from that of vitamin D_3 with λ_{max} 290, 280 and 272 while its dihydro derivative (dihydrotachysterol) spectrum is shifted to give λ_{max} 260.5, 251 and 242.5 nm.

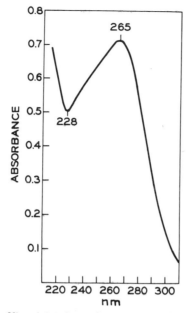

Fig. 20. Ultraviolet absorption spectrum of vitamin D_3.

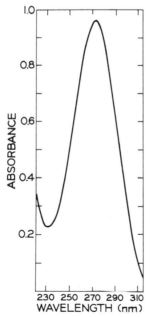

Fig. 21. Ultraviolet absorption spectrum of 5,6-*trans*-D_3 (Reproduced with the kind permission of the publisher, Holick *et al.*, 1972d.)

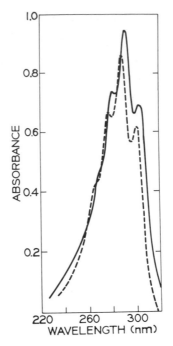

Fig. 22. Ultraviolet absorption spectra of (——) isotachysterol and (- - -) isovitamin D_3.

D. GAS-LIQUID CHROMATOGRAPHY FOR VITAMIN D AND ANALOGS

The fortuitous observation (Ziffer *et al.*, 1960) that vitamin D pyrolizes in the gas chromatograph provides the vitamin D chemist with yet another technique for differentiating the 5,6-*cis* triene system of vitamin D from all of its other isomers. Although it had been known for a long time that vitamin D undergoes a thermal cyclization reaction yielding pyro and isopyro vitamin D, Ziffer *et al.* (1960) were the first to demonstrate that vitamin D also cyclizes in the gas chromatograph to yield two peaks with a relative ratio of approximately 2/1 (Fig. 23). They identified the larger peak as the isopyro isomer and the smaller peak as the pyro isomer of the vitamin.

Even though it has been observed that 5,6-*trans*-vitamin D isomerizes to isotachysterol during gas–liquid chromatography (Nair *et al.*, 1968) isotachysterol and isovitamin D do not undergo thermal change. Therefore, each of these isomers chromatographs as one homogeneous compound in comparison to the two products observed for vitamin D.

This unique property of the 5,6-*cis* triene for vitamin D has recently been used to further substantiate the ultraviolet absorption data concerning the 5,6-*cis* triene structure of vitamin D metabolites. 25-OH-D$_3$ (Blunt and DeLuca, 1968; Holick and DeLuca, 1972), 25-OH-D$_2$ (Suda *et al.*, 1969), 24,25-(OH)$_2$D$_3$ (Suda *et al.*, 1970a; Holick *et al.*, 1972c) all demonstrate the pyro and isopyro isomers on gas–liquid chromatography.

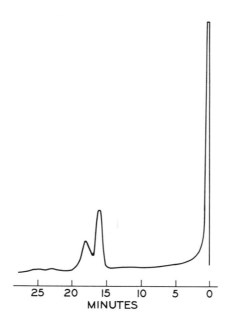

Fig. 23. Gas–liquid chromatography of vitamin D$_3$.

E. CHROMATOGRAPHY OF THE POLAR METABOLITES OF 25-OH-D$_3$

It will not be the purpose of this section to review all of the extraction and chromatographic methods used for separating vitamin D and its metabolites, but rather bring into focus techniques developed subsequent to the previous review on this subject (DeLuca *et al.*, 1969).

The investigation into the more polar metabolites of vitamin D led Ponchon and DeLuca (1969) to develop a silicic acid chromatographic system which resolved their peak IV fraction from rat plasma into six components. A year later Suda *et al.* (1970b,c) examined the peak V fractions after silicic acid chromatography of a plasma extract from chicks given 2.5 µg [1,2-^{3}H]-vitamin D$_3$ and found it to be heterogeneous. Furthermore they found that the peak Va fraction contained at least two metabolites while the peak Vc region included at least five different compounds when they were chromatographed on a liquid–liquid partition column (Suda *et al.,* 1970b,c).

In 1971 a powerful new chromatographic system using Sephadex LH-20

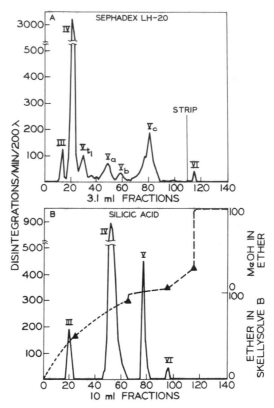

Fig. 24. Comparison of the chromatography of a lipid extract from plasma of rats that received 2.5 µg ^{3}H-vitamin D$_3$ intraperitoneally 24 hours earlier. (A) Sephadex LH-20 (CHCl$_3$: Skellysolve B 65 : 35), (B) Silicic acid (25 g), (——) radioactivity, (- - -) gradient. (Reproduced with the kind permission of the publisher, Holick and DeLuca, 1971.)

packed in and developed with a mixed solvent of chloroform and Skellysolve B was introduced (Holick and DeLuca, 1971). This system offered many advantages over silicic acid adsorption chromatography. These columns are simple to develop since only one solvent is needed throughout the chromatography and the volume of solvent used is about 30% of that needed for silicic acid chromatography. Besides being easy to prepare, the same column may be used repeatedly, while a silicic acid column can only be used once before it is discarded. In a mixed solvent system of chloroform : Skellysolve B (1 : 1) vitamin D is separated from 25-hydroxy vitamin D. As the percentage of chloroform is decreased and the percentage of Skellysolve B increased, the retention volumes for vitamin D_3 relative to 25-OH-D_3 increase. A solvent system of 65:35 chloroform : Skellysolve B is especially useful for studies of vitamin D metabolites more polar than 25-OH-D_3. Figure 24 illustrates the capability of this chromatographic system in the resolution of various vitamin D_3 metabolites in rat plasma as compared to silicic acid chromatography. The peak V region which appears to be homogeneous on silicic acid separates into four distinct peaks, V_{t_1}, 24,25-$(OH)_2 D_3$, Vb and 25,26-$(OH)_2 D_3$-1,25-$(OH)_2 D_3$ or Vc on the Sephadex system. This system however has a disadvantage that it will not resolve 1,25-$(OH)_2 D_3$ from 25,26-$(OH)_2 D_3$. Haussler and Rasmussen (1972) have proposed treatment with periodate before chromatography to distinguish between these two metabolites since 25,26-$(OH)_2 D_3$ is periodate sensitive while 1,25-$(OH)_2 D_3$ is not.

F. THE USE OF NMR FOR IDENTIFYING VITAMIN D METABOLITES

The nuclear magnetic resonance (nmr) spectra of the peak IV metabolites generated from both vitamin D_2 and vitamin D_3 were extremely useful in deducing that the additional hydroxyl function was on carbon 25. The location of the hydroxyl group at carbon 25 for the vitamin D_3 metabolite was verified by 100 Hz nmr spectrum of the metabolite (Fig. 25), which exhibited a strong singlet at δ = 1.20 ppm as in 25-hydroxy-cholesterol, and an absence of the doublet at δ = 0.87 ppm (J = 6.5 Hz), due to the secondary C-26,C-27 methyl groups as found in vitamin D_3 (Blunt et al., 1968). The nmr spectrum of the peak IV metabolite generated from vitamin D_2 showed an intense singlet δ = 1.24 ppm, representing the two methyl groups at C-25 and two doublets at 0.79 ppm (J = 6.5 Hz) and 0.81 ppm (J = 7.0 Hz), represented the two remaining methyl constituents of the side chain, namely C-21 and C-28. When compared to the nmr spectrum of vitamin D_2, which had two doublets at 0.87 ppm (J = 7.0 Hz) and 0.98 ppm (J = 6.0 Hz), it was clear that the elimination of these two doublets which correspond to the two methyl groups can only be explained by a hydroxyl constituent on C-25.

Vitamin D compounds and hence metabolites have peaks at δ = 4.81 and 5.03 ppm characteristic of the C_{19} methylene group which allows clear identification of this grouping in metabolites. Of additional importance are the doublets at δ = 6.02 ppm (J = 11.5 Hz) and δ = 6.24 ppm (J = 10.5 Hz) due to the protons on C-6 and C-7. These can also be used in structural identification (Blunt et al., 1969). The use of nmr for structural identification of vitamin D metabolites is limited, however. Metabolites more polar than 25-OH-D_3, which have been

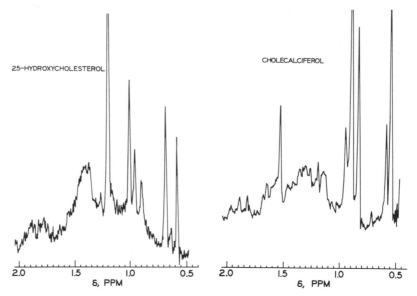

25-HYDROXYCHOLESTEROL

CHOLECALCIFEROL

Fig. 25. Nuclear magnetic resonance spectra (at 100 Hz) of cholecalciferol and 25-hydroxycholecalciferol. (Reproduced with the kind permission of the publisher, Blunt *et al.*, 1968.)

isolated are in such small amounts that nmr is not a practical procedure for structural identification.

VII. DISCUSSION

The new developments in our understanding of the functional metabolism of vitamin D and its regulation have opened a variety of new approaches to old problems of bone disease on one hand and more theoretical problems of structure-function relationship with regard to vitamin D on the other. The realization that $1\alpha,25\text{-}(OH)_2D_3$ is at least one of the metabolically active forms of the vitamin strongly indicates that the question of what portions of the vitamin D molecule are essential to activity must be re-examined using 1-hydroxy and 25-hydroxy analogs. In addition, it is evident that the vitamin has more than one target of action, i.e. intestinal calcium absorption, mobilization of calcium from bone, possibly calcification of bone and renal tubular reabsorption of ions. Analogs must be tested for activity in all these systems before a complete understanding of the structure-function relationship can be achieved.

The fact that vitamin D must be metabolized to active form(s) before it can function opens new and exciting avenues in the management of a number of metabolic bone diseases. Because 25-OH-D_3 is made in liver, there may be an obvious relationship between a defect in the vitamin D 25 hydroxylase system and bone disease related to hepatic difficulties. Of even greater significance is the fact that 25-OH-D_3 must be converted in kidney to $1\alpha,25$-$(OH)_2D_3$ before it can function to stimulate intestinal calcium absorption or bone calcium mobilization. Perhaps the osteodystrophy found in patients suffering from chronic renal disease can be attributed to a failure to produce $1,25$-$(OH)_2D_3$. Because the synthesis of $1,25$-$(OH)_2D_3$ is regulated by parathyroid hormone and inorganic phosphorus levels suggests that hypoparathyroid patients and patients suffering from vitamin D resistant rickets would greatly benefit from administration of $1,25$-$(OH)_2D_3$ or an analog.

The inroads made in our understanding of vitamin D metabolism have produced a new profile for the calcium homeostatic mechanisms and the regulation of intestinal calcium absorption. The breakthroughs achieved in these investigations will likely carry through to an understanding of the molecular mechanism of intestinal calcium transport in the near future.

Finally, the methods and approaches used in the elucidation of the vitamin D pathways may be applied to other physiologically active compounds. These possibilities will undoubtedly be closely scrutinized in the near future.

ACKNOWLEDGEMENT

Some of the original work described in this review was possible by a grant from the U.S.P.H.S. No. AM-15512 and the Harry Steenbock Research Fund of the Wisconsin Alumni Research Foundation.

REFERENCES

Askew, F. A., Bourdillon, R. B., Bruce, H. M., Jenkins, R. G. C. and Webster, T. A. (1931). *Proc. Roy. Soc.* **B107**, 76-90.

Bauer, G. C. H., Carlsson, A. and Lindquist, B. (1955). *Kungl. Fysiograf. Sallskapets I Lund. Forhandlingar* **25**, 3-18.

Bhattacharyya, M. H. and DeLuca, H. F. (1973). *J. Biol. Chem.* **248**, 2969-2973.

Blunt, J. W. and DeLuca, H. F. (1969). *Biochemistry* **8**, 671-675.

Blunt, J. W., DeLuca, H. F. and Schnoes, H. K. (1968). *Biochemistry* **7**, 3317-3322.

Bolton, I. J., Harrison, R. G. and Lythgoe, B. (1970). *Chem. Comm.* 1512-1513.

Boucher, R. V. (1944). *J. Nutr.* **27**, 403-413.

Boyle, I. T., Gray, R. W. and DeLuca, H. F. (1971) *Proc. Nat. Acad. Sci. USA* **68**, 2131-2134.

Boyle, I. T., Miravet, L., Gray, R. W., Holick, M. F. and DeLuca, H. F. (1972a). *Endocrinology* **90**, 605-608.

Boyle, I. T., Gray, R. W., Omdahl, J. L. and DeLuca, H. F. (1972b). *In* 'Endocrinology 1971' (S. Taylor, ed.), pp. 468-476. Wm. Heinemann Medical Books Ltd., London.

Bruck, P. R., Clark, R. D., Davidson, R. S., Gunther, W. H. H., Littlewood, P. S. and Lithgoe, B. (1967). *J. Chem. Soc.* 2529-2533.

Callow, R. K., Kodicek, E. and Thomson, G. A. (1966). *Proc. Roy. Soc.* **B164**, 1-20.

Campbell, J. A., Squires, D. M. and Babcock, J. C. (1969). *Steroids* **13**, 567-577.

Carlsson, A. (1952). *Acta Physiol. Scand.* **26**, 212-220.

Chen. P. S., Jr. and Bosmann, H. B. (1964). *J. Nutr.* **83**, 133-139.

Cousins, R. J., DeLuca, H. F., Suda, T., Chen, T. and Tanaka, Y. (1970a). *Biochemistry* **9**, 1453-1459.

Cousins, R. J., DeLuca, H. F. and Gray, R. W. (1970b). *Biochemistry* **9**, 3649-3652.

Dawson, T. M., Dixon, J., Lythgoe, B. and Siddigoi, I. A. (1970). *Chem. Comm.* 992-993.

DeLuca, H. F. (1967). *Vitamins and Hormones* **25**, 315-367.

DeLuca, H. F. (1972). *In* 'Calcium, Parathyroid Hormone and the Calcitonins' (R. V. Talmage and P. L. Munson, eds.), pp. 221-235. Excerpta Medica, Amsterdam.

DeLuca, H. F. and Suttie, J. W. (1970). 'The Fat-Soluble Vitamins'. University of Wisconsin Press, Madison.

DeLuca, H. F., Weller, M., Blunt, J. W. and Neville, P. F. (1968). *Arch. Biochem. Biophys.* **124**, 122-128.

DeLuca, H. F., Zile, M. H. and Neville, P. F. (1969). *In* 'Lipid Chromatographic Analysis' (G. V. Marinetti, ed.) Vol. 2, pp. 345-457. Marcel Dekker Inc., New York.

Dimroth, K. and Poland, J. (1939). *Berdt Ver Volkshyg Uber die Ultraviolettbestrahlung* **72**, 187-190.

Drescher, D., DeLuca, H. F. and Imrie, M. H. (1969). *Arch. Biochem. Biophys.* **130**, 657-661.

Fairbanks, B. W. and Mitchell, H. H. (1936). *J. Nutr.* **11**, 551-572.

Fraser, D. R. and Kodicek, E. (1970). *Nature, Lond.* **228**, 764-766.

Frolik, C. A. and DeLuca, H. F. (1971). *Arch. Biochem. Biophys.* **147**, 143-147.

Frolik, C. A. and DeLuca, H. F. (1972). *J. Clin. Invest.* **51**, 2900-2906.

Galante, L., MacAuley, S. J., Colston, K. W. and MacIntyre, I. (1972a). *Lancet* i, 985-988.

Galante, L., Colston, K. W., MacAuley, S. J. and MacIntyre, I. (1972b). *Nature, Lond.* **238**, 271-273.

Garabedian, M., Holick, M. F., DeLuca, H. F. and Boyle, I. T. (1972). *Proc. Nat. Acad. Sci. USA* **69**, 1673-1676.

Grab, W. (1936). *Hoppe-Seyler's Z. Physiol. Chem.* **243**, 63-89.

Gray, R., Boyle, I. and DeLuca, H. F. (1971). *Science, N.Y.* **172**, 1232-1234.

Halkes, S. J. and van Vliet, N. P. (1969). *Recl. Trav. Chim. Pays-Bas.* **88**, 1080-1083.

Hallick, R. B. and DeLuca, H. F. (1971). *J. Biol. Chem.* **246**, 5733-5738.

Hallick, R. B. and DeLuca, H. F. (1972). *J. Biol. Chem.* **247**, 91-97.

Harrison, H. E. and Harrison, H. C. (1972). *J. Clin. Invest.* **51**, 1919-1922.

Harrison, H. E., Harrison, H. C. and Lifschitz, F. (1968). *In* 'Parathyroid Hormone and Thyrocalcitonin (Calcitonin)' (R. V. Talmage and L. F. Belanger, eds.), pp. 455-460. Excerpta Medica, Amsterdam.

Harrison, R. G. and Lythgoe, B. (1970). *Chem. Comm.* 1513-1514.
Haslewood, G. A. D. (1939). *Biochem. J.* 33, 454-456.
Haussler, M. R. and Rasmussen, H. (1972). *J. Biol. Chem.* 247, 2328-2335.
Haussler, M. R., Myrtle, J. F. and Norman, A. W. (1968). *J. Biol. Chem.* 243, 4055-4064.
Haussler, M. R., Boyce, D. W., Littledike, E. T. and Rasmussen, H. (1971). *Proc. Nat. Acad. Sci. USA* 68, 177-181.
Hess, A. F., Weinstock, M. and Helman, F. D. (1925). *J. Biol. Chem.* 63, 305-308.
Holick, M. F. and DeLuca, H. F. (1971). *J. Lipid Res.* 12, 460-465.
Holick, M. F., Schnoes, H. K. and DeLuca, H. F. (1971a). *Proc. Nat. Acad. Sci. USA* 68, 803-804.
Holick, M. F., Schnoes, H. K., DeLuca, H. F., Suda, T. and Cousins, R. J. (1971b). *Biochemistry* 10, 2799-2804.
Holick, M. F., Garabedian, M. and DeLuca, H. F. (1972a). *Science, N.Y.* 176, 1146-1147.
Holick, M. F., Garabedian, M. and DeLuca, H. F. (1972b). *Science, N.Y.* 176, 1247-1248.
Holick, M. F., Schones, H. K., DeLuca, H. F., Gray, R. W., Boyle, I. T. and Suda, T. (1972c). *Biochemistry* 11, 4251-4255.
Holick, M. F., Garabedian, M. and DeLuca, H. F. (1972d). *Biochemistry* 11, 2715-2719.
Holick, M. F., Semmler, E., Schnoes, H. K. and DeLuca, H. F. (1973a). *Science*, 180, 190-191.
Holick, M. F., DeLuca, H. F., Kasten, P. M. and Korycka, M. B. (1973b). *Science*, 180, 064-966.
Horsting, M. and DeLuca, H. F. (1969). *Biochem. Biophys. Res. Commun.* 36, 251-256.
Huldshinsky, K. (1919). *Deutsche Medizinische Wochenschrift* 45, 712-713.
Hunt, R. D., Garcia, F. G. and Hegsted, D. M. (1967). *Lab. Animal Care* 17, 222-234.
Imrie, M. H., Neville, P. F., Snellgrove, A. W. and DeLuca, H. F. (1967). *Arch. Biochem. Biophys.* 120, 525-532.
Inhoffen, H. H. (1960). *Angervandte Chemie* 72, 875-926.
Inhoffen, H. H., Bruckner, K. and Grundel, R. (1954). *Ber.* 87, 1-12.
Kennedy, J. W., III and Talmage, R. V. (1972). *In* 'Calcium, Parathyroid Hormone and the Calcitonins' (R. V. Talmage and P. L. Munson, eds.), pp. 407-415. Excerpta Medica, Amsterdam.
Lawson, D. E. M., Wilson, P. W. and Kodicek, E. (1969a). *Biochem. J.* 115, 269-277.
Lawson, D. E. M., Wilson, P. W., Barker, D. C. and Kodicek, E. (1969b). *Biochem. J.* 115, 263-268.
Lawson, D. E. M., Fraser, D. R., Kodicek, E., Morris, H. R. and Williams, D. H. (1971). *Nature, Lond.* 230, 228-230.
Lund, J. and DeLuca, H. F. (1966). *J. Lipid Res.* 7, 739-744.
Lund, J. DeLuca, H. F. and Horsting, M. (1967). *Arch. Biochem. Biophys.* 120, 513-517.
McCollum, E. V., Simmonds, N., Becker, J. E. and Shipley, P. G. (1922). *J. Biol. Chem.* 53, 293-312.
McDonald, F. G. (1936). *J. Biol. Chem.* 144, lxv.
Mellanby, E. (1919a). *Lancet* 1, 407-412.

Mellanby, E. (1919b). *J. Physiol.* **52**, liii.
Murry, T. K., Day, T. C. and Kodicek, E. (1966). *Biochem. J.* **98**, 293-297.
Myrtle, J. F. and Norman, A. W. (1971). *Science, N.Y.* **171**, 79-82.
Nair, P. P. and de Leon, S. (1968). *Arch. Biochem. Biophys.* **128**, 663-672.
Neville, P. F. and DeLuca, H. F. (1966). *Biochemistry* **5**, 2201-2207.
Nicolaysen, R. and Eeg-Larsen, N. (1953). *Vitamins and Hormones* **11**, 29–60.
Nicolaysen, R., Eeg-Larson, N. and Malm, O. J. (1953). *Physiol. Rev.* **33**, 424-444.
Norman, A. W. (1968). *Biol. Rev.* **43**, 97-137.
Norman, A. W., Midgett, R. J., Myrtle, J. F. and Nowicki, H. G. (1971a). *Biochem. Biophys. Res. Commun.* **42**, 1082-1087.
Norman, A. W., Myrtle, J. F., Midgett, R. J. Nowicki, H. G., Williams, V. and Popjak, G. (1971b). *Science, N.Y.* **173**, 51-54.
Omdahl, J. L. and DeLuca, H. F. (1971). *Science, N.Y.* **174**, 949-951.
Omdahl, J. L. and DeLuca, H. F. (1972). *J. Biol. Chem.* **247**, 5520–5526.
Omdahl, J. L. and DeLuca, H. F. (1973). *Physiol. Rev.* **53**, 327-372.
Omdahl, J., Holick, M., Suda, T., Tanaka, Y. and DeLuca, H. F. (1971). *Biochemistry* **10**, 2935-2940.
Omdahl, J. L., Gray, R. W., Boyle, I. T., Knutson, J. and DeLuca, H F. (1972). *Nature (New Biology)* **237**, 63-64.
Pelc, B. and Kodicek, E. (1971). *J. Chem. Soc.* (C) 3415-3418.
Ponchon, G. and DeLuca, H. F. (1969a). *J. Nutr.* **99**, 157-167.
Ponchon, G. and DeLuca, H. F. (1969b). *J. Clin. Invest.* **48**, 1273-1279.
Ponchon, G., Kennan, A. L. and DeLuca, H. F. (1969). *J. Clin. Invest.* **48**, 2032-2037.
Rasmussen, H., Wong, M., Bikle, D. and Goodman, D. B. P. (1972). *J. Clin. Invest.* **51**, 2502-2504.
Roborgh, J. R. and DeMan, T. J. (1960). *Biochem. Pharmacol.* **3**, 277-282.
Rosenberg, H. R. (1942). 'Chemistry and Physiology of the Vitamins'. Interscience Publishers Inc., New York.
Rottensten, K. V. (1938). *Biochem. J.* **32**, 1285-1292.
Schenck, F. (1937). *Naturwissenschaften* **25**, 159.
Sebrell, W. H., Jr. and Harris, R. S. (1954). 'The Vitamins' Vol. II, 1st Ed., pp. 131-266. Academic Press, New York and London.
Sebrell, W. H., Jr. and Harris, R. S. (1971). 'The Vitamins' Vol. III (2nd Ed.), pp. 155-301, Academic Press, New York and London.
Semmler, E. J., Holick, M. F., Schnoes, H. K. and DeLuca, H. F. (1972). *Tetrahedron Lett.* **40**, 4147-4150.
Steenbock, H. and Black, A. (1924). *J. Biol. Chem.* **61**, 405-422.
Steenbock, H., Kletzien, S. W. F. and Halpin, J. G. (1932). *J. Biol. Chem.* **97**, 249-264.
Suda, T., DeLuca, H. F., Schnoes, H. and Blunt, J. W. (1969). *Biochem. Biophys. Res. Commun.* **35**, 182-185.
Suda, T., DeLuca, H. F. and Tanaka, Y. (1970a). *J. Nutr.* **100**, 1049-1052.
Suda, T., DeLuca, H. F., Schnoes, H. K., Ponchon, G., Tanaka, Y. and Holick, M. F. (1970b). *Biochemistry* **9**, 2917-2922.
Suda, T., DeLuca, H. F., Schnoes, H. K., Tanaka, Y. and Holick, M. F. (1970c). *Biochemistry* **9**, 4776-4780.
Suda, T., Hallick, R. B., DeLuca, H. F. and Schnoes, H. K. (1970d). *Biochemistry* **9**, 1651-1657.

Suda, T., DeLuca, H. F. and Hallick, R. B. (1971). *Anal. Biochem.* **43**, 139-146.

Talmage, R. V., Anderson, J. J. B. and Cooper, C. W. (1972). *Endocrinology* **90**, 1185-1191,

Tanaka, Y. and DeLuca, H. F. (1971). *Arch. Biochem. Biophys.* **146**, 574-578.

Tanaka, Y., DeLuca, H. F., Omdahl, J. and Holick, M. F. (1971). *Proc. Nat. Acad. Sci. USA* **68**, 1286-1288.

Tanaka, Y. and DeLuca, H. F. (1973). *Arch. Biochem. Biophys.* **156**, 566-574.

Trummel, C. L., Raisz, L. G., Hallick, R. B. and DeLuca, H. F. (1971). *Biochem. Biophys. Res. Commun.* **44**, 1096-1101.

Verloop, A., Koevoet, A. L. and Havinga, E. (1955). *Recl. Trav. Chim. Pays-Bas.* **74**, 1125-1130.

Verloop, A., Koevoet, A. L., VanMoorsellar, R. and Havinga, E. (1959). *Recl. Trav. Chim. Pays-Bas.* **78**, 1004-1015.

von Werder, F. (1939). *Hoppe-Seyler's Z. Physiol. Chem.* **260**, 119-134.

Waddell, J. (1934). *J. Biol. Chem.* **105**, 711-739.

Wasserman, R. H. (1963). *In* 'The Transfer of Calcium and Strontium Across Biological Membranes' (R. H. Wasserman, ed.), pp. 211-228. Academic Press, New York and London.

Wasserman, R. H. and Taylor, A. N. (1972). *Ann. Rev. Biochem.* **41**, 179-202.

Windaus, A., Linsert, O., Lüttringhaus, A. and Weidlich, G. (1932). *Ann.* **492**, 226-241.

Windaus, A., Lettre, H. and Schenck, F. (1935). *Ann.* **520**, 98-106.

Windaus, A., Schenck, F. and von Werder, F. (1936). *Hoppe-Seyler's Z. Physiol. Chem.* **241**, 100-103.

Windaus, A. and Trautman, G. (1937). *Hoppe-Seyler's Z. Physiol. Chem.* **247**, 185-188.

Ziffer, H., VandenHeuvel, W. J. A., Haahti, E. O. A. and Horning, E. C. (1960). *Chem. Comm.* **82**, 6411-6412.

EFFECTS OF CORTICOSTEROIDS ON CONNECTIVE TISSUE AND FIBROBLASTS

S. NACHT and P. GARZÓN

Vick Divisions Research and Development, One Bradford Road,
Mount Vernon, New York, U.S.A. and
Depto. Bioquimica, Facultad de Medicina, Universidad de Guadalajara,
Guadalajara, Jalisco, Mexico

I. INTRODUCTION

The connective tissue has long been recognized as an important 'target tissue' for hormones, both in normal and in pathologic conditions. As early as 1939, Zuckerman demonstrated that estrone injections in monkeys induced changes in the mucin and water content of their perigenital skin, while shortly thereafter Menkin (1940) reported that adrenal cortex extracts were able to inhibit the inflammatory response of rabbit skin to leukotaxine injections.

Years later, when pure corticosteroids became available, it was found that cortisone injections inhibited the spread of India ink in the skin of the mouse (Opsahl, 1949), and in 1953 Dixon and Bywaters demonstrated in human subjects that injections of cortisone acetate or hydrocortisone acetate into the inflamed joints of rheumatoid arthritics produced symptomatic relief and resulted in the appearance of synovial fluid of higher viscosity.

A vast amount of information has been accumulated since then on the influence of hormones on the connective tissue cells, and many studies have been published on the cellular metabolism of specific hormones, the steroids and sterols in particular (Dougherty and Berliner, 1968). Despite this knowledge, neither the mechanism by which hormones act as chemical messengers nor the manner in which the cells of the connective tissue interpret the message can yet be fully explained.

The purpose of this review is to illustrate the multitudinous effects that the corticosteroids can elicit on the different components of the connective tissue and to emphasize the usefulness of the fibroblast as an experimental target cell for the *in vitro* study of corticosteroid action, correlating the results obtained by this procedure with the effects induced by these compounds *in vivo*. Techniques currently employed in steroid research are described and selected aspects of steroid biochemistry are discussed.

II. THE CONNECTIVE TISSUE

The connective tissue is ubiquitously distributed in the organism and consists of a variety of cells and fibers embedded in an amorphous jelly-like matrix called ground substance, which fills the spaces between the cells, the fibers and the vasculature, and which contains the tissue fluid and diffusible metabolites. The combination of cells and their matrix is called mesenchyme (from the Greek Mesos, middle; enchyme, infusion), a term introduced by D. Hertwig in 1883 to designate tissue derived from cells of an early embryonic layer, the mesoderm.

Six types of cells account for the majority of the cellular population of the connective tissue: fat cells, mast cells, lymphocytes, eosinophils, a small number of phagocytic cells, and the fibroblast which is the most common one by far.

The fibers are entirely extracellular and composed of a particular protein called collagen.

The possible general functions of the connective tissue and its cells have been reviewed elsewhere (Hall, 1963; Wagner and Smith, 1967; Schubert and Hamerman, 1968), and they will not be discussed here.

A. MORPHOLOGY OF FIBROBLASTS

It is now convenient to describe briefly the normal morphology of fibroblasts to understand better the changes induced on these cells by the corticosteroids.

Fibroblasts are actively secreting cells found in the connective tissue of any portion of the body. Their characteristic feature is the stellate or spindle shape of their cytoplasm which contains an oval nucleus. Cinematographic studies have shown that fibroblasts can drastically change their cytoplasmic configuration depending on the substances present in the environment (Schneebeli *et al.*, 1968a,b). The cytoplasm may elongate into slender processes which extend between bundles of collagen fibrils (Porter, 1964). Studies of fibroblast cell structure evidenced a prominent Golgi apparatus and a very extensive and granular ergastoplasm, particularly in fibroblasts found in young connective tissue (Ross and Benditt, 1961; Rhodin, 1967).

B. COLLAGEN

The collagen fibers in connective tissue are one of the principal structural elements of the animal body; they are very flexible but they resist longitudinal stretching and possess great tensile strength (Berliner and Nabors, 1967). They also form the structures that separate or connect organs and, in general, hold the body together. This fibrous character is easily discernible in tendons, where the fibers display a parallel array, and in the corium of the skin where they are closely interwoven. For many years, collagen's fibrous nature and water insolubility discouraged protein chemists from its study, in spite of the increasing interest in rheumatic diseases and, consequently, in connective tissue chemistry.

But the discovery that a water-soluble collagen, called tropocollagen, could be separated from some rapidly growing tissues (Gross et al., 1955; Jackson and Fessler, 1955) and the development of electron microscopic techniques stimulated and helped to elucidate the nature of the collagenous fiber.

Collagen fibers vary in diameter depending on the tissue they originate from: in loose connective tissue fibers one micron in diameter can be observed, while they range from 10 to 50 microns in the skin and diameters of up to several hundred microns are noticed in tendons.

Finer fibrils arranged in parallel bundles can be distinguished with the electron microscope. They are uniform in diameter but of variable length, and they present a cross-striation pattern periodically repeated every 640 Å, corresponding to each tropocollagen unit junction. A tropocollagen unit has a molecular weight of about 300,000 and consists of a cable of three protofibril chains of the same length (Rhodin, 1967).

Three amino acids unusual in proteins can be found in collagen: 4-hydroxy-proline, δ-hydroxylysine, and small amounts of 3-hydroxyproline (Tristam and Smith, 1963). Glycine accounts for one third of the total amino acids while proline, hydroxyproline, and alanine make up another one third. This elevated proportion of glycine and alanine, amino acids that have the smallest side chains, allows close packing of the peptide chains while the steric limitations imposed by the pyrrolidine ring in proline and hydroxyproline must certainly influence the overall chain configuration.

If not formal periodicity, collagen has a discernible recurrence of certain sequences of amino acids. Glycine appears regularly every third residue in each polypeptide chain, frequently followed by proline or hydroxyproline. These sequences are found in the crystalline, non-polar regions of the molecule, visible as interbands in electron micrographs, and comprising 50-60% of the basic collagen molecule (Seifter *et al.*, 1964). Polar regions, on the other hand, are amorphous and rich in glutamic acid, aspartic acid, and lysine.

A soluble preparation called gelatin, containing varying amounts of smaller molecular species, is obtained by heat denaturation of collagen. Analysis of gelatin has shown that at least 21 of the 78 residues of glutamic acid, present per 1,000 amino acid residues, are in peptide linkage through their δ-carboxyl groups.

A unique feature of the collagen molecule is the occurrence of hexoses attached to a simple hydroxylysine residue in each peptide chain in an *o*-glycosidic linkage. Untreated tropocollagen presents another peculiarity, namely the presence of aldehydes yet uncharacterized, although there is evidence that they may be amino aldehydes corresponding to glycine, lysine, alanine and aspartic acid. α-Glutaryl peptide bonds are also usually present in the polypeptide backbone. Ester linkages between aspartic and glutamic residues and hydroxyl groups of unidentified residues have also been found in collagen; these bonds have been implicated in the formation of collagen strands.

Fibroblasts have been recognized as the source of collagen, both when its synthesis was studied *in vitro* in tissue cultures, as well as *in vivo* during the process of healing.

In a review on cellular differentiation and tissue culture techniques, Bloom (1937) discussed studies performed by several investigators on fibroblasts which led to the conclusion that these cells can make connective tissue fibers both *in vivo* and in *in vitro* cultures, a property shared by other cellular components of the connective tissue like reticular cells, smooth muscle cells, perivascular cells, osteoblasts and chondroblasts.

Jackson and Smith (1957) and Kuwabara (1959) demonstrated that connective tissue cells in tissue culture produce collagen; fiber formation was measured by the increase in hydroxyproline content and by the incorporation of added ^{14}C-proline into collagen as ^{14}C-hydroxyproline. Fibrogenic capacity has also been found in mouse fibroblasts of the LLC-M1 strain (Hull, 1953) and Merchant and Kahn (1958) published a very conclusive study on the synthesis of collagenous fibers by fibroblasts NCTC-929 grown as a suspension. Electron microscopic preparations of fibers accumulated in the medium evidenced the presence of fibrils with a periodicity of 640 Å and collagen was identified in these structures by enzymatic procedures. Furthermore, collagen antibodies were found to inhibit the formation of intracellular substance in cultured fibroblasts (Robbins *et al.*, 1955) and the presence of soluble collagen was later demonstrated in chick embryo fibroblasts by immunofluorescence techniques (Mancini *et al.*, 1965a,b).

Autoradiography and electron microscopy studies revealed that the endoplasmic reticulum produces collagen fiber precursors. When collagen biosynthesis, as measured by the conversion of proline into hydroxyproline, was expressed per unit number of cells, faster rate of formation was found in cultures at the proliferative stage than at the stationary growth phase (Prockop et al., 1962; Goldberg and Green, 1964; Porter, 1964; Davies and Priest, 1967; Davies et al., 1968; Gribble et al., 1969; Kretsinger et al., 1964).

But, in spite of the progress made in the understanding of the synthetic process and on the relationship between cellular growth stage and collagen synthesis, the mechanism of fibrilligenesis is still poorly understood (Kuwabara, 1959; Castor and Muirden, 1964). Cell synchronizing techniques have not yet been utilized for these purposes although the study of the biochemical events taking place in synchronized cultures could help to define at which stage of the cell cycle collagen synthesis takes place.

C. GROUND SUBSTANCE

The amorphous portion of the connective tissue called ground substance is not a substance in the chemical sense of the word, but a complex mixture of many components, and it has different composition in connective tissues from different parts of the body.

It is not only the matrix in which the collagen fibers and connective tissue cells are embedded, but also the medium from where the cells receive their nutrients, and into which they unload their waste products, thus acting as a connecting path between the bloodstream and the other cells of the body. In addition, the ground substance seems to be the main habitat of the polysaccharides characteristic of connective tissue.

Hyaluronic acid, chondroitin sulfate, dermatan sulfate, keratan sulfate, haparan sulfate and heparin have been identified in ground substance; these compounds are not present as free polysaccharides, but are bound to proteins by covalent bonds (Schubert and Hamerman, 1968).

Although some investigators claim that the mast cell is the main originator of ground substance components (Sylven, 1945; Asboe-Hansen and Iversen, 1951; Asboe-Hansen, 1954, 1967), the fibroblast is presently recognized as the cell responsible for the formation of ground substance (Gersh and Catchpole, 1949; Curran, 1953; Taylor and Saunders, 1957; Kennedy, 1960; Crane, 1962).

In 1932, Parker described for the first time the secretion by fibroblast-like cells of an acidic substance, later identified as hyaluronic acid, into the culture media. The same compound was also found in embryonic skeletal muscle.

Layton (1951a,b) was able to measure the incorporation of radio labeled sulfate into connective tissue both using an in vitro model and in vivo trials, and

Grossfeld *et al.* (1957) demonstrated that freshly explanted embryonic tissues could synthesize chondroitin sulfate.

Trace amounts of galactosamine were identified in mucopolysaccharides isolated from the culture media in which human dermal fibroblasts were grown (Castor *et al.*, 1962), but the main substance produced by fibroblasts strains in tissue culture is hyaluronic acid (Castor, 1959; Hamerman and Green, 1963; Shimizu *et al.*, 1965).

Normal skin fibroblasts produce 0.06 μg of mucopolysaccharides per tissue culture plate (100 mm diameter) containing ca. 12×10^6 cells. Skin fibroblasts isolated from patients with cystic fibrosis, Hurler syndrome and with Margau syndrome produce nine times more mucopolysaccharides than those from normal individuals (Matalon and Dorfman, 1966, 1968a,b). Normal fibroblasts produce hyaluronic acid of higher molecular weight than that secreted by fibroblasts isolated from patients with rheumatoid arthritis (Castor and Prince, 1964a,b). The evidence obtained indicates rapid incorporation of $^{35}SO_4$ and $4\text{-}^{14}C$-glucosamine into the Golgi organelle of fibroblasts, which then transfer the mucopolysaccharides to the intercellular matrix by emeyocytosis. It has also been demonstrated that during the first six days of wound repair, mucopolysaccharide synthesis is increased; thereafter, there is an increase in collagen content as well as in tensional resistance (Nabors and Berliner, 1969).

III. EXPERIMENTAL TECHNIQUES AND FINDINGS

Tissue slices and minces, organ cultures and primary organ explants grown in balanced culture media, as well as cell-free extracts, have been widely used to explore the effects of hormones on morphological, physiological and biochemical parameters. Intact animals and organ perfusion techniques have also been utilized for the same purposes, but since these procedures exceed the scope of this review, they will not be discussed.

In 1907, Harrison succeeded in maintaining for a short time nerve cells from the spinal cord of a frog in a drop of clotted lymph. Thus he may be credited as the founder of tissue culture methodology. Cell culture procedures were greatly improved by the development of appropriate glassware (Carrel, 1923) and more efficient culture media (Eagle, 1959). The availability of better techniques and micromethods stimulated the study of the responses of individual cell lines to hormones to the point that almost 15,000 articles on tissue culture research were published until 1950 (Murray and Kopech, 1953). Clear demonstration of the increasing interest in the use of cell culture techniques is the review by Dawson and Dryden (1967) on 'Tissue Culture and the Effects of Drugs' in which the authors were able to cite nearly 4,000 articles published only in the 17-year span from 1950 to 1967.

The widespread application of tissue culture techniques to the study of mechanisms of drug action has been facilitated by the development of sophisticated equipment and required the aid of computerized data processing systems to assist with the interpretation of results from complex investigations. Moore and Glick (1967) forecasted the development of cell culture studies from 1966 until the year 2000 predicting that tissue culture research will play a vital role in the future progress of medicine.

However, it should be noted that *in vivo* conditions cannot always be duplicated by cells grown *in vitro* since, due to the mechanical separation required by this technique, the cells in culture lose the tridimensional framework provided by the original tissue they derive from. Besides, when cells multiply *in vitro*, the growth-regulatory mechanisms which exist in the intact animal may not be operational.

The need for careful optimization of culture conditions to obtain adequate survival of the cells and good multiplication rates was demonstrated by Earle *et al.* in 1954. When these investigators inoculated a culture medium with an amount of a certain cell suspension equivalent to 100,000 to 500,000 nuclei, all the cells proliferated. An inoculum equivalent to 10,000 to 50,000 nuclei resulted in only 64% of the cells proliferating while when the inoculum was reduced to only 600 nuclei no proliferation was obtained, all the cells dying rapidly.

In spite of these limitations, an adequate *in vitro* system can often provide useful qualitative and quantitative data to correlate with information obtained from *in vivo* experiments (Schindler, 1969).

Dougherty and Schneebeli (1950) conducted pioneering studies on the anti-inflammatory properties of corticosteroids using an experimental inflammation model produced by antigen-antibody reaction. They evaluated the effects of a wide range of cortisone acetate dosages in this model by performing differential counts and by investigating morphological cell modifications in loose connective tissue stained by the May Grünwald-Giemsa technique. Inhibition of the inflammatory process was found to be proportional to the amounts of steroid administered within a certain range; very low cortisone dosages failed to induce inhibition while high ones seemed to have deleterious effects (Dougherty, 1951). Such biphasic effects on steroid action were later confirmed by different investigators and established the criteria for dose-response studies on other compounds.

The study of the biochemical modifications induced in different cells by steroids has been greatly facilitated by the use of cell-synchronizing techniques, time-lapse cinematography, radioactively labelled precursors and autoradiography (Doniach and Pelc, 1950), making feasible the evaluation of cell life span, morphological and biochemical changes and cellular localization of steroids.

The sequence of biological events which occur at different stages of the cell cycle has been the subject of extensive reviews (Baserga, 1965, 1968; Nachtwey and Cameron, 1968) and will be partially discussed later on.

A great deal of attention has been paid to the possible correlation between the *in vivo* anti-inflammatory properties of steroids and their capacity for inhibiting cell growth *in vitro*, but for such a comparison to be a valid one, the effects of steroids on cell fuction have to be studied both in the intact organism and in tissue culture, on the same type of cells. This problem was solved by the discovery of the biological role of fibroblasts in inflammatory processes and in wound repair, which led to the development of an *in vitro* biological assay to evaluate the relative anti-inflammatory properties of naturally occurring as well as synthetic steroids (Berliner and Ruhmann, 1967; Ruhmann and Berliner, 1967). A satisfactory correlation between the *in vitro* relative potency of corticosteroids and their clinical efficacy has been found (Jaffe *et al.*, 1963; Cline, 1967; Ruhmann and Berliner, 1967; Berliner and Nabors, 1968; Brotherton and Andrews, 1970; Brotherton, 1971a,b).

A. STEROID INHIBITION OF FIBROBLAST GROWTH

Steroids affect most mammalian cells in tissue culture and numerous investigators have demonstrated the growth-inhibitory properties of gluco-corticoids on fibroblasts from different sources (Holden and Adams, 1957; Grossfeld, 1958; Nowell, 1961; Grosser *et al.*, 1962).

Cortisol, at a concentration of 100 μg/ml, completely inhibited the growth of fibroblasts derived from chick embryo; only slight inhibition was found when 50 μg/ml were used, but restriction in growth could be demonstrated even at dosages as low as 0.3 μg/ml (Kaufman *et al.*, 1953). Grossfeld and Ragan (1954) confirmed this effect using chick heart fibroblasts but concentrations of cortisol between 200 and 500 μg/ml were required to inhibit these cells. This inhibition was reversible, disappearing when the steroid was removed from the culture medium.

Geiger *et al.* (1956) reported also reversible inhibition of growth on dog fibroblasts by cortisone at concentrations ranging from 10 to 100 μg/ml, an effect which is directly proportional to the concentration of steroid used (Wellington and Moon, 1961).

The time of exposure to the steroid is an important factor in the evaluation of cell growth-inhibitory properties; Cox and Macleod (1962), using L-cell and various human epithelial cell lines, found that the effect of prednisolone was maximal after 40 or more hours of incubation.

That inhibition of growth was not the only cellular effect of corticosteroids was demonstrated by Guillete and Bushbaum in 1955; these investigators found marked cytological changes in chick and mouse fibroblasts that had been exposed to concentrations of compound 'S' of Reichstein (17α-hydroxy-11-deoxycorticosterone) of 35 to 70 µg/ml. While testing several different steroids, Arpels *et al.* (1964) could not demonstrate acute toxicity, as evidenced by inhibition of cell growth, for all of them, but after 3 to 7 days of exposure some degree of cell damage was found in all cell lines and at all the steroid concentrations used.

In 1960, Perlman and co-workers showed that small amounts of progesterone, testosterone, and androstenedione had toxic effects on fibroblast growth. Later on, Perlman *et al.* (1962) studied the effects of fluorinated and non-fluorinated steroids as well as of different progesterone derivatives and concluded that the addition of a fluorine atom to the molecule increases its toxicity, an effect which is independent on the presence of other chemical substituents in the steroid structure.

Fibroblasts NCTC-929 were much more sensitive to fluorinated steroids than to the non-fluorinated parent compounds, while derivatives of progesterone proved to be more toxic than those from corticosteroids. These same authors also demonstrated that tissue cultures from various cell lines differ in their sensitivity to the growth-inhibitory effect of adrenal steroids.

Berliner observed that the same steroid can be metabolized in different ways by different types of cells and proposed (1964, 1965) that the sensitivity of a specific cell line to a certain steroid may depend on the toxicity of the metabolites produced rather than on that of the parent compound.

Biswas *et al.* (1964) trying to correlate chemical structure with biologic activity, tested ninety-nine steroids for growth inhibitory properties on cultured fibroblasts from chick heart embryos; thirty-six of these compounds exhibited toxicity which could not be related to their molecular structure, although the absolute stereochemical configurations were not taken into consideration, a factor that later on was demonstrated to influence steroid action.

Rozen and Chernin (1965) studied the effects of cortisol and cortisone on monolayer cultures of connective tissue, finding that these compounds exerted a dichotomic effect depending on the concentration utilized: they stimulated cell growth at low dosages while higher ones were inhibitory. Similar results were later reported by Rasche and Ulmer (1968) using prednisolone. The possible physiologic significance of this biphasic mode of action was investigated by Undritsov *et al.* (1965) using rat fibroblasts obtained from ribs and femurs; cells were allowed to grow for 48 hours in media containing cortisol acetate in concentrations from 0.03 to 0.3 µg/ml. The steroid was then removed by changing the media and the rate of cell growth was measured three to five days later. Stimulation of growth was found at low cortisol concentration (0.03 µg/ml), corresponding to those present in the tissue fluid under conditions of physiological rest or mild stress; but when the steroid content was increased to 0.3 µg/ml, comparable to situations of severe stress, cellular growth was inhibited.

When cortisone acetate was added at a 0.035 μg/ml concentration, it increased the growth rate of the culture by ca. 38%, while when 12 μg/ml were used, growth decreased by 40% as compared to controls. So, dualism of effects was obtained with both steroids, but while similar concentrations of cortisol and cortisone were able to stimulate cellular growth rate, thirty times higher concentration of 11-keto than of 11-hydroxy compounds were needed to elicit inhibition.

Evidence was thus accumulating on the importance of the chemical structure of the 11-position in the steroid molecule on the overall pharmacologic properties of the compound (Bush, 1956). Berliner and Dougherty (1961) investigated the biological activity of different 11β-hydroxy steroids, and later Berliner and Ruhmann (1966) compared these results with those obtained with 11-keto compounds. Inhibition of growth was studied on fibroblasts from strain L-929 in monolayer cultures, at steroid concentrations ranging from 0.1 to 10 μg/ml. Cortisol, methylcortisol, prednisolone and corticosterone inhibited fibroblast growth at the lowest dosage tested. 11-Deoxycortisol and 11-deoxycorticosterone exhibited some inhibitory activity when added at 1 μg/ml, and the reduction observed in cellular proliferation rates was intermediate between those obtained with 11β-hydroxy and 11-keto compounds. On the other hand, 11-dehydrocorticosterone failed to produce any effect even at concentrations of 10 μg/ml. The chemical structures of the compounds studied are presented in Fig. 1 for comparison. As an extension of the studies on the effects of steroid concentration and of specific functional group substitutions on the fibroblast growth inhibition potency of steroid hormones, Ruhmann and Berliner (1965, 1967) tested different cortisol and cortisone derivatives, as well as several halogenated synthetic steroids. These authors had already demonstrated that even relatively inactive steroids can inhibit cell proliferation at concentrations of 25 μg/ml or higher, but in the experiments designed to establish the correlation between the *in vitro* fibroblast assay and topical anti-inflammatory potency *in vivo,* the compounds were tested at 0.1 ng/ml to 1 μg/ml concentrations (10^{-9} to 10^{-6} M), well within physiological limits, and therefore fulfilling an essential requirement for the validity of a bioassay.

Table 1 presents the steroids studied with their structural formulas and compares the potency ratios obtained *in vitro* by the fibroblast assay with those measured *in vivo* by different techniques. In all cases, the activity of cortisol (the most potent naturally occurring compound) was adopted as unity.

Several relationships between chemical structure and fibroblast growth inhibitory activity became evident from these studies. Decrease in activity is associated with the lack of an α-OH group at the C-17 position, as is obvious from the comparison of corticosterone and cortisol, but the influence of the 11β-hydroxy group was proven to be overriding since cortisone, a steroid that only differs from cortisol in the C-11 position, is totally devoid of *in vitro* inhibitory properties, in spite of retaining the 17α-OH configuration. In fact, as will be discussed later, cortisone can even stimulate fibroblast growth *in vitro*.

This should not be regarded as an inconsistency between the fibroblast assay and the various other *in vivo* tests, since Berliner and Dougherty (1961) had previously indicated that cortisone, when administered parenterally, only has anti-inflammatory activity in those tissues where it can be converted to cortisol,

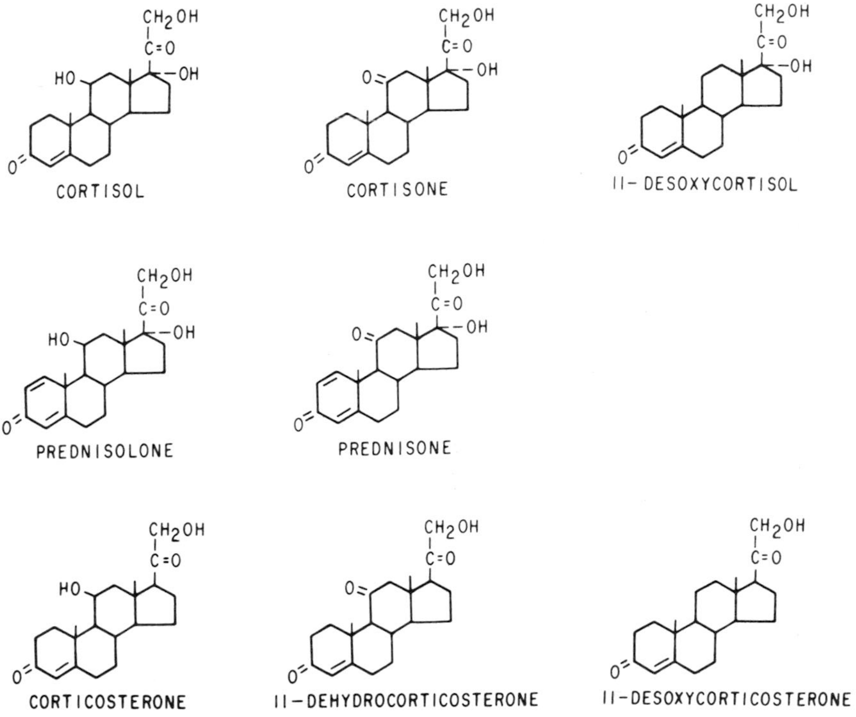

Fig. 1. Structure of some of the steroids studied for inhibitory properties of fibroblast growth.

being totally inactive when applied topically (Schlagel, 1965; Goldman *et al.*, 1952a,b). The activity of the 11β-OH dehydrogenase system (and hence, the biotransformation of cortisol and cortisone) is minimal in cultured fibroblasts, as demonstrated by Berliner and Ruhmann (1966), and consequently the fibroblast assay is a more objective test for steroid anti-inflammatory potency that those in which enzymic transformations may result in an apparent increase or decrease in biologic activity.

Introduction of an additional double bond between C-1 and C-2 results in the

Table 1. *Comparison of structural formulae and relative potencies of several steroids by different bioassays. (1) Tonelli et al. (1965); (2) Lerner et al. (1964a); (3) Lerner et al. (1964b); (4) Schlagel (1965); (5) Scher (1961); (6) Sawyer (1962). (From Ruhmann and Berliner, 1967.)*

STEROID	STRUCTURAL FORMULA	POTENCY RATIOS				
		FIBROBLAST ASSAY (Average of >2 Determinations)	TOPICAL ANTIPHLOGISTIC TEST (1)	ANTIGRANULOMA ACTIVITY (2,3)	THYMUS INVOLUTION ASSAY (1,2,3)	TOPICAL CLINICAL EVALUATION (4,5,6)
CORTISONE			0.58		0.62	
CORTICOSTERONE		0.48	0.33		0.17	
CORTISOL		1.0	1.0	1.0	1.0	1.0
PREDNISOLONE		1.7	3.4	2.7	4.0 4.1	2.0
DEXAMETHASONE		7.5	38.0	104.0	47.0 83	10.0
11-DESOXYFLURAN-DRENOLONE		7.8				
PARAMETHASONE		11.3		63.6	45.1	
Δ^1, 9,11-DICHLOROCORTISONE ACETATE		14.2				
TETRAHYDROTRIAMCINOLONE ACETONIDE		19.4				
Δ^1, 9,11-DICHLOROCORTISONE 16,17-ACETONIDE		43.7	23.2		<1	
TRIAMCINOLONE ACETONIDE		156.0		48.5	37.7	40.0
FLUOCINOLONE ACETONIDE		440.0		446.0	263.0	160.0

compound known as prednisolone and almost doubles the potency of the steroid, both *in vitro* as well as *in vivo*.

But the most striking increases in activity are obtained by the addition of halogens at C-6, C-9 or both positions. Thus, dexamethasone, paramethasone and dichlorisone are between 7 and 10 times more potent than cortisol. These activities could be increased even further by introduction of a 16, 17-acetonide group; some of these steroids are listed in the lower part of Table I, and as can be seen, resulted in compounds 100 to 500 times more potent than cortisol. Cortisol concentrations higher than 20 μg/ml are needed to demonstrate inhibition of fibroblast growth, but less than 0.2 μg/ml of fluocinolone acetonide was enough to induce a significant decrease in growth rate.

Using a system similar to this, Wieser and Taifour (1969) measured the relative potencies of prednisolone and betamethasone for inhibiting the proliferation of mouse L-cell cultures; they found that inhibition linearly increased with steroid concentration in the culture within the range studied (0.01 to 1,000 μg/ml), and that betamethasone was 10 times more potent than prednisolone, results that agree well with those described previously.

Brotherton (1971a,b) used the fibroblast assay to study a similar series of steroids derived from corticosterone. Her conclusions about the structural requirements for the molecule to have biologic activity were in complete agreement with those stated before; namely that the presence of an 11β-OH, a 3-keto and a 20-keto groups and a 4,5-double bond were essential while potency was increased by the introduction of an additional double bond at C-1 and 6α and/or a 9α-halogen.

Each corticosterone derivative tested was slightly less potent than its equivalent in the cortisol series, indicating that although the 17α-OH group is not an obligatory requirement for anti-inflammatory activity, it exerts some favourable influence (Brotherton and Andrews, 1970).

The presence of an ester group at C-21 or C-17 or the formation of an acetonide across the C-16 and C-17 atoms substantially increases the potency of topical steroids. This may be partially due to the protection of the C-21 hydroxyl group from enzymic removal, as suggested by Berliner (1967), but also to the more favourable lipid: water partition coefficient of the resulting compound, which facilitates the penetration of the steroid into the skin across the stratum corneum and into the cultured fibroblast, through its cellular membrane, since in both cases the main diffusional barrier is of lipophillic nature.

Results obtained for glucocorticoid activity by different *in vivo* techniques like the topical antiphlogistic test (Tonelli *et al.*, 1965) antigranuloma activity (Lerner *et al.*, 1964a,b), and thymus involution assay (Tonelli *et al.*, 1965; Scher, 1961; Sawyer, 1962) do not correlate as well as the *in vitro* fibroblast assay with topical anti-inflammatory activity in man.

It is also interesting to note that Rasche and Ulmer (1970) found that, while glucocorticoids inhibited growth when added to fibroblast cultures, mineralo-corticoids had no effect; when the same compounds were tested on epithelial cell cultures, the glucocorticoids were inhibitory only at high dosages and the mineralocorticoids enhanced growth at all the concentrations used. These findings support the specificity of the fibroblast assay for determining anti-inflammatory potency.

In conclusion, the inhibitory effect that certain corticosteroids possess on fibroblast growth can be related to their topical anti-inflammatory action *in vivo*, a property that has been used to develop a very useful and valid procedure for the *in vitro* evaluation of such pharmacologic properties.

B. STEROID ENHANCEMENT OF FIBROBLAST GROWTH

As it was mentioned above, when Berliner and Ruhmann (1966) studied the effect of several 11-keto steroids (cortisone, 2-methylcortisone, prednisone, and 11-dehydrocorticosterone) on fibroblast growth, they could not detect any inhibition even at concentrations as high as 10 μg/ml of medium. On the contrary, cells cultured in the presence of cortisone (1 μg/ml) evidenced higher growth rates than controls and this stimulation was still significant at 0.01 μg/ml steroid concentration (Fig. 2). An oxygen function at the C-11 position is necessary for the compound to have growth stimulating properties, since when 11-deoxy-cortisol was assayed, inhibition was found at all the concentrations studied.

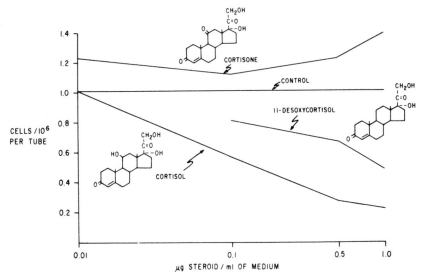

Fig. 2. Effect of cortisol, cortisone and 11-deoxycortisol on fibroblast growth. (From Ruhmann and Berliner, 1967.)

It is known that high doses of cortisone administered subcutaneously to mice can induce changes in fibroblast morphology and even fibroblastolysis (Dougherty, 1951), in spite of the total lack of anti inflammatory activity of this steroid when topically applied. This duality of effects suggests the possibility that 11-keto compounds may elicit biphasic responses of the type discussed earlier depending on the steroid dosages used.

C. INTRACELLULAR LOCALIZATION OF STEROID HORMONES

The availability of radiolabeled steroids and the introduction of auto-radiography techniques (Doniach and Pelc, 1950) encouraged investigators interested in hormone research to study the intracellular localization of specific steroids. Tritium labeled estrone and cortisol were detected in cytoplasm of renal tubular cells incubated with these steroids, incorporated into the microsomal fraction (Williams and Baba, 1967), and Litvack and Baserga (1964) reported that, when hepatocytes were exposed to ^{3}H-cortisol, 15 times more radioactivity accumulated in the nucleus than in the cytoplasm.

Garzón and Berliner (1970) attempted to correlate the intracellular localization of cortisol and fluocinolone acetonide with their different anti-inflammatory potencies and fibroblast growth inhibitory properties, by incubating cells for 48 hours in the presence of tritiated steroid and then studying the distribution of the label by autoradiography. The results demonstrated that while cortisol is preferentially retained in the cytoplasm as opposed to the nucleus, in a ratio of about 10:1, almost all the fluocinolone acetonide was located in the nucleus. Moreover, radioactivity tracks could also be found in the newly formed nucleus of cells in anaphase, but none were detected in the cytoplasm that separated the nuclei of the future daughter cells. Not all the cells incorporated the same amount of radioactivity, suggesting that those with less labeled material are either daughter cells or that there is a stage in the cell cycle which is specially receptive to steroids.

It is possible that the greater biologic activity of fluocinolone acetonide, as compared to that of cortisol, may be due to its preferential localization in the nucleus. Further studies on the intracellular distribution of other anti-inflammatory steroids could provide enough information to hypothesize biochemical mechanisms that would explain this steroid effect.

D. STEROID EFFECTS ON GROUND SUBSTANCE AND COLLAGEN SYNTHESIS

In 1951 Layton observed that cortisone inhibited $^{35}SO_4$ incorporation into connective tissue and concluded that this was a reflection of a decrease in chondroitin sulfate synthesis. Measurement of $^{35}SO_4$ uptake became then a very popular technique to evaluate the effects of corticosteroids on polysaccharide formation (Boström, 1953; Clark and Umbreit, 1954; Lash and Whitehouse, 1961) although this method is not free of possible pitfalls (Schubert and Hamerman, 1968).

But, working with cells in tissue culture, Castor (1962) and Castor and Prince (1964a) showed that cortisol depressed the total synthesis of mucopolysaccharides as well as the rate of synthesis per cell.

Several anti-inflammatory drugs, at concentrations at which they did not affect cell proliferation, were later found to inhibit glucosamine incorporation into acid mucopolysaccharides in fibroblast cultures (Kalbhen et al., 1967) as well as total mucopolysaccharide synthesis (Karzel and Domenjoz, 1969). Yaron and Castor (1969) demonstrated that the addition of either living or dead leukocytes to fibroblast cultures derived from human synovial tissue stimulates the production of hyaluronic acid and glucose uptake by the fibroblasts. This stimulatory effect can be prevented by the addition of 1 μg/ml hydrocortisone acetate to the medium (Yaron et al., 1970).

During inflammatory processes in vivo, overproduction of mucopolysaccharides by fibroblasts could be the result of leukocyte interaction, since both types of cells are in close vicinity, and the anti-inflammatory effects of corticosteroids may be related, at least in part, to their ability for preventing this stimulation.

Castor et al. (1971) reported that human synovial cell strains obtained from rheumatoid arthritis patients not only grow more slowly than normal cells, and produce hyaluronate polymers smaller than those from normal cultures, but they are relatively unresponsive to the suppressive effects of cortisol on hyaluronic acid synthesis.

Corticosteroids also affect the synthesis of collagen. Castor (1965) reported that cortisol induced changes in the ultrastructural characteristics of cultured fibroblasts, and in the concomitant synthesis of collagen, that resembled those associated with fibrogenesis in vivo during the anabolic phase of inflammatory reactions. Human connective tissue cells derived from synovial membrane and grown in monolayer cultures are capable of producing collagen for several months after removal from the donor, and the collagen formed has the same amino acid composition as that of collagen formed in vivo; when cortisol was added to the medium at a concentration of 1 μg/ml, a significant inhibition of collagen formation was observed (Castor and Muirden, 1964). In experiments performed with five different primary cell strains of human connective tissue for several months, these authors demonstrated that the steroid effects are persistent, not cumulative, and not subject to spontaneous reversal. However, removal of the steroid from the culture medium, even after prolonged exposure, resulted in a prompt reversal of hormone effects. Similar results had been previously reported by Gerarde and Jones (1953) using fibroblast cultures obtained from cortisone-treated embryos; prolonged inhibition of growth and collagen production was observed only when these cells were cultured in medium containing cortisone and not in the absence of steroid. Prednisolone and methyl-prednisolone produced essentially the same effects obtained with cortisol (Castor and Prince, 1964b) while observations made on cultured cells treated with 0.02% fluocinolone acetonide revealed the development of numerous cytoplasmic dense bodies, as well as a decrease in the formation of collagen (Panagiotis and Berliner, 1966).

Recent evidence has been published which suggests that corticosteroids may inhibit collagen biosynthesis by interfering with the formation of its polypeptide precursors (Uitto *et al.*, 1971).

E. STEROID EFFECTS ON THE CELL CYCLE

Three distinct stages have been identified in the normal cell cycle by studying the incorporation of radioactive precursors into cellular components: the post-mitotic or pre-duplicating state (G_1) which lasts from the late telophase until the beginning of the synthesis of DNA; the DNA synthetic or duplicating state (S), and the pre-mitotic or post-duplicating state (G_2) extending from the end of the 'S' stage to the early prophase, when the next mitosis takes place. Autoradiographic cytophotometry and time-lapse cinemicrography techniques have been utilized to evaluate the duration of each stage as well as the rates at which protein, DNA and RNA are synthesized (Stanners and Till, 1960; Killander and Zetterberg, 1965; Zetterberg and Killander, 1965a,b). It was found that G_1, S, and G_2 periods are eight, seven, and three hours long, respectively, while mitosis takes one hour for completion. That these are only mean times and not absolutely fixed ones at which certain events take place, it is obvious; otherwise, all the cells in a clone should always be at the same stage and undergo mitosis simultaneously. The duration of each stage in individual cells deviates slightly from the average values and, as a consequence, cells in any living organism or tissue culture are randomly distributed, at any given time, between the different possible cell stages. Under these conditions, it is difficult to ascribe a biochemical event or a pharmacologic effect to any specific stage of the cell cycle; instead, synchronously-growing cultures would reveal metabolic activities that take place in cell populations at the onset of cell division.

Such synchronized cultures can be obtained by treating the cells with metabolic inhibitors or by separating those cells which are in a certain phase of the cycle from the rest of the population. Among the variety of methods to induce cells into synchronism, the use of excess thymidine has been found convenient to inhibit DNA synthesis (Xeros, 1962). Thymidine possibly interferes with the reduction of cytidine to deoxycytidine (Reichard *et al.*, 1961; Morris and Fischer, 1963; Morris *et al.*, 1963), thus the cells are arrested either at the boundary between the G_1 and S periods or somewhere during the S stage

(Studzinsky and Lambert, 1969; Lambert and Studzinsky, 1969). Figure 3 illustrates the different stages of the cell cycle and the point of blockade with thymidine.

Addition of thymidine to fibroblast cultures results in the synchronization of almost 70% of the cells (Fig. 4) although this number decreases after the first filial generation (Garzón and Berliner, 1968; Schneebeli *et al.,* 1968a; Berliner and Garzón, 1969).

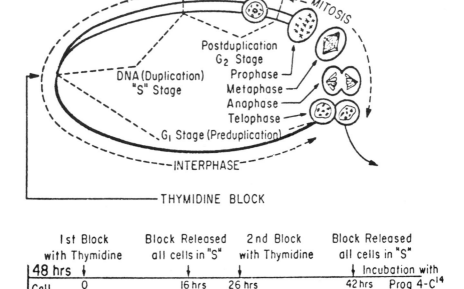

Fig. 3. Different stages on the cell cycle and point of blockade with thymidine utilized for cell synchronization. (From Berliner and Garzón, 1969.)

To study the effects of steroids on cell cycle, cortisol and fluocinolone acetonide were added at concentrations ranging from 0.01 μg/ml to 10 μg/ml of medium to replicate fibroblast cultures at the time of inoculation (Berliner and Ruhmann, 1966). The cells were grown on cover-slips in Leighton tubes and, for each dose of steroid used, trypan blue exclusion tests were performed for 120 hours to evaluate cell viability (McLimans *et al.,* 1957) and cell counts and mitotic indices were determined. In the control cultures more than 96% of the cells were found to remain viable throughout the experimental period and a generation time of 19.2 hours was consistently measured; this time increased to

26 hours when cortisol was added at a 0.01 µg/ml concentration and to 50 hours at a steroid concentration of 1.0 µg/ml. Cultures containing 0.01 µg/ml of fluocinolone acetonide exhibited a generation time of 31 hours.

Mitotic indices significantly below the control values were determined with both steroids and the addition to the medium of either one of them at concentrations between 1 and 10 µg/ml resulted in a profound increase in cell mortality.

Kollmorgen and Griffin (1969, 1970), Griffin and Ber (1969) and Yuan et al. (1967) also reported prolonged generation times when cells were exposed to steroids, while inhibition of mitosis has been found by Pearson and Eliel (1952);

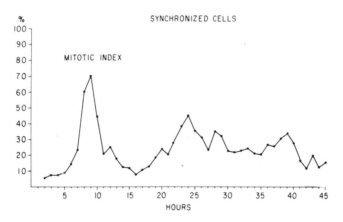

Fig. 4. Degree of cell synchrony induced by thymidine indicating the decrease in synchrony after the first generation time. (From Berliner and Garzón, 1969.)

Yuan et al. (1967); Bullough and Laurence (1968a,b,c) and Bullough et al. (1968).

The sustaining or preserving effects that physiologic concentrations of cortisol exert on diploid and heteroploid cells in monolayer cultures, as reported by several investigators (Dougherty and Schneebeli, 1955; Wheeler et al., 1961; Arpels et al., 1964; Omura et al., 1967; Schneebeli et al., 1968), can be partially ascribed to the ability of this steroid for lengthening cell life span while decreasing its rate of division.

Since short-term exposure of asynchronized or synchronic cell cultures to cortisol or fluocinolone acetate at concentrations of 0.1 µg/ml does not affect the synthesis of DNA nor the duration of the S period and, nevertheless, the mitotic index decreased, it follows then that either the G_1 or the G_2 or both stages have to be extended. Kollmorgen and Griffin (1969) measured the fraction of the total cell population that remains in the proliferative part of the cell cycle in cultures containing 1.7 μg/ml of cortisol. They found that fifteen hours after addition of the steroid 94% of the cells were in the proliferative pool, retained at the G_1 stage, as determined by continuous labeling with ^3H-thymidine, while the mitotic index had dropped to half of that in the control cells. These data indicate synchronization, at least partial, of the cells, but this was not verified removing the steroid from the media and allowing the cells to progress throughout the remaining phases of the cycle.

When unbalanced fibroblast growth is induced by adding thymidine (6 mMol), the cells usually reach mitosis about 9.5 hours after removal of the synchronizing agent (Fig. 4); if the cells are exposed to fluocinolone acetonide (0.1 μg/ml) immediately after synchronization, a delay in the occurrence of the

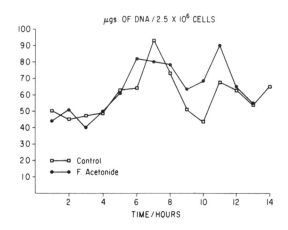

Fig. 5. Synthesis of DNA in synchronized fibroblasts with and without steroid added to the medium. (From Berliner and Garzón, 1969.)

mitotic peak is observed without a significant change in the amount of DNA synthesized (Fig. 5).

Since, as it has been discussed above, thymidine blocks the cells at the interphase between G_1 and S stages, and no effects can be detected on the latter one upon removal of the obstructing agent, the delay in the mitotic peak must be attributed to a prolongation of G_2 due to the presence of steroid (Garzón and Berliner, 1969). This conclusion received further support from data published by Kang et al. (1968), who found similar delay in the mean duration of the G_2 phase in cells treated for 12 hours with progesterone or testosterone (0.1 μg/ml); autoradiography studies performed on these cells led these authors to postulate that chromosome breakage may be induced by these steroids during the last part of the S stage.

F. EFFECTS OF STEROIDS ON NUCLEIC ACIDS AND ΓΠOTEIN SYNTHESIS

Cell systems do not remain inactive after division, but they synthesize macromolecules during interphase. RNA and protein synthesis take place during the G_1, G_2, and S stages, but DNA is synthesized only in the latter one; during mitosis, protein synthesis is reduced to a minimum and RNA is formed only at early prophase and late telophase (Baserga, 1965, 1968). The nuclear mass of the average cell in the population remains practically constant during the G_1 period but it doubles during the S and G_2 stages; the amount of cytoplasmic protein increases throughout the interphase but the rate of accumulation is slower during the S phase than at the G_1 one.

The study of the biochemical events occurring at specific stages of the cell cycle was facilitated by the introduction of cell synchronizing techniques. When unbalanced growth is induced by the addition of a synchronizing agent, a two to three-fold increase in cell volume, protein and RNA content occurs, but the cells return to normal following the removal of the inhibitor.

The addition of steroid hormones possessing growth-inhibitory properties to fibroblast cultures produces morphological changes (rounding up), decrease in pinocytotic activity and in collagen and ground substance production, and delay in the frequency of mitosis (Rasche and Ulmer, 1969). These effects can be attributed to severe alterations in the synthesis of macromolecules needed for cell division to take place.

When physiologic concentrations of the naturally occurring steroid cortisol or of the most potent synthetic steroid, fluocinolone acetonide, were added to either asynchronous or synchronous fibroblast cultures, no effect was observed either on ^{3}H-thymidine uptake or on total DNA cell content (Fig. 6) (Garzón and Berliner, 1968, 1969) but when steroid concentrations larger than 10 $\mu g/ml$ were used, the incorporation of ^{3}H-thymidine was depressed.

Studies were also performed in which synchronized cultures were pulse-labeled at different stages during the cell cycle; measurements of DNA content and of radioactivity per cell evidenced no effect of either cortisol or fluocinolone acetonide on the S phase, but these experiments could not be followed for more than one cell generation due to a decrease in cell viability (Garzón and Berliner, 1969). From these data it was concluded that cortisol does not interfere with the DNA biosynthetic pathway, but it simply reduces the number of cells capable of incorporating thymidine.

Results previously obtained by Pratt and Aronow (1966) with the same strain of fibroblast disagree with those just described. These authors found a decrease in RNA and DNA synthesis as early as six hours after adding physiologic amounts of glucocorticoids to the cultures, but no effect could be detected on protein synthesis during the first 24 hours of cell exposure to steroids. Kemper *et al.* (1969a,b), later analyzed DNA and RNA content in nuclei isolated from untreated fibroblasts and from cells exposed to steroids. No decrease in DNA synthesis with respect to that of RNA could be detected in the steroid-treated cells nor could inhibition of synthesis be induced by direct addition of high levels of glucocorticoids to nuclear suspensions derived from untreated cells.

On the other hand, Peck *et al.* (1967) reported that short-term *in vitro* exposure of cells to cortisol, inhibits collagen and, in general, protein synthesis and decreases RNA content within five hours, but no significant alterations could be detected on DNA metabolism.

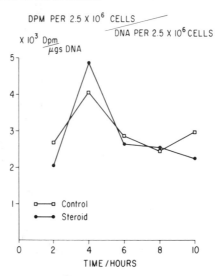

Fig. 6. Relationship between ^{3}H-Thymidine incorporation and DNA content in synchronized fibroblasts in the presence or absence of steroid. (From Berliner and Garzón, 1969.)

No obvious changes in fibroblast morphology or in DNA, RNA, and protein cell content were observed by Phihl and Ecker (1965) after exposure of the cultures to prednisolone, but Melnykovich *et al.* (1969) reported a slight increase in leucine content and a decrease in ^{3}H-thymidine incorporation into the trichloroacetic acid-insoluble fraction obtained from synchronized cells after treatment with 0.5 μg/ml of prednisolone.

G. STEROID HORMONES AND CELL ENZYMES

Whenever cells are exposed to steroids, two different types of enzymatic phenomena can be observed: some cellular enzymes may be repressed or activated and, on the other hand, the steroids themselves may undergo enzymatic transformation.

Induction of alkaline phosphatase by prednisolone was demonstrated using cultured epithelial cells (Cox and Macleod, 1961, 1962; Cox and Pontecorvo, 1961), maximum increase in activity occurring three days after steroid addition (Griffin and Cox, 1966a,b); this effect seems to be directly related to the modal chromosome number (Griffin and Cox, 1967). Waters and Summer (1969, 1970) reported that alkaline phosphatase activity in skin fibroblasts is induced without concomitant increase in protein synthesis or decrease in the rate of cell multiplication and occurs after the culture has reached confluency and maximal rate of protein and DNA synthesis.

When the effects of fluocinolone acetonide on acid phosphatase, sulfatase and phosphodiesterase were studied, both in synchronized and in asynchronic cells, acid phosphatase activity as measured by the hydrolysis of p-nitrophenyl phosphate seemed to be the most sensitive to steroid treatment, decreasing in both types of cultures even though the actual enzyme concentration per cell was augmented. Houck *et al.* (1968) found that when monolayer cultures of fibroblasts were exposed to cortisol, proteolytic and collagenolytic activities which the cells did not possess before, appeared as soon as 4 hours after addition of the steroid.

The use of steroid hormones as enzymatic substrate in growing cultures of human uterine fibroblasts (Swim and Parker, 1958; Sweat *et al.*, 1958; Berliner *et al.*, 1970), human skin fibroblasts (Garzón and Berliner, 1970), and mouse fibroblasts (Berliner *et al.*, 1958; Gallegos and Berliner, 1965; Berliner and Ruhmann, 1966; Garzón and Berliner, 1968, 1969, 1970; Berliner and Garzón 1969) evidenced that all the cells used had the capability of transforming enzymatically these hormones into metabolites which were less toxic to the cells or with lower biologic activity.

Table 2 summarizes the enzymatic synthesis or biotransformation of steroids known to occur in human uterine and skin fibroblasts and in the established strains of fibroblasts U-12-72 and L-929. Some of these reactions could only be detected when studied in synchronic cultures because they occur in such small proportion compared to the rest that, in asynchronous cells the amount of metabolite produced at any given time is below the detection limit; the C-21 hydroxylase, responsible for the biotransformation of progesterone into deoxy-corticosterone, is a typical example of an enzyme that was identified in fibroblasts using cell synchronizing techniques (Berliner and Garzón, 1969).

From the inspection of this table, it is evident that fibroblasts have enzymes which can hydroxylate steroids at the C-6 and C-21 positions, cleave side chains at C-17, hydrogenate $\Delta^{4,5}$-double bonds and convert a C-20 carbonyl group into a C-20 hydroxyl function; they also possess Δ^5-3-hydroxy dehydrogenase activity. All these enzymatic processes are present in fibroblasts from different origins but quantitative differences are found, e.g. the production of 20α-hydroxy-4-pregnen-3-one from progesterone is larger in mouse fibroblasts than in those from humans.

Table 2. *Formation and metabolism of steroids by fibroblasts.*

Precursors	Products
Acetate	Cholesterol
Pregnenolone	4-Pregnene-3,20-dione (Progesterone)
Dehydroepiandrosterone	4-Androstene-3,20-dione (Androstenedione)
Estrone	Estradiol
Estradiol	Estrone
Progesterone	21-hydroxy-4-pregnene-3,20-dione (DOC)
Progesterone	6β-hydroxy-4-pregnene-3,20-dione
Progesterone	20α-hydroxy-4-pregnen-3-one
Progesterone	20β-hydroxy-4-pregnen-3-one
Progesterone	5α-pregnane-3,20-dione
Progesterone	5β-pregnane-3,20-dione
Progesterone	20α-hydroxy-5α-pregnan-3-one

Furthermore, the rate at which a given steroid is metabolized by a serially subcultured fibroblast is a function of the anatomical site of the primary explant: skin cells derived from sex organs metabolize testosterone more actively than those originated from non-sex skin (Pinsky *et al.*, 1971; Mulay *et al.*, 1972) but this difference disappeared when cells obtained from patients with testicular feminization syndrome were studied (Pinsky *et al.*, 1971) indicating that the genetic deficiency responsible for the metabolic abnormality continues to express itself in the subcultured fibroblasts.

The biotransformations that progesterone undergoes when added to fibroblast cultures and their relationship with the life cycle of synchronized cells have received special attention (Garzón and Berliner, 1968, 1969, 1970). The results obtained evidenced that in synchronic cultures the same phenomena take place as in asynchronous cells; but, in the former, the biochemical expression of a specific enzyme system appears in an abrupt fashion, due to the majority of the cells reaching simultaneously the stage at which the enzyme is synthesized or triggered. Most enzymatic activities appear during the last part of the S phase and increase markedly during the G_2 stage; a typical example is the 20α-steroid dehydrogenase and $\Delta^{4,5}$-reductase which convert progesterone into both α and β isomers of 5-pregnane-3,20-dione.

In agreement with these findings, Halvorson *et al.* (1963), after studying the activities of various enzymes throughout the life cycle of a cell, concluded that enzyme biosynthesis is not a random or continuous process occurring during the whole interphase and mitotic periods, but that there is a particular stage for each

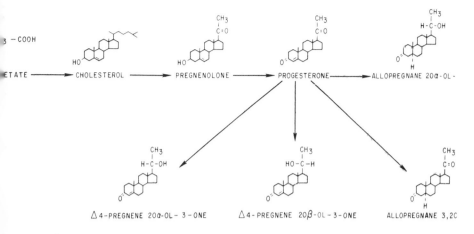

Fig. 7. Biotransformations of progesterone and pregnenolone by fibroblasts. Note: the transformation of cholesterol into pregnenolone has not yet been demonstrated.

enzyme at which its synthesis is induced, maintained at a constant rate or repressed.

The fibroblasts ability for transforming progesterone into less active products, evident particularly at the S and G_2 stages of cell cycle, is an indication of a self-controlling detoxication mechanism which operates by the induction of enzymes, probably adaptive ones.

IV. CONCLUSIONS

As has been indicated throughout the present review, corticosteroids have versatile effects on the cellular components of the connective tissue: they can inhibit cell growth or stimulate it; they can repress mucopolysaccharides and collagen synthesis; they probably affect DNA and RNA synthesis; they clearly modify the duration of cell cycle; they can induce or de-repress intracellular enzymes and, at the same time, they undergo biotransformations resulting in metabolites sometimes more, but usually less, biologically active than the parent compound.

Nevertheless, their pharmacologic activity as anti-inflammatory agents cannot as yet be ascribed with certainty to any given effect. Whether this action is a consequence of a stabilizing effect on cellular membranes or of an inhibition in water transport and on the release of acid hydrolases, is still highly speculative.

It also remains to be demonstrated if the effects that steroids have on fibroblasts, or at least some of them, are mediated by cyclic AMP, since adenyl cyclase has been recently identified in these cells and found to have similar properties to those described in other systems (Rao *et al.*, 1971). Furthermore, it is surprising to realize how little attention the intracellular distribution of corticosteroids has received.

This lack of conclusive information in some basic areas of steroid research is undoubtedly a reflection of the complexities of a biological system such as the connective tissue, constituted by a variety of cellular and extracellular components, some of them still not totally defined, but is also due to the unavailability of good experimental models representative of human disease states like rheumatoid arthritis.

In this respect, the fibroblast has proven to be so far the best available model for *in vitro* studies, since not only is it a natural target cell for steroid action, but it also renders itself able to be grown in tissue culture under defined and reproducible conditions, and human explants, both normal and pathologic, can be easily obtained.

In addition, determination of steroid potency by a technique which utilized fibroblast culture counts ('the fibroblast assay') has been demonstrated to be reproducible and to correlate well with the *in vivo* anti-inflammatory properties of the compound.

As was discussed above, there is presently evidence that serially subcultured fibroblasts derived from patients with genetic enzyme deficiencies retain the abnormality even after several cell generations. Full utilization of this approach should facilitate the understanding of such inborn disorders and may eventually lead to the development of appropriate treatments.

In conclusion, the main purpose of this review has been to summarize briefly the present state of various lines of research on the effects that corticosteroids may induce on the different components of the connective tissue, specially the fibroblast, and to emphasize some of the controversial points and possible aspects for further investigation.

REFERENCES

Arpels, C., Babcock, V. I. and Southern, C. M. (1964). *Proc. Soc. Exp. Biol. Med.* **115**, 102.

Asboe-Hansen, G. (ed.) (1954). *In* 'Connective Tissue in Health and Disease', p. 351. Munksgaard, Copenhagen.

Asboe-Hansen, G. (1967). *In* 'Connective Tissue', C.I.O.M.S. Symposium (R. E. Tunbridge, ed.), p. 30. Blackwell, Oxford.

Asboe-Hansen, G. and Iversen, K. (1951). *Acta Endocrinol.* **8**, 90.

Baserga, R. (1965). *Cancer Res.* **25**, 581.

Baserga, R. (1968). *Cell. Tissue Kinet.* **1**, 167.

Berliner, D. L. (1964). *Ann. N.Y. Acad. Sci.* **116**, 1078.

Berliner, D. L. (1965). *Cancer Res.* **25**, 1085.

Berliner, D. L. (1967). Symposium on Inflammation and Corticosteroids. Tokyo, p. 3.
Berliner, D. L., Bartley, M. H., Kenner, G. H. and Jee, W. S. S. (1970) *Br. J. Derm.* 82, Suppl. 6, 53.
Berliner, D. L. and Dougherty, T. F. (1961). *Pharmacol. Rev.* 13, 329.
Berliner, D. L. and Garzón, P. (1969). *Steroids* 14, 409.
Berliner, D. L., Grosser, B. I. and Dougherty, T. F. (1958). *Arch. Biochem. Biophys.* 77, 81.
Berliner, D. L. and Nabors, Jr., C. J. (1967). *J.R.E.S.* 4, 284.
Berliner, D. L. and Nabors, Jr., C. J. (1968). *Top Pharm. Sci.* 1, 99.
Berliner, D. L. and Ruhmann, A. G. (1966). *Endocrinology* 78, 373.
Berliner, D. L. and Ruhmann, A. G. (1967). *J. Invest. Dermat.* 49, 117.
Biswas, S., Macdougall, J. D. and Cook, R. P. (1964). *Brit. J. Exp. Path.* 45, 13.
Bloom, W. (1937). *Phys. Rev.* 17, 589.
Boström, H. (1953). *Arkiv. f. Kemi* 6, 43.
Brotherton, J. (1971a). *J. Endocrin.* 49, XV.
Brotherton, J. (1971b). *Cytobios.* 3, 225.
Brotherton, J. and Andrews, I. (1970). Personal communication.
Bullough, W. S., Homan, J. D. and Laurence, E. B. (1968). *J. Endocrin.* 41, 453.
Bullough, W. S. and Laurence, E. B. (1968a). *Europ. J. Cancer* 4, 587.
Bullough, W. S. and Laurence, E. B. (1968b). *Europ. J. Cancer* 4, 607.
Bullough, W. S. and Laurence, E. B. (1968c). *Nature, Lond.* 220, 134.
Bush, I. E. (1956). *Experientia*, 12, 325.
Carrel, A. (1923). *Expt. Med.* 38, 407.
Castor, C. W. (1959). *Arth. Rheum.* 2, 259.
Castor, C. W. (1962). *J. Lab. Clin. Med.* 60, 788.
Castor, C. W. (1965). *J. Lab. Clin. Med.* 65, 490.
Castor, C. W., Dorstewitz, E. L., Rowe, K. and Ritchie, J. C. (1971). *J. Lab. Clin. Med.* 77, 65.
Castor, C. W. and Muirden, K. D. (1964). *Lab. Invest.* 13, 560.
Castor, C. W., Prince, R. K. and Dorstewitz, E. L. (1962). *Lab. Invest.* 11, 703.
Castor, C. W. and Prince, R. K. (1964a). *Biochim. Biophys. Acta.* 83, 165.
Castor, C. W. and Prince, R. K. (1964b). *J. Lab. Clin. Med.* 64, 847.
Clark, I. and Umbreit, W. W. (1954). *Proc. Soc. Exp. Biol. Med.* 86, 558.
Cline, M. J. (1967). *Blood* 30, 176.
Cox, R. P. and Macleod, C. M. (1961). *Nature, Lond.* 190, 85.
Cox, R. P. and Macleod, C. M. (1962). *J. Gen. Physiol.* 45, 439.
Cox, R. P. and Pontecorvo, G. (1961). *Proc. Nat. Acad. Sci. U.S.A.* 47, 839.
Crane, W. A. J. (1962), *J. Pathol. Bacteriol.* 83, 183.
Curran, R. C. (1953). *J. Pathol. Bacteriol.* 66, 271.
Davies, L. M. and Priest, R. E. (1967). *Fed. Proc.* 26, 300.
Davies, L. M., Priest, J. H. and Priest, R. E. (1968). *Science N.Y.* 159, 91.
Dawson, M. and Dryden, W. F. (1967). *J. Pharm. Sci.* 56, 545.
Doniach, I. and Pelc, S. R. (1950). *Brit. J. Radiol.* 23, 184.
Dougherty, T. F. (1951). *Fed. Proc.* 10, 36.
Dougherty, T. F. and Berliner, D. L. (1968). *In* 'Treatise on Collagen'. (G. N. Ramachandran, ed.), p. 367. Academic Press, London and New York.
Dougherty, T. F. and Schneebeli, G. L. (1950). *Proc. Soc. Exp. Biol. Med.* 75, 854.
Dougherty, T. F. and Schneebeli, G. L. (1955). *Ann. N.Y. Acad. Sci.* 61, 328.

Eagle, H. (1959). *Science, N.Y.* **122**, 501.

Earle, W. R., Bryant, J. C. and Schilling, E. L. (1954). *Ann. N.Y. Acad. Sci.* **58**, 1000.

Gallegos, A. J. and Berliner, D. L. (1965). *J. R.E.S.* **14**, 8.

Garzón, P. and Berliner, D. L. (1968). Fifth Annual National Meeting of the R.E.S. Vol. 5(6).

Garzón, P. and Berliner, D. L. (1969). Fifty-first Meeting of the Endocrine Society, p. 78.

Garzón, P. and Berliner, D. L. (1970a). *J. Reticuloeudothel. Soc.* **7**, 397.

Garzón, P. and Berliner, D. L. (1970b). *In* Proc. 7th Pan-American Congress Endocrinol., Sao Paulo, Brazil, August 1970. 'Recent Advances in Endocrinology' (Excerpta Medica International Congress Series No. 238), p. 153.

Gerarde, H. W. and Jones, M. (1953). *J. Biol. Chem.* **201**, 553.

Geiger, R. S., Dingwall, J. A. and Andrus, W. D. (1956). *Am. J. Med. Sci.* **231**, 427.

Gersh, L. and Catchpole, H. R. (1949). *Am. J. Anat.* **85**, 457.

Goldberg, H. and Green, H. (1964). *J. Cell. Biol.* **22**, 227.

Goldman, L., Preston, R. and Rockwell, E. (1952a). *J. Invest. Derm.* **18**, 89.

Goldman, L., Thompson, R. G. and Trice, E. R. (1952b). *Arch. Dermat. Syphil.* **65**, 177.

Gribble, T. J., Comstock, J. P. and Udenfriend, S. (1969). *Arch. Biochem. Biophys.* **129**, 308.

Griffin, M. J. and Ber, R. (1969). *J. Cell, Biol.* **40**, 397.

Griffin, M. J. and Cox, R. P. (1966a). *J. Cell. Biol.* **29**, 1.

Griffin, M. J. and Cox, R. P. (1966b), *Proc. Nat. Acad. Sci. U.S.A.* **56**, 946.

Griffin, M. J. and Cox, R. P. (1967). *J. Cell Sci.* **2**, 545.

Gross, J., Highberger, J. H. and Schmitt, F. O. (1955). *Proc. Nat. Acad. Sci. U.S.A.* **41**, 1.

Grosser, B. I., Swat, M. L., Berliner, D. L. and Dougherty, T. F. (1962). *Arch. Biochem. Biophys.* **96**, 259.

Grossfeld, H. (1958). *Endocrinology* **65**, 777.

Grossfeld, H., Meyer, K., Godman, G. and Linker, A. (1957). *J. Biophys. Biochem. Cytol,* **3**, 391.

Grossfeld, H. and Ragan, C. (1954). *Proc. Soc. Exp. Biol. Med.* **86**, 63.

Guillete, R. and Bushbaum, R. (1955). *Proc. Soc. Exp. Biol. Med.* **89**, 146.

Hall, D. A. (1963). 'International Review of Connective Tissue Research'. Academic Press, New York and London.

Halvorson, H. O., Winderman, S. and Gorman, J. (1963). *Biochim. Biophys. Acta.* **67**, 42.

Hamerman, D. and Green, H. (1963). Tenth International Session of the American Rheumatologists Association, Boston.

Harrison, R. G. (1907). *Anat. Record* **1**, 116.

Holden, M. and Adams, L. B. (1957). *Proc. Soc. Exp. Biol. Med.* **95**, 364.

Houck, J. C., Sharma, V. K. and Patel, Y. M. (1968). *Biochem. Pharmacol.* **17**, 2081.

Hull, R. N. (1953). *Science, N.Y.* **117**, 223.

Jackson, D. S. and Fessler, J. H. (1955). *Nature, Lond.* **176**, 69.

Jackson, S. F. and Smith, R. H. (1957). *J. Biophysic. Biochem. Cytol.* **3**, 897.

Jaffe, J. J., Fisher, G. A. and Welch, A. D. (1963). *Biochem. Pharmacol.* **12**, 1081.

Kalbhen, D. A., Karzel, K. and Domenjoz, R. (1967). *Med. Pharmacol. Exper.* **16**, 185.

Kang, V. S., Kang, H. S. and Park, S. D. (1968). *Canad. J. Genet. Cytol.* **10**, 299.

Karzel, K. and Domenjoz, R. (1969). *Pharmacology* **2**, 302.

Karzel, K., Kalbhen, D. A. and Domenjoz, R. (1969). *Pharmacology* **2**, 295.

Kaufman, N., Masson, E. J. and Kinney, T. D. (1953). *Am. J. Pathol.* **29**, 761.

Kemper, B., Pratt, W. B. and Aronow, L. (1969a). *Molec. Pharmacol.* **5**, 507.

Kemper, B., Pratt, W. B. and Aronow, L. (1969b). *Proc. West. Pharmacol. Soc.* **12**, 69.

Kennedy, J. S. (1960). *J. Path. Bact.* **80**, 359.

Killander, D. and Zetterberg, A. (1965). *Exp. Cell Res.* **38**, 272.

Kollmorgen, G. M. and Griffin, M. J. (1969). *Cell Tissue Kinet.* **2**, 111.

Kollmorgen, G. M. and Griffin, M. J. (1970). *Ann. Okla. Acad. Sci.* **1970**, 66.

Kretsinger, R., Manner, G., Gould, B. and Rich, A. (1964). *Nature, Lond.* **202**, 438.

Kuwabara, H. (1959). *Japan J. Exp. Med.* **29**, 627.

Lambert, W. C. and Studzinsky, G. P. (1969). *J. Cell. Physiol.* **73**, 261.

Lash, J. W. and Whitehouse, M. W. (1961). *Lab. Invest.* **10**, 388.

Layton, L. L. (1951a). *Proc. Soc. Exp. Biol. Med.* **76**, 596.

Layton, L. L. (1951b). *Arch. Biochem. Biophys.* **32**, 224.

Lerner, L. J., Bianchi, A., Turkheiner, A. R., Singer, F. M. and Borman, A. (1964a). *Ann. N.Y. Acad. Sci.* **116**, 1071.

Lerner, L. J., Turkheiner, A. R., Bianchi, A., Singer, F. M. and Borman, A. (1964b). *Proc. Soc. Exp. Biol. Med.* **116**, 385.

Litvack, R. M. and Baserga, R. (1964). *Exp. Cell Res.* **33**, 540.

Mancini, R. E., Marquet, J., Paz, M. A. and Vilar, O. (1965a). *Proc. Soc. Exp. Biol. Med.* **119**, 656.

Mancini, R. E., Vilar, O., Davidson, O. W. and Berquet, J. (1965b). *Proc. Soc. Exp. Biol. Med.* **118**, 346.

Matalon, R. and Dorfman, A. (1966). *Proc. Nat. Acad. Sci. U.S.A.* **56**, 1310.

Matalon, R. and Dorfman, A. (1968a). *Biochem. Biophys. Res. Commun.* **32**, 150.

Matalon, R. and Dorfman, A. (1968b). *Biochem. Biophys. Res. Commun.* **33**, 954.

McLimans, W. F., Underwood, G. E., Slater, E. A., Davis, E. V. and Siem, R. A. (1957). *J. Immunol.* **78**, 104.

Melnykovich, G., Swayze, M. A. and Bishop, C. (1969). *Biochim. Biophys. Acta* **184**, 672.

Menkin, V. (1940). *Am. J. Physiol.* **129**, 691.

Merchant, D. J. and Kahn, R. H. (1958). *Proc. Soc. Exp. Biol. Med.* **97**, 359.

Moore, G. E. and Glick, J. L. (1967). *Surg. Clin. North. Amer.* **47**, 1315.

Morris, N. R. and Fischer, G. A. (1963). *Biochim. Biophys. Acta* **68**, 84.

Morris, N. R., Reichard, P. and Fischer, G. A. (1963). *Biochim. Biophys. Acta* **68**, 93.

Mulay, S., Finkelberg, R., Pinsky, L. and Solomon, S. (1972). *J. Clin. Endocr.* **34**, 133.

Murray, M. R. and Kopech, G. (1953). 'A Bibliography of the Research in Tissue Culture'. Academic Press, New York and London.

Nabors, C. J. Jr. and Berliner, D. L. (1969). *J. Invest. Dermat.* **52**, 465.

Nachtwey, D. S. and Cameron, I. L. (1968). *Methods in Cell Physiol.* **3**, 213.

Nowell, P. C. (1961). *Cancer, Res.* **21**, 1518.
Omura, E. F., Schwartz, M. S., Jahiel, R. I. and Kilbourne, E. D. (1967). *Proc. Soc. Exp. Biol. Med.* **125**, 447.
Opsahl, J. C. (1949). *Yale J. Biol. Med.* **22**, 115.
Panagiotis, N. M. and Berliner, D. L. (1966). *Anat. Record* **1954**, 391.
Pearson, O. H. and Eliel, L. P. (1952). *Proc. 2nd Nat. Cancer Conf.* **1952**, 1504.
Peck, W. A., Brandt, J. and Miller, I. (1967). *Proc. Nat. Acad. Sci. U.S.A.* **57**, 1599.
Perlman, D., Giuffre, N. A., Brindle, S. A. and Pan, S. C. (1962). *Proc. Soc. Exp. Biol. Med.* **111**, 623.
Perlman, D., Jackson, P. W., Giuffre, N. A. and Fried, J. (1960). *Canad. J. Biochem. Physiol.* **38**, 393.
Phihl, A. and Eker, P. (1965). *Biochem. Pharmacol.* **14**, 1065.
Pinsky, L., Mulay, S., Weksberg, R. and Solomon, S. (1971). *In vitro,* **6**, 393.
Porter, K. R. (1964). *Biophysic. J.* **4**, 167.
Pratt, W. B. and Aronow, L. (1966). *J. Biol. Chem.* **241**, 5244.
Prockop, D. J., Peterkofsky, B. and Udenfriend, S. (1962). *J. Biol. Chem.* **237**, 1581.
Rao, G. J. S., Del Monte, M. and Nadler, H. L. (1971). *Nature New Biol.* **232**, 253.
Rasche, B. and Ulmer, W. T. (1968). *Z. Zellforsch.* **84**, 506.
Rasche, B. and Ulmer, W. T. (1969). *Z. ges. exp. Med.* **149**, 316.
Rasche, B. and Ulmer, W. T. (1970). *Z. ges. exp. Med.* **152**, 42.
Reichard, P., Canellakis, Z. N. and Canellakis, E. S. (1961). *J. Biol. Chem.* **236**, 2514.
Rhodin, J. A. G. (1967). *In* 'The Connective Tissue'. International Academy of Pathological Monograph. (B. M. Wagner and D. E. Smith, eds), p. 1. Williams and Wilkins, Baltimore.
Robbins, G. P., Cooper, J. A. D. and Alt, H. L. (1955). *Endocrinology* **56**, 161.
Ross, R. and Benditt, E. P. (1961). *J. Biophys. Biochem. Cytol.* **11**, 677.
Rozen, V. B. and Chernin, L. S. (1965). *Fed. Proc. (Transl. Suppl.)* **24**, 861.
Ruhmann, A. G. and Berliner, D. L. (1965a). *Proc. Fed. Amer. Soc. Exp. Biol.* **24**, 575.
Ruhmann, A. G. and Berliner, D. L. (1965b). *Endocrinology* **76**, 916.
Ruhmann, A. G. and Berliner, D. L. (1967). *J. Invest. Derm.* **49**, 123.
Sawyer, W. C. (1962). *Ann. Allergy* **20**, 330.
Scher, R. K. (1961). *Curr. Ther. Res.* **3**, 361.
Schindler, R. (1969). *Ann. Rev. Pharmacol.* **9**, 393.
Schlagel, C. A. (1965). *J. Pharm. Sci.* **54**, 335.
Schneebeli, G. L., Garzón, P., Berliner, D. L. and Dougherty, T. F. (1968a). *Fifth Ann. Natl. Meet. R.E.S.* **5**, 557.
Schneebeli, G., Garzón, P., Gallegos, A. J. and Berliner, D. L. (1968b). *8a. Reunión Annual Soc. de Nut. y. Endoc.,* p. 45.
Schubert, M. and Hamerman, D. (1968). 'A Primer on Connective Tissue Biochemistry'. Lea and Febiger, Philadelphia.
Seifter, S., Franzblan, C., Harper, E. and Gallop, P. M. (1964). *In* 'Structure and Function of Connective Skeletal Tissue'. *Proc. Advan. Study Inst.* St. Andrews, organized under the auspices of NATO, p. 21. Butterworths, London.
Shimizu, Y., McCann, D. S. and Keech, M. K. (1965). *J. Lab. Clin. Med.* **65**, 286.

Stanners, C. P. and Till, J. E. (1960). *Biochim. Biophys. Acta* **37**, 406.
Studzinsky, G. P. and Lambert, W. C. (1969). *J. Cell. Physiol.* **73**, 109.
Sweat, M. L., Grosser, B. K., Berliner, D. L., Swim, H. E., Nabors, Jr., C. J. and Dougherty, T. F. (1958). *Biochim. Biophys. Acta* **28**, 591.
Swim, H. E. and Parker, R. F. (1958). *Arch. Biochem. Biophys.* **78**, 46.
Sylven, B. (1945). *Acta. Radiol. (Suppl.)* **59**, 1.
Taylor, H. E. and Saunders, A. M. (1957). *Am. J. Path.* **33**, 525.
Tonelli, G., Thibault, L. and Ringler, I. (1965). *Endocrinology* **77**, 625.
Tristam, G. R. and Smith, R. H. (1963). *Advan. Protein Chem.* **18**, 227.
Uitto, J., Teir, H., Peltokallio, P. and Mustakallio, K. K. (1971). *Acta Endocr. (Suppl.)* **155**, 146.
Undritsov, M. I., Rozen, V. B. and Chernin, L. S. (1956). *Fed. Proc.* **24**, 248.
Wagner, B. M. and Smith, D. E. (1967). 'The Connective Tissue'. International Academy Pathological Monograph. Williams and Wilkins, Baltimore.
Waters, M. D. and Summer, G. K. (1969). *Biochim. Biophys. Acta* **177**, 650.
Waters, M. D. and Summer, G. K. (1970). *Proc. Soc. Exp. Biol. Med.* **133**, 926.
Wellington, J. S. and Moon, H. D. (1961). *Proc. Soc. Exp. Biol. Med.* **107**, 556.
Wheeler, C. W., Vltarvic, E. J. and Canby, C. M. (1961). *J. Invest. Derm.* **36**, 89.
Wieser, O. and Taifour, A. H. (1969). *Experientia* **25**, 841.
Williams, M. A. and Baba, W. I. (1967). *J. Endocrin.* **39**, 543.
Xeros, N. (1962). *Nature, Lond.* **194**, 682.
Yaron, M. and Castor, C. W. (1969). *Arthr. Rheum.* **12**, 365.
Yaron, M., Yaron, I., Allalouf, D. and Joshua, H. (1970). *Israel J. Med. Sci.* **6**, 308.
Yuan, G. C., Chang, S., Little, J. B. and Cornil, G. S. (1967). *J. of Gerontol.* **22**, 174.
Zetterberg, A. and Killander, D. (1965a). *Exp. Cell. Res.* **39**, 22.
Zetterberg, A. and Killander, D. (1965b). *Exp. Cell. Res.* **40**. 1.
Zuckerman, S. (1939). *J. Endocrinol.* **1**, 147.

INTERACTIONS BETWEEN THE PROSTAGLANDINS AND STEROID HORMONES

JANE E. SHAW and STEPHEN A. TILLSON

ALZA Research, 950 Page Mill Road, Palo Alto, California, U.S.A.

I. INTRODUCTION

The prostaglandins constitute a large family of C_{20} unsaturated hydroxy carboxylic fatty acids, which no biologist can afford to ignore if concerned with mechanisms involved in the control of cellular function, or in interpreting the response of a tissue to varying stimuli. Many articles have appeared over the last decade in both the scientific and lay press, which have emphasized the multiplicity of actions which these compounds exhibit, and their potential use in clinical medicine. In consequence, most biologists are by now well acquainted with the ability of these compounds to modify reproductive, alimentary and vascular smooth muscle, platelet function, the inflammatory process, and formation of adenosine $3'5'$-monophosphate (cyclic AMP) in various tissues; for reviews of these areas the reader is referred to Bergström *et al.*, 1968; Ramwell and Shaw, 1970; Horton, 1969; Pharriss *et al.*, 1972 and the Proceedings of a recent meeting of the New York Academy of Sciences (*Ann. N.Y. Acad. Sci. 180, 1971*).

The widespread distribution of prostaglandins throughout the animal kingdom is a consequence of their ready formation from the ubiquitous C_{20} polyunsaturated fatty acids (Fig. 1); the latter possess both structural and functional properties, which implies that the event of their metabolism to form the prostaglandins—even if we ignore the pharmacological potency of the prostaglandins themselves—would lead to perturbations in biological systems. At present, however, the precise mechanism whereby mechanical, hormonal or neural stimulation of tissues leads to increased prostaglandin formation eludes clarification.

Attempts have been made to extrapolate results obtained with high concentrations of prostaglandins in pharmacological test systems to *in vivo* situations and thereby identify a biological role for the naturally occurring compounds; this has led to much speculation as to the importance of these

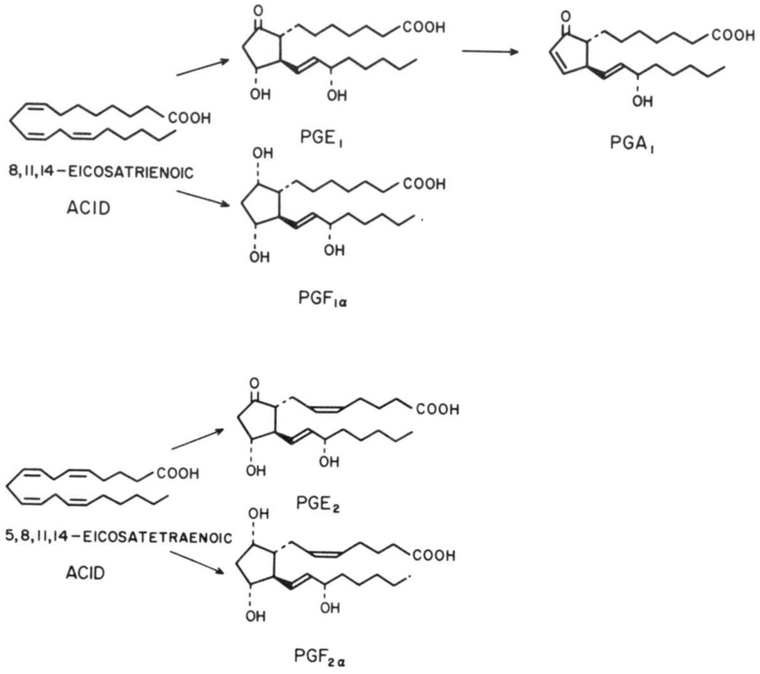

Fig. 1. Biosynthesis of PGE$_1$, PGF$_1\alpha$, and PGE$_2$ and PGF$_2\alpha$ from 8, 11, 14, licosatrienoic acid and 5, 8, 11, 14 licosatetranoic (arachidonic) acid.

compounds, and in certain instances confusion has arisen when results obtained *in vivo* have not agreed with *in vitro* investigations. Perhaps the classical example is the ovary, where *in vivo*, in certain species, the prostaglandins are luteolytic, while *in vitro* they are effective luteotrophic agents. Such differences have now been reconciled by implying more than one site of action for the prostaglandins in this tissue.

The prostaglandins exhibit such a number of actions that undesirable side effects, primarily stimulation of the gastrointestinal tract and modification of platelet aggregation and red cell deformability are likely to curtail their clinical

application following systemic administration. Furthermore, since the prostaglandins are rapidly removed from the circulation by lungs and liver, prolonged
administration is required to maintain an effect. Such rapid metabolism of
circulating prostaglandins would also tend to negate the probability that the
endogenous compounds are blood borne prior to manifestation of a physiological effect, and it is currently envisaged that prostaglandins produced within a
localized part of a cell can either modify different subcellular structures, or
adjacent cells within the same tissue (Änggard, 1971). However, the role which
endogenous prostaglandins play in modifying tissue function, still awaits
sensitive and specific methods of assay, for confusion is further compounded by
the multiplicity of compounds with qualitatively similar, but quantitatively
variable actions.

An impressive body of information is now available indicating that the
prostaglandins modify cyclic AMP formation in many tissues, and can thereby
increase or attenuate hormonal responses. This nucleotide is now accepted as the
intracellular mediator of the action of many polypeptides, including the trophic
hormones, which implies that by modifying tissue cyclic AMP levels, prostaglandins can potentially alter steroid formation at the cellular level.

While exploring the interactions between the steroids and prostaglandins in
this chapter, we will continually refer to the vasoactive properties of the
prostaglandins. In general, the compounds are hypotensive agents, though
prostaglandin $F_2\alpha$ ($PGF_2\alpha$) is vasoconstrictor in certain species (Bergström *et
al.*, 1968). It has been suggested that formation of endogenous prostaglandins in
a particular tissue may be responsible for the appearance of hyperemia
associated with tissue activation. Evidence for such a role for the prostaglandins
has been accrued in adipose tissue (Lewis and Matthews, 1969) and skeletal
muscle (Beck *et al.*, 1968), and has been suggested for the adrenal gland (Maier
and Staehelin, 1968; Grant, 1968). In addition, the prostaglandins can exert
certain physiological effects by redistributing blood flow within a gland, as
exemplified in the kidney (Lee *et al.*, 1971), an effect which could result from
the known differential action of the prostaglandins on vessels of varying
diameters (Strong and Bohr, 1968).

II. EFFECT OF PROSTAGLANDINS ON STEROID PRODUCTION

Pharmacologically active agents can modify the production of steroids by
affecting (i) the activity of the hypothalamus, and thereby the release of the
trophic hormone releasing factors, (ii) the cells of the anterior pituitary, either
by a direct effect on trophic hormone synthesis or release, or by modifying the
response of these cells to the action of the hypothalamic releasing factors, or (iii)
the function of the endocrine glands, the target tissues of the trophic hormones.

A. EFFECT OF PROSTAGLANDINS ON THE HYPOTHALAMUS

There is little evidence available describing specific effects of prostaglandins on release of trophic hormone releasing factors from the hypothalamus. There is, however, data available implicating prostaglandins in the normal functioning of central nervous tissue. Thus, prostaglandins which have been identified in extracts of central nervous tissue of different species can effectively modify the activity of individual neurones in the cerebrum and cerebellum following iontophoretic application. In addition, prostaglandins modify food intake and temperature regulation following direct injection into the hypothalamus (Scaramuzzi et al., 1971; Baile et al., 1968; Feldberg and Saxena, 1971). In view of the importance of the hypophyseal/pituitary portal vessels, and the pronounced effects of prostaglandins on both peripheral and cerebral vasculature (Yamamoto et al., 1972), it has been suggested that the functionality of these central vessels may well be modified by the prostaglandins (Flack et al., 1971).

Indirect evidence, indicating that prostaglandins can modify steroid output from the adrenal gland via an effect on the central nervous system arose from the work of Peng et al. (1972); using the intact rat, they demonstrated that prostaglandin E_1 (PGE_1) (0.125-4 μg i.v.) increased plasma corticosterone and depleted adrenal ascorbic acid and cholesterol. That these effects were mediated via adrenocorticotrophic hormone (ACTH) release was deduced from the finding that hypophysectomy abolished this effect of PGE_1. However, the use of morphine and pentobarbitone (which depress higher centers in the brain, but not trophic hormone release) indicated that PGE_1 was unlikely to affect the anterior pituitary directly, but was possibly stimulating ACTH release by an effect on higher centers in the brain.

B. EFFECT OF PROSTAGLANDINS ON THE ANTERIOR PITUITARY

There is now data available which describes the effects of prostaglandins on the content and release of trophic hormones from the pituitary both *in vivo* and *in vitro*. The initial observations of Zor et al. (1969, 1970) studying rat anterior pituitaries incubated in Krebs–Ringer bicarbonate indicated that several of the prostaglandins would increase adenyl cyclase activity and cyclic AMP accumulation in this preparation, but they could not detect any change in the release of luteotrophic hormone (LH). This result was substantiated *in vivo* by Pharriss et al. (1968) who found that $PGF_2\alpha$, administered to rats under conditions which curtailed ovarian luteal function, did not affect the LH content of the pituitary. However, Labhsetwar (1970) has reported that the pituitary content of LH was significantly ($P < 0.05$) higher in rats treated with racemic $PGF_2\alpha$ (0.5 or 1 mg b.i.d.) when compared with 8 day pregnant control rats; furthermore, the pituitary LH content of $PGF_2\alpha$-treated rats was higher than that of pseudo-pregnant, cycling or ovariectomized animals. The discrepancy between these studies should be resolved by further experiments directed towards measurement of changes in circulating LH following administration of prostaglandins.

In the previous section (IIA) we described the stimulatory effect of PGE_1 on ACTH release *in vivo*, as possibly mediated via an effect of the prostaglandins on the hypothalamus or higher centers of the C.N.S. However, Vale *et al.* (1971) using rat hemi-pituitaries incubated *in vitro* have demonstrated that PGF_1 (2.8 x 10^{-6} M), but not $PGF_2\alpha$, will modify the activity of the pituitary directly and stimulate release of both ACTH and TSH. In this effect, PGE_1 produces a similar response to that seen following depolarization of the cells by increasing the potassium content of the media to 30 mM. Further direct effects of prostaglandins on synthesis and release of anterior pituitary hormones have been described with respect to growth hormone (McLeod and Lehymeyer, 1972; Hertelendy *et al.*, 1971; Ito *et al.*, 1971), but to date there is no reported study concerning the effect of prostaglandins on follicle stimulating hormone (FSH) release either *in vitro* or *in vivo*. With respect to other anterior pituitary hormones, Gutknecht's findings that $PGF_2\alpha$ administration did not suppress lactation in the rat (Gutknecht *et al.*, 1969) indicated that this prostaglandin was unlikely to inhibit release of prolactin, while McLeod *et al.* (1971) could detect no effect of prostaglandin on release of prolactin from rat anterior pituitaries incubated *in vitro*. *In vivo* serum prolactin was increased following administration of $PGF_2\alpha$ 0.3 mg i.p. b.i.d. on day 18 of pregnancy in the rat, but this effect was considered secondary to a luteolytic effect which resulted in decreased plasma progesterone levels (Deis and Vermouth, 1972). Thus, the data available would indicate that administration of prostaglandins *in vivo* may well modify the activity of certain cells of the anterior pituitary.

With the recent availability of inhibitors of both prostaglandin synthesis and action, attention has also been focused on the function of the prostaglandins which are endogenous to the pituitary gland. Recent interest has been aroused in the non-steroidal group of anti-inflammatory compounds, including aspirin and indomethacin for they have been shown to inhibit the biosynthesis of prostaglandins from their essential fatty acid precursors (Vane, 1971). Use of these compounds *in vivo* therefore permits one to study the effect of depletion of endogenous prostaglandins on tissue function. Thus, Orczyk and Behrman (1972) have demonstrated that indomethacin (9.5 mg/kg b.i.d. for 56 hr), after a primary dose of pregnant mares' serum (PMS) decreased the PGF content of the pituitary glands of rats some 3-fold, when compared with PMS treated rats, and 6-fold when compared with control animals; the prostaglandin content of the hypothalamus was also depressed. These effects of indomethacin were associated with inhibition of ovulation, which was partially reversed by administration of LH, but not by prostaglandin. From these results the inference was drawn, that the endogenous prostaglandins of the hypothalamus or pituitary may be involved in the release of LH prior to ovulation. Armstrong and Grinwich (1972) have also reported that indomethacin administered prior to the ovulation-inducing surge of LH will result in inhibition of follicular luteinization and progesterone secretion in immature PMS primed rats, again indicating a pituitary-blocking action, though in these studies pituitary prostaglandin content was not measured. However, these workers extended their observations to show that indomethacin would also block ovulation when given 30 minutes after the expected pre-ovulatory surge of LH, an effect which could not be overcome by exogenous LH, and indicated an additional blocking effect of indomethacin at the ovarian level; once again the implication is that the endogenous prostaglandins, this time within the ovary, play some essential role in tissue function, in this instance, ovulation.

C. EFFECT OF PROSTAGLANDINS ON STEROID BIOSYNTHESIS

It is now widely accepted that the large molecular weight polypeptide hormones modify tissue function by altering the intracellular concentration of the nucleotide cyclic AMP. Briefly, the polypeptide hormones are thought to recognize and interact with a specific receptor on the outside of the plasma membrane, which activates change in the membrane and eventually leads to modification of the enzyme adenyl cyclase which is located on the inner side of the plasma membrane. This enzyme catalyzes the conversion of adenosine triphosphate (ATP) to cyclic AMP, which in turn is susceptible to hydrolysis by phosphodiesterase, but initially exerts its physiological effect by combination with a cytoplasmic protein and subsequent activation of a protein kinase; the subsequent physiological manifestations attributed to the hormone then depend upon the genetic differentiation of the cell. We therefore have the concept of specificity of hormone action built in at the level of the outer surface of the plasma membrane, followed by the formation of a common intracellular mediator (cyclic AMP).

(a) *Adrenal.* In the adrenal gland, ACTH is considered to promote steroidogenesis by increasing cyclic AMP formation, and there is no evidence to date indicating that ACTH itself even enters the adrenal cell. Similarly, although a direct effect of prostaglandins on cyclic AMP formation in adrenal tissue has not been reported, it is known that in acutely hypophysectomized rats, prostaglandins will increase corticosterone synthesis and release (Flack and Ramwell, 1972). The same studies revealed that cycloheximide blocked this steroidogenic action of the prostaglandins, indicating an effect prior to pregnenolone formation. It is conceivable that in this tissue the prostaglandins could act by a vascular mechanism. Indeed, it has been suggested that functional hyperemia associated with ACTH stimulation results from formation of endogenous prostaglandins using the fatty acids liberated from the adrenals rich supply of cholesterol esters (Grant, 1968; Maier and Staehelin, 1968). However, it has been demonstrated that PGE_1 and prostaglandin E_2 (PGE_2), albeit at high concentrations (100 $\mu g/g$ tissue) will effectively increase synthesis of aldosterone, corticosterone, and cortisol in minced beef adrenals (Saruta and Kaplan, 1971) which would imply a direct action of prostaglandins on the steroidogenic process. In addition, in the autotransplanted adrenal gland of the sodium deficient sheep, it was possible to demonstrate an increase in blood flow during prostaglandin infusion, associated with a concomitant decrease in aldosterone secretion and no change in corticosterone and cortisol secretion (Blair-West et al., 1971). However these results were somewhat inconsistent, for in a total of 21 studies, intra-arterial infusion of PGE_1 (2-20 mg/ml, for 15-60 min) did not modify ACTH release (as reflected in consistent basal steroid values), but in only one third of the experiments was there a marked fall in aldosterone secretion.

Thus, the results would indicate that the stimulatory effect of prostaglandins seen on steroidogenesis in vitro are not always reflected in in vivo observations, and more studies are required to determine not only the site of action of pharmacological doses of prostaglandins in the adrenal gland, but also the function of these compounds which are endogenous to the gland.

The in vivo studies in rats involving cycloheximide indicate that the stimulatory action of prostaglandins on adrenal steroidogenesis in the rat, is prior to pregnenolone formation. To date there is little evidence to indicate that prostaglandins can modify cyclic AMP action. Neither PGE_2 nor $PGF_2\alpha$ cause swelling of adrenal mitochondria or alter the conversion of 11-deoxycorticosterone to corticosterone as effected by isocitrate or succinate. A comparison of the effect of prostaglandins with that of ACTH and cyclic AMP in promoting steroidogenesis in vitro, with respect to the onset and duration of response and the maxima attained would infer that one site of prostaglandin action could indeed be associated with changes in cyclic AMP formation, though this remains to be confirmed (Flack and Ramwell, 1972).

(b) *Testes.* The first investigation reporting an interrelationship between prostaglandins and testicular steroid secretion was by Eik-Nes (1969); he demonstrated that intra-arterial infusion of PGE_2 (11 $\mu g/min$) augmented testosterone secretion induced by human chorionic gonadotrophin (HCG) or cyclic AMP infusion in the dog.

Since secretion of steroid hormones from the testis does depend on its arterial irrigation (Eik-Nes, 1964), infused prostaglandins could act by a vascular mechanism. Free and Jaffe (1972) reported that intra-testicular and testicular arterial infusions of PGE_1, PGE_2, or $PGF_2\alpha$ in conscious rats increased venous pressure and reduced the blood flow and arterial side pressure in testes; PGE_1 had the greatest effect in depressing blood flow and spontaneous oscillations in blood flow. The depression of spontaneous oscillations was attributed to be a response of the smooth muscle of the testicular capsule, and supports the *in vitro* data of Hargrove *et al.* (1971). In the halothane anesthetized rat, $PGF_2\alpha$ produced a highly significant decrease in blood flow (P < 0.005) and reduced testicular testosterone secretion (P < 0.1). Whether this effect of $PGF_2\alpha$ on steroid secretion results from initial changes in blood flow, or from a direct effect on the secreting cells remains to be determined (Free and Tillson, submitted for publication). Thus, in the testes, as well as in the ovary and adrenal, it is possible that initial effects of the postaglandins on the vasculature of the gland mask and thus confuse the interpretation of the direct effects of these compounds on cellular secretion. PGE_1 decreased the amplitude and rate of contractions in a dose-dependent manner, as well as the tone of the rabbit testis *in vitro* (Hargrove *et al.*, 1971); further use of this model showed that prostaglandin $F_1\alpha(PGF_1\alpha)$ increased the rate of contraction and the overall tone. At lower concentrations of $PGF_1\alpha$ the amplitude increased, but above 71 nM the amplitude was decreased (Johnson *et al.*, 1971). Ellis and Baptista (1969) proposed a scheme which incorporates a relationship between lipid peroxidation and androgen synthesis. They reported that prostaglandin A_1 (PGA_1) diminished conversion of progesterone to androgens and increased lipid peroxidation in minced rat testicular tissue. In addition, PGE_1 significantly (P < 0.05) reduced testosterone production when compared with control samples, but a physiological interpretation of these results is difficult due to the high concentrations of prostaglandin added (1 mg/5 ml incubation mixture). Thus, in the testes it appears that prostaglandins can modify secretory blood flow and smooth muscle function, which may result from a single or multiple action.

(c) *Placenta.* It has been demonstrated that the prostaglandin can increase adenyl cyclase activity in human term placental homogenates, PGE_1 being the most potent of the compounds tested (Satoh and Ryan, 1972). This finding, together with the knowledge that prostaglandins are also biosynthesized in human placenta (Russell, 1971; Nakano *et al.*, 1971) is of interest since currently there are no described trophic or regulating factors for placental function. Liggins *et al.* (1972) have indicated that in sheep, dexamethasone infusion into the fetus increases the $PGF_2\alpha$ content of the maternal placenta. However, Schwarzel *et al.* (1973) have indicated that none of the prostaglandins so far tested have any effect on estrogen biosynthesis in placenta *in vitro*. The evidence to date would indicate that the formation of $PGF_2\alpha$ in maternal placenta would facilitate parturition via a direct effect on the uterine myometrium.

(d) *Ovary.* Pharriss and Wyngarden (1969) reported that $PGF_2\alpha$ would mimic LH activity in ovarian minces and that progesterone synthesis was increased some 30-150% during 60 minute incubation; this increase agrees with the data published for LII stimulation of rat ovaries *in vitro* (Armstrong *et al.*, 1964). Similarly, Bedwani and Horton (1968) reported that when minced rabbit ovaries were incubated with HCG, PMS or PGE_1 (1 $\mu g/ml$) there was an increase in 20α-hydroxypregn-4-en-3-one. Further confirmation of the *in vitro* luteotrophic action of the prostaglandins was provided by Speroff and Ramwell (1970) who demonstrated that PGE_2 was more active than PGE_1, PGA_1, or $PGF_2\alpha$ in stimulating progesterone synthesis in bovine luteal slices, and that on a molar basis PGE_2 was approximately half as active as LH. However, $PGF_2\alpha$ did not augment the steroidogenic response to saturating concentrations of LH (Pharriss and Wyngarden 1969; Speroff and Ramwell, 1970).

It has been reported that the response of bovine or rabbit corpora lutea to LH is probably mediated through cyclic AMP (Marsh *et al.*, 1966; Dorrington and Baggett, 1969). An effect of prostaglandins on steroid synthesis, was shown by Marsh (1970); using pregnant bovine luteal homogenates, PGE_2 activated the adenyl cyclase system and increased cyclic AMP and progesterone levels.

Studies comparing the action of prostaglandins in different glands with that of the appropriate trophic hormone have been performed, concerning the time course of the steroid response, the maximum increase in adenyl cyclase activity attained, and possible synergism between the hormone and prostaglandin, but to date little inference can be drawn as to the significance of the finding that relatively high concentrations of the prostaglandins so non-specifically modify cyclic AMP formation in so many tissues. The latter is of course in marked contrast to the concept of hormone specificity as delineated at the beginning of this section. One can demonstrate increased cyclic AMP formation in intact and broken cell preparations, and stimulation of adenyl cyclase activity in relatively pure preparations, but there is no conclusive evidence as to whether the prostaglandins interact with the enzyme directly, or modify its action by interfering with the required ionic environment, or simply exert some perturbation in a cooperative membrane which results in a number of effects, one of which may be changes in adenyl cyclase activity (Rabinowitz *et al.*, 1971). The latter explanation is attractive, since it offers a possible explanation for the means whereby prostaglandins can modify cyclic AMP levels in so many tissues including those of such divergent function as the target tissues of the trophic hormones, human placenta (Satoh and Ryan, 1972), thyroid (Zor *et al.*, 1969), neuroblastoma cells (Gilman and Nirenberg, 1971), platelets (Shio *et al.*, 1972), and turkey erythrocytes (Shaw *et al.*, 1971). In addition, such a single mechanism of action may well explain the diverse pharmacological effects evident during prolonged prostaglandin infusion.

The knowledge that the same prostaglandins which can effectively modify cyclic AMP formation, are also present in the tissues themselves, and, furthermore, that the biosynthesis and release of these compounds are modified on hormonal stimulation (Ramwell and Shaw, 1970) has led to the concept that the endogenous prostaglandins may be an integral part of the sequence whereby a hormone activates adenyl cyclase. Experimental support for such a role for prostaglandins in the ovary can be derived from several sources. Firstly, Kuehl *et al.* (1970) have demonstrated that 7-oxa-13-prostynoic acid, an inhibitor of prostaglandin action in several systems blocks stimulation of cyclic AMP formation induced by PGE_1, PGE_2, or LH in the mouse ovary, in a competitive manner; secondly, Chasalow and Pharriss (1972) have recently shown that in the rat ovary, LH will stimulate prostaglandin biosynthesis and thirdly, the *in vivo* results of Armstrong and Grinwich (1972) show that indomethacin, an inhibitor of prostaglandin biosynthesis, blocks ovulation, an effect which cannot be overcome by administration of exogenous LH and which infers an important role for the endogenous prostaglandins in ovarian function.

To avoid potential confusion, perhaps it should be mentioned here, that in certain tissues the prostaglandins can effectively *inhibit* hormonal stimulation of cyclic AMP formation (including toad bladder, kidney, and adipocytes), an effect which is almost certainly associated with decreased adenyl cyclase formation (see Ramwell and Shaw, 1970). To date, there is no basis on which it can be predicted as to whether the prostaglandins will increase or decrease cyclic AMP formation.

Having established that the prostaglandins are luteotrophic *in vitro*, the results obtained *in vivo* contrast rather markedly and indicate that at least one of the prostaglandins, namely $PGF_2\alpha$, is luteolytic in various species (Fig. 2). Thus, $PGF_2\alpha$ was initially shown to shorten the life span of the corpus luteum of pseudopregnant rats (Pharriss *et al.*, 1968). That the effect was evident in pseudopregnant animals, in the absence of fetus or placenta, implicated the ovary as a potential site of action for $PGF_2\alpha$. These studies were confirmed in guinea pigs (Blatchley and Donovan, 1969), hamsters (Gutknecht *et al.*, 1971a), sheep ovarian transplants (Goding *et al.*, 1971), and early pregnant rhesus monkeys (Kirton *et al.*, 1970), in addition, the luteolytic effect correlated with decreased progesterone levels in ovarian venous blood of pregnant rats (Behrman *et al.*, 1971a), peripheral plasma of pregnant hamsters (Gutknecht *et al.,* 1971a), and rhesus monkeys (when $PGF_2\alpha$ was administered on day 11, 12, or 13 post-ovulation, Kirton *et al.*, 1970). Antifertility effects of $PGF_2\alpha$ in hamsters were obtained by administration on days 5-7 of pregnancy, and could be reversed by subcutaneous administration of progesterone (Gutknecht *et al.*, 1971a).

It is now considered that this effect of $PGF_2\alpha$ may be mediated via a constrictor effect on the ovarian venous vasculature. Thus, $PGF_2\alpha$ is known to be vasoconstrictor in various species (Ducharme *et al.*, 1968), and has been shown to reduce blood flow through the ovary; such an effect could limit substrate availability and result in the noted decrease in progesterone release and increased formation of metabolite. This luteolytic effect of $PGF_2\alpha$ has been oxplored and suggests the possibility that this compound may be the endogenous uterine luteolytic factor in many mammalian species. The evidence supporting such a conclusion has recently been summarized (Pharriss et al., 1972; McCracken et al., 1972).

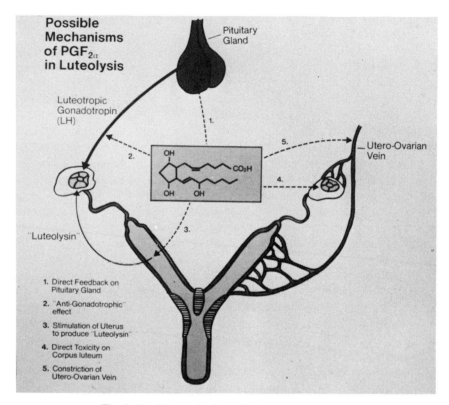

Fig. 2. Possible mechanisms of PGF_{2a} in Luteolysis.

The apparent conflict between demonstration of a luteotrophic effect of the prostaglandins *in vitro* and luteolytic effect *in vivo* is thus resolved by definition of more than one site of action for the same compound in the same tissue. This is exemplified by the work of Behrman *et al.* (1972) who administered $PGF_2\alpha$ *in vivo* to early pregnant rats; ovarian secretion of progesterone was decreased, and that of 20α-hydroxy progesterone was increased. However, when ovarian tissue from the same animals was then incubated *in vitro*, total progesterone synthesis increased. Furthermore, evidence indicating that the luteolytic effect of the prostaglandins is not the only effect to be seen following administration of prostaglandins *in vivo* has previously been demonstrated by Behrman *et al.*

(1971b); using hypophysectomized pseudo-pregnant rats in which progesterone secretion was decreased by some 50% they were able to increase ovarian progesterone synthesis by some 23% with $PGF_2\alpha$. Furthermore, while these workers confirmed that $PGF_2\alpha$ alone would decrease progesterone synthesis in intact pseudo-pregnant rats, concomitant administration of LH with $PGF_2\alpha$ prevented this fall which implied that $PGF_2\alpha$ may interfere with the action of circulating LH at the ovarian level.

Again, if we consider the possible role for endogenous prostaglandins in the ovary, rather than effects seen following use of these compounds as pharmacological agents, we see that not only is the trophic hormone (LH) capable of stimulating prostaglandin biosynthesis in the tissue, but that inhibitors of both prostaglandin biosynthesis (indomethacin) and prostaglandin action (7-oxa-13-prostynoic acid) modify the response of the tissue to trophic hormone stimulation. Thus, Armstrong and Grinwich (1972), report that indomethacin administered *in vivo* can inhibit ovulation induced by either endogenous or exogenous LH, while Kuehl *et al.* (1970) report that 7-oxa-13-prostynoic acid inhibits cyclic AMP formation induced by both LH and prostaglandin in mouse ovary. From the latter observations has arisen the suggestion that prostaglandins may form part of an essential link between the hormone receptor and adenyl cyclase, a possibility which requires further investigation in this and other tissues.

All observations so far described for the ovary have pertained to the luteal phase of development. To date, no effects of prostaglandins on release of FSH from the pituitary have been described, and it is reported that in rats, administration of $PGF_2\alpha$ has no effect on plasma estrogen levels (Behrman *et al.*, 1972).

Recently, much attention has focussed on the use of prostaglandins for termination of pregnancy. It is currently envisaged that such an effect results from the profound smooth muscle stimulating effect of the prostaglandins on the uterine musculature, possibly in conjunction with release of oxytocin from the pituitary (Gillespie *et al.*, 1972) or an enhancement of the effect of circulating oxytocin in stimulating uterine smooth muscle. Speroff *et al.* (1971) have measured maternal free plasma steroids during infusion of prostaglandins for induction of abortion in the human and report a decrease in estriol and estradiol prior to expulsion of the fetus, while a significant decrease in progesterone secretion was not evident until the abortion had been completed. This result was interpreted to imply initial fetal embarrassment probably as a result of the hypoxia induced by uterine contractions, rather than impairment of luteal or placental function. In addition, it has been reported that intravenous infusion of prostaglandins does not affect peripheral plasma concentrations of estrogens, progesterone, or 17-hydroxy progesterone in the human. Furthermore, the results of Speroff *et al.* (1972) and Newton and Collins (1972) show no, or variable changes in chorionic gonadotrophins during infusion of $PGF_2\alpha$ for termination of pregnancy. To date therefore, we know that in various tissues *in vitro* the prostaglandins can mimic the action of the trophic hormones, and promote steroidogenesis via activation of adenyl cyclase and increased cyclic AMP formation. It has not been demonstrated that the prostaglandins have any effect on phosphodiesterase activity or on cyclic AMP action, with the possible exception of inhibition by PGE_1 of cyclic AMP induced increase in gastric secretion (Shaw and Ramwell, 1968). The interpretation of this latter effect is in question however, since it appears likely that cyclic AMP itself has little effect on gastric secretion, but potentiates hormone action, and thus the site of action of inhibitors must be interpreted with caution (Main and Whittle, 1972). To date, there are few, if any, reported intracellular effects of the prostaglandins which cannot be explained by modification of intracellular cyclic AMP levels, with the possible exception of a finding that PGE_1 may function as a calcium 'ionophore' in isolated mitochondria (Kirtland and Baum, 1972).

Thus, the site of action of the prostaglandins would appear to be localized at the membrane level, and yet in contrast to the trophic hormones, the prostaglandins appear to penetrate cells with ease.

The *in vivo* data would indicate that in subhuman primates $PGF_2\alpha$ may function as an abortifacient by inducing luteolysis. Whether such a mechanism pertains in humans remains to be demonstrated, but the evidence to date would indicate that the prostaglandins are effective in inducing labor, both prematurely and at term, by a direct effect on the uterine musculature.

III. EFFECT OF PROSTAGLANDINS ON STEROID ACTION

The steroids, like the prostaglandins, are small and rather simple molecules which, however, modify numerous biochemical responses in their target tissues; the end product of their action is usually a change in growth and differentiation processes. Their specificity of action is controlled by the presence of a binding protein within the cytoplasm of the cells of the target tissue, with which the steroid must bind for effective interaction with a specific receptor located in the cell nucleus. In such a manner, the steroids induce changes in gene expression which is subsequently reflected in induction of protein synthesis some hours after the steroids have initially entered the cell. The cytoplasmic binding protein has been characterized for estrogen (in the uterus) for cortisol (in the liver and lymphoid cells) and for progesterone, dihydrotestosterone and aldosterone in their respective target tissues. The cytoplasmic receptor proteins for the steroids all bear certain similarities in that when prepared in the presence of 0.3 MK^+ they sediment at 4S; if K^+ is omitted they sediment at 7-8S, and the specificity appears to be in the nuclear receptor for the steroid-protein complex. To date, the only reported interaction of prostaglandins with this process is the finding that $PGF_2\alpha$ in the rabbit reduces the concentration of estrogen receptor in both the corpus luteum and in the uterus. In comparison with the steroids, the effects of the prostaglandins at the cellular level are manifest with very different characteristics. Firstly, the prostaglandins have an action which is rapid in onset and decay; secondly, with the possible exception of adipocytes (Kuehl et al., 1970), no tissue has yielded a specific prostaglandin receptor, and finally, there is little tissue specificity for the prostaglandins. To date, there is no reported study concerning effect of prostaglandins on estrogen, progesterone, or glucocorticoid action. Herman and Edelman (1968) reported that PGE_1 (2.5 x 10^{-7} M) neither potentiated nor reduced the effect of a submaximal dose of aldosterone on short circuit current in the toad bladder. There are however, many cited reports of prostaglandins modifying steroid action, effects which result from changes in endogenous steroid production. Instances were quoted in section IIC, including the ability of prostaglandins to reduce androgen formation and thereby increase lipid peroxidation in the testes (Ellis and Baptista, 1969). Similarly, PGE_2 has an inhibiting effect on steroid esterification in skin (Ziboh and Hsia, 1972), and it has been suggested that this effect may be responsible for the ability of PGE's to alleviate the scaly lesions in skin associated with essential fatty acid deficiency.

IV. EFFECT OF PROSTAGLANDINS ON STEROID METABOLISM

The fate of secreted steroid hormones is inactivation of the hormone by the liver and kidney. Inactivation occurs primarily by conjugation of the steroid to a β-glucosiduronate or a sulfate ester which is followed by elimination via the urinary or biliary systems. Evidence showing an effect of prostaglandin directly on steroid metabolism either, in these specific organs, or by shifts in urinary steroid metabolites, has not to our knowledge been reported.

V. EFFECT OF STEROIDS ON PROSTAGLANDIN DYNAMICS

The precise mechanism of prostaglandin action in any particular situation remains to be defined. However, there are reported instances where in vivo administration of steroids modifies a subsequent response to prostaglandins, measured either in vivo or in vitro. Thus, Hawkins et al. (1968) have reported that variation in sensitivity of the isolated rat uterus to prostaglandins could be correlated with the stage of the estrus cycle of the rat from which the uterus was removed; the uterus from an animal in estrus was the least responsive to the prostaglandins. This situation could be mimicked by administration of steroids to the ovariectomized animal; estrogen administration producing a uterine state which showed little response to the prostaglandin; conversely, progesterone administration produced a more responsive tissue. The mechanism of this steroid modification of prostaglandin action was not defined. Similarly, Bygdeman (1967) reported that the sensitivity of isolated strips of human myometrium to PGE and PGF compounds was different for pregnant and non-pregnant tissue. Also, in sheep it has now been shown that the PGF content of peripheral plasma peaks at approximately the time of ovulation (Caldwell *et al.*, 1972). In the sheep, this effect (a) was not seen if the animal was immunized against estradiol and (b) could be mimicked in the ovariectomized animal by estrogen administration following progesterone injections. Such evidence has been used to support the contention that $PGF_2\alpha$ is the luteolytic factor in subhuman primates. The effect of estrogen on $PGF_2\alpha$ formation in maternal placenta of the ewe, and the possible involvement of this in the regulation of patients was discussed in section IIC.

In the rabbit, where estrogen is a luteotrophic agent, administration of 17β-estradiol can overcome the luteolytic effect of infused $PGF_2\alpha$ (Gutknecht *et al.*, 1971b; Pharriss *et al.*, 1972). Similarly, in the rat where LH is the predominate luteotrophic factor, progesterone is the steroid which can protect against the luteolytic effect of infused $PGF_2\alpha$ (Pharriss *et al.* 1968).

There is little data yet available regarding urinary excretion of total prostaglandins in animals or humans, and to date there is no reported study concerning the effect of extirpation of various glands on this process. The knowledge that virtually every organ can biosynthesize and metabolize the prostaglandins would indicate that single gland extirpation will not lead to dramatic changes in prostaglandin excretion such as can be seen for the steroids following, for example, adrenalectomy.

VI. CONCLUSIONS

It has become apparent that the prostaglandins can modify more than one function within the same tissue. For example, in adrenal, testes, and ovary one can elicit a change in blood flow by infusion of the prostaglandins. In addition, when using ovarian tissue *in vitro* one can stimulate steroidogenesis, an effect which can be mimicked *in vivo* under the appropriate conditions. However, in some species in the intact animal, certain prostaglandins can decrease ovarian blood flow, an effect which is considered to be responsible for the observed luteolytic effect.

Undoubtedly, there is more than one site of action for applied prostaglandins in any particular tissue, a fact which illustrates the necessity for use of single cell types, when conducting studies concerned with the mechanism of action of the prostaglandins; for example in homogenates of adipose tissue, prostaglandins produce an increase in cyclic AMP levels, while in isolated adipocytes the compounds effectively decrease intracellular cyclic AMP levels previously elevated by the lipolytic hormones. These results indicate that prostaglandins could effectively decrease cyclic AMP in adipocytes and increase cyclic AMP in another component of adipose tissue (Butcher and Baird, 1968).

Many of the actions of the prostaglandins have now been identified with changes in intracellular cyclic AMP levels (Shaw et al., 1971). Whether these changes result from direct interaction of prostaglandins with the adenyl cyclase system or whether changes in cyclic AMP levels result from a more non-specific interaction of prostaglandins with the plasma membrane of cells remains to be determined. That the latter may pertain is indicated by the finding firstly, that prostaglandins do not modify adenyl cyclase activity in fragmented adipocytes (though they can effectively reduce cyclic AMP formation in the intact cell) and secondly, that prostaglandins can also modify other plasma membrane enzymes including adenylate kinase and ATPase prepared from human platelet and red cells or rat liver mitochondria (Johnson and Ramwell, 1973).

The role for calcium in the action of prostaglandins has received much attention but has not as yet been defined; calcium is required for manifestation of the pharmacological effects of the prostaglandins, it is important in the regulation of adenyl cyclase activity, and a recent publication indicates that when using inner membranes prepared from mitochondria, PGE_1 functions as an ionophore for calcium (Kirtland and Baum, 1972).

Elucidation of the precise mechanism of action of pharmacological doses of the prostaglandins, together with the knowledge that aspirin and indomethacin are efficient inhibitors of prostaglandin biosynthesis, should lead to the possibility of manipulation and control of the endogenous prostaglandins with concomitant modification of tissue function, including those tissues associated with the release and action of steroids. Such an approach has many advantages for it would not be accompanied by the unwanted side effects which result from systemic administration of the natural prostaglandins.

REFERENCES

Änggård, E. (1971). *Ann. N.Y. Acad. Sci.* **180**, 200-217.

Armstrong, D. T., O'Brien, J. and Greep, R. O. (1964). *Endocrinology* **75**, 488.

Armstrong, D. T. and Grinwich, D. L. (1972). *Prostaglandins* **1** 21.

Baile, C. A., Martin, F. H. and Simpson, C. W. (1972). *Fed. Proc. Fed. Am. Soc. Exp. Biol.* **31**, 397 Abst.

Beck, L., Pollard, A. A., Harbo, J. N. and Silver, T. M. (1968). *In* 'Prostaglandin Symposium, Worcester Foundation for Experimental Biology, (P. W. Ramwell and J. E. Shaw, eds.), pp. 295-307, Interscience, New York.

Bedwani, J. R. and Horton, E. W. (1968). *Life Sci.* **7**, 389-393.

Behrman, H. R., Yoshinaga, K., Wyman, H. and Greep, R. O. (1971a). *Am. J. Physiol.* **221**, 189-193.

Behrman, H. R., Yoshinaga, K. and Greep, R. O. (1971b). *Ann. N.Y. Acad. Sci.* **180**, 426-435.

Behrman, H. R., Orczyk, G. P. and Greep, R. O. (1972). *Prostaglandins* **1**, 245-258.

Bergström, S., Carlson, L. A. and Weeks, J. R. (1968). *Pharmacol. Rev.* **20**, 1-48.

Blair-West, J., Coghlan, J. P., Denton, D. A., Funder, J. W., Scoggins, B. and Wright, R. D. (1971). *Endocrinology* **88**, 367-371.

Blatchley, F. R. and Donovan B. T. (1969). *Nature, Lond.* **221**, 1065-1066.

Butcher, R. W. and Baird, C. E. (1968). *J. Biol. Chem.* **243**, 1713-1717.

Bygdeman, M. (1967). *In* 'Nobel Symposium, Vol. 2. Prostaglandins' (S. Bergström and B. Samuelsson eds.,) pp. 71-77, Almquist and Wiksell, Stockholm.

Caldwell, B. V., Tillson, S. A., Brock, W. A. and Speroff, L. (1972). *Prostaglandins* **1(3)**, 217-228.

Chasalow, F. and Pharriss, B. (1972). *Fed. Proc. Fed. Am. Soc. Exp. Biol.* **31**, 545 Abst.

Deis, R. P. and Vermouth, N. T. (1972). *Abst. Int. Cong. Endocrinology 4th*, 1972, Abst. 481.

Dorrington, J. H. and Baggett, B. (1969). *Endocrinology* **84**, 989.

Du Charme, D. W., Weeks, J. R. and Montgomery, R. G. (1968). *J. Pharm. Exp. Therapeutics* **160**, 1-10.

Eik-Nes, K. B. (1964). *Can. J. Physiol. Pharmacol.* **42**, 671.

Eik-Nes, K. B. (1969). *Gen. Comp. Endo. Supp.* **2**, 87.

Ellis, L. C. and Baptista, M. H. (1969). *In* 'Radiation Biology of the Fetal and Juvenile Mammal' (M. R. Sikov and D. P. Mahlum, eds.). U.S. Atomic Energy Commission, Division of Technicial Information, pp. 963-974.

Feldberg, W. and Saxena, P. N. (1971). *J. Physiol., Lond.* **217**, 547-556.

Flack, J. D., Ramwell, P. W. and Shaw, J. E. (1971). *In* 'Current Topics in Experimental Endocrinology' (L. Martini and V. H. T. James, eds.), Vol. 1, pp. 199-228, Academic Press, New York and London.

Flack, J. D. and Ramwell, P. W. (1972). *Endocrinology* **90**, 371-377.

Free, M. J. and Jaffe, R. A. (1972). *Am. J. Physiol.* **223**, 241-248.

Free, M. J. and Tillson, S. A. (1973). *Endocrinology* **93**, 874-879.

Gillespie, A., Brummer, H. C. and Chard, T. (1972). *Br. Med. J.* **1**, 543-544.

Gilman, A. G. and Nirenberg, M. (1971). *Nature, Lond.* **234**, 356-358.

Goding, J. R., Baird, D. T., Cumming, I. A. and McCracken, J. A. (1971). *In* 'Karolinska Symposia on Research Methods in Reproductive Endocrinology, 4th Symposium: Perfusion Techniques' (E. Diczfalusy, ed.). Bogtrykkeriet Forum, Copenhagen, pp. 169-199.

Grant, J. K. (1968). *J. Endocrinol.* **41**, 111-135.

Gutknecht, G. D., Cornette, J. C. and Pharriss, B. B. (1969). *Biol. Reprod.* **1**, 367-371.

Gutknecht, G. D., Wyngarden, L. J. and Pharriss, B. B. (1971a) *Proc. Soc. Exp. Biol. Med.* **136**, 1151-1157.

Gutknecht, G. D., Duncan, G. W. and Wyngarden, L. J. (1971b). *Biol. Reprod.* **5**, 87.

Hargrove, J. L., Johnson, J. M. and Ellis, L. C. (1971). *Proc. Soc. Exp. Biol. Med.* **136**, 958-961.

Hawkins, R. A., Jessup, R. and Ramwell, P. W. (1968). *In* 'Prostaglandin Symposium of the Worcester Foundation for Experimental Biology' (P. W. Ramwell and J. E. Shaw, eds.), pp. 11-19, Interscience, New York.

Herman, T. S. and Edelman, I. S. (1968). 'Proc. Int. Union Physiol. Sci., Vol. 7, 24th Int. Congress, (Washington, 1968)', Abst. 188.

Hertelendy, F., Peake, G. and Todd, H. (1971). *Biochem. biophys. Res. Commun.* **44**, 253-260.

Horton, E. W. (1969). *Physiol. Rev.* **49**, 122-161.

Ito, H., Momose, G., Katayama, T., Takagishi, H., Ito, L., Nakajima, H. and Takei, Y. (1971). *J. Clin. Endocrin. Metab.* **32**, 857-859.

Johnson, M. and Ramwell, P. W. (1973). *In* 'Advances in the Biosciences, **9**, International Conference on Prostaglandins, 1972 (S. Bergstrom, ed.), pp. 205-217, Pergamon Press, Oxford.

Johnson, J. M., Hargrove, J. L. and Ellis, L. C. (1971). *Proc. Soc. Exp. Biol. Med.* **138**, 378-381.

Kirtland, S. J. and Baum, H. (1972). *Nature New Biol.* **236**, 47-49.

Kirton, K. T., Pharriss, B. B. and Forbes, A. D. (1970). *Proc. Soc. Exp. Biol. Med.* **133**, 314-316.

Kuehl, F. A., Humes, J. L., Tarnoff, J., Cirillo, V. J. and Ham, E. A. (1970). *Science, N.Y.* **169**, 883-886.

Labhsetwar, A. P. (1970). *J. Reprod. Fert.* **23**, 155-159.

Lee, J., Kannegiesser, H., O'Toole, J. and Westura, E. (1971). *Ann. N.Y. Acad. Sci.* **180**, 218-240.

Lewis, G. P. and Matthews, J. (1969). *J. Physiol., Lond.* **202**, 95-96.

Liggins, G. C., Grieves, S. A., Kendall, J. Z. and Knox, B. S. (1972). *J. Reprod. Fertil. (suppl.)* **16**, 85-103.

McCracken, J. A., Carlson, J. C., Glew, M. E., Goding, J. R., Baird, D. T., Green, K. and Samuelsson, B. (1972). *Nature New Biol.* **238**, 129-134.

MacLeod, R. M., Lehmeyer, J. E. and Fontham, E. H. (1971). *Fed. Proc.* **30**, 533 Abst.

MacLeod, R. M. and Lehmeyer, J. E. (1972). *Clin. Res.* **18**, 366.

Maier, R. and Staehelin, M. (1968). *Acta Endocrinol. (Copenhagen)* **58**, 619.

Main, I. H. M. and Whittle, B. J. R. (1972). *Brit. J. Pharmacol.* **44**, 331-332.

Marsh, J. M., Butcher, R. W., Savard, K. and Sutherland, E. W. (1966). *J. Biol. Chem.* **241**, 5436-5440.

Marsh, J. M. (1970). *F.E.B.S. Lett.* **7**, 283-286.

Nakano, J., Montague, B. and Darrow, B. (1971). *Biochem. Pharmacol.* **20**, 2512-2514.

Newton, J. R. and Collins, W. P. (1972). International Conference on Prostaglandins, 1972, Abst. 113.

Orczyk, G. P. and Behrman, H. R. (1972). *Prostaglandins* **1**, 3-20.

Peng, T. C., Six, K. M. and Munson, P. L. (1972). *Endocrinol.* **86**, 202-206.

Pharriss, B. B., Wyngarden, L. J. and Gutknecht, G. D. (1968). *In* 'Gonadotrophins' (E. Rosenberg, ed.) pp. 121-129. Geron-x Inc., Los Altos, California.

Pharriss, B. B. and Wyngarden, L. J. (1969). *Proc. Soc. Exp. Biol. Med.* **130**, 92-94.

Pharriss, B. B., Tillson, S. A. and Erickson, R. R. (1972). *Recent Prog. in Horm. Res.* **28**, 51-89.

Rabinowitz, I., Ramwell, P. W. and Davison, P. (1971). *Nature New Biol.* **233**, 88-90.

Ramwell, P. W. and Shaw, J. E. (1970) *Recent Prog. Horm. Res.* **26**, 139-187.

Russell, P. T. (1971). *J. Am. Oil Chem. Soc.* **48**, 94A.

Saruta, T. and Kaplan, N. M. (1971). *Clin. Res.* **19**, 69.

Satoh, K. and Ryan, K. J. (1972). *J. Clin. Invest.* **51**, 456-458.

Scaramuzzi, O. E., Baile, C. A. and Mayer, J. (1971). *Experientia* **27**, 256-257.

Shaw, J. E. and Ramwell, P. W. (1968). *In* 'Prostaglandin Symposium of the Worcester Foundation for Experimental Biology' (P. W. Ramwell and J. E. Shaw, eds), pp. 55-66, Interscience, New York.

Shaw, J. E., Gibson, W., Jessup, S. and Ramwell, P. W. (1971). *Ann. N.Y. Acad. Sci.* **180**, 241-260.

Schwarzel, W. C., Kruggel, W. G. and Brodie, H. J. (1973). *Endocrinol.* **92**, 866-880.

Shio, H., Ramwell, P. W. and Jessup, S. J. (1972). *Prostaglandins* **1**, 29-36.

Speroff, L. and Ramwell, P. W. (1970). *J. Clin. Endocrin.* **30**, 345-350.

Speroff, L., Brock, W. A., Caldwell, B. V., Anderson, G. G. and Hobbins, J. C. (1971). *In* 'Abstracts, 18th Annual Meeting, Soc. Gynec. Invest., Phoenix 1971', p. 16.

Speroff, L., Caldwell, B. V., Brock, W. A., Anderson, G. G. and Hobbins, J. C. *J. Clin. Endocrin. and Metabolism* **34**, 531-536.

Strong, C. G. and Bohr, D. F. (1968). *In* 'Prostaglandin Symposium of the Worcester Foundation of Experimental Biology' (P. W. Ramwell and J. E. Shaw, eds.), pp. 225-245. Interscience, New York.

Vale, W., Rivier, C. and Guillemin. R. (1971). *Fed. Proc.* **30**, 363.

Vane, J. R. (1971). *Nature New Biol.* **231**, 232-235.

Yamamoto, L., Feindel, W., Wolfe, L. and Hodge, C. (1972). *Ann. R. Coll. Phys. Surg. Can.* **5**, 64.

Ziboh, V. A. and Hsia, S. L. (1972). *J. Lipid Res.* **13**, 458-467.

Zor, U., Kaneko, T., Schneider, H. P. G., McCann, S. M., Lowe, I. P., Bloom, G., Borland, B. and Field, J. B. (1969). *Proc. Natn. Acad. Sci.* **63**, 918-925.

Zor, U., Kaneko, T., Schneider, H. P. G., McCann, S. M. and Field, J. B. (1970). *J. Biol. Chem.* **245**, 2883-2888.

STEROID HORMONES AND BREAST CANCER

D. C. WILLIAMS

The Marie Curie Memorial Foundation, The Chart, Oxted, Surrey, England

I. INTRODUCTION

It has been recognized for many years that, at least in their initial stages, some human tumours which arise from hormone sensitive tissues retain some of the original characteristics of the cells from which they were derived. In certain cases tumours, arising from organs which are normally dependent upon hormones for growth and function, may themselves be influenced by these substances until this facility is eventually lost by the normal de-differentiation process which appears to be common to all malignant growth. However, in many cases there is a considerable period of hormone sensitivity as the tumour develops and this effect can often be exploited as the basis for therapy. Ultimately, this advantage is usually lost and the tumour becomes autonomous. In general, the better differentiated the tumour and the more hormone sensitive the original parent tissue, the more likely is a favourable response to hormone therapy. It is perhaps surprising that although hormonal control is widespread throughout the body, relatively few tumours arising from hormone sensitive organs are subject to prolonged treatment by hormonal therapy.

In practice these seem to be limited to breast and prostatic tumours and perhaps to some testicular tumours and tumours of the female reproduction system. It is proposed briefly to discuss the main methods by which the steroid hormone environment of human breast tumours in particular may be modified, giving some idea of the statistical effectiveness of each treatment and to indicate some of the newer and prospective modes of hormone therapy and diagnosis. Relevant review articles will be quoted for reference but a formal review of the extensive literature on the subject will not be attempted. Cancer of the breast has been chosen to illustrate the clinical effects of hormone treatment because very much more data is available on the treatment of this type of malignancy than any other hormone sensitive tumours. Thus statistically significant results of hormonal therapy are more readily obtained in this form of cancer.

Carcinoma of the female breast is generally regarded as the first type of malignant tumour to have shown sensitivity to hormones. The proposal that oophorectomy should be used as a treatment for advanced breast cancer appears to have been made as early as 1889 by Schinzinger, but the paper of Beatson (1896) is the first published result of such treatment. The technique increased in popularity at the beginning of the century, but interest declined presumably because the objective response rate was, in general, poor and of brief duration. Interest in the hormonal response of human tumours was revived by the classical work of Huggins and his colleagues.

Carcinoma of the breast is the most widespread malignancy in the female and may account for as much as 25% of total female cancer. There is, however, wide variation in incidence of breast cancer in different parts of the world. The extremes which are usually quoted are Japanese women, in which the incidence is about 3.3 per 100,000 and British women at some 36.3 per 100,000, which even when age adjustment is made for expectation of life in the two countries, represents a mortality rate of six to one. There are wide variations in many other countries, but the examples quoted may be more readily accepted since fairly complete records are available. Suggestions for this variation have included nutrition, racial variation, environment, child bearing rate, availability of medical supervision and hormone levels, but no firm conclusion seems possible at present. It is perhaps interesting to note in passing that a similar difference in the death rate from uterine cancer between Japan and the other countries is not shown, but there appears to be a very considerable difference in age specific death rate.

It is a sad fact that, although breast cancer is such a common disease and the site so easily accessible for diagnosis, the death rate from this disease has remained largely unchanged over the past two or three decades. This suggests that this disease is not, in general, diagnosed sufficiently early to prevent metastatic spread and it would seem that cancer education and improved adjuvant therapy should help to improve the prognosis.

Endocrine treatment appears to be most effective in those patients having slow growing tumours. Tumours which have well differentiated structures, which is sometimes a sign of retained hormone sensitivity, offer a better prognosis than do rapidly metastasising anaplastic tumours. A long period between original diagnosis and recurrence of symptoms is also generally a good sign. Beyond these broad generalizations very little information can be gained, either from histological or clinical examination, as to the response of a particular tumour to therapy. It would seem desirable that some form of biochemical test should be evolved for this purpose, but, although much work has been done in this direction, there is no reliable test at the present time. The best methods for patient evaluation at present appear to be based on clinical experience supported by histological data and results from previous therapy. The specific estimation of hormone secretion levels or those of enzymes involved in hormone metabolism (see below) has so far been somewhat disappointing.

It is a matter of clinical experience that tumours may respond either to oestrogen or to androgen therapy depending on the tumour-host relationship of a particular patient. In practice attempts have been made to relate effects of therapy to the menstrual status of the patient. The relationship does not, however, seem to be a simple one and in order to remove this complication the Co-operative Breast Cancer Group of the Cancer Chemotherapy National Service Centre subdivided patients in their trials according to their past menstrual history (Segaloff et al., 1962).

The whole question of the interaction of hormone sensitive tumours with the endocrine status of the host is a fascinating one which remains to be resolved. There is a great deal of data from experimental tumours which suggests that tumours having different hormone responses can coexist in the same species and even in the same animal (e.g. see Gardner, 1962). It has also been shown that mammary tumours, differing in hormonal specificity, can be induced by a given chemical carcinogen (Williams, 1965). It seems likely that, in a proportion of cases, tumours consist of a mixed population of cells some of which are hormone sensitive, and can be controlled by hormone treatment, but that the insensitive cells become increasingly dominant on prolonged treatment so that the tumour eventually becomes autonomous.

II. THE EXAMINATION OF HUMAN BREAST TUMOURS IN TISSUE CULTURE

The gradual realization that the animal tumour is, at best, a poor tool for investigation of many aspects of human cancer has stimulated interest in alternative procedures. One of the more important of these is a realistic method of culturing cancer *in vitro*. It is now possible to grow practically all human carcinomas with a fair degree of reproducibility but the mammary carcinoma has presented considerable difficulty, probably due to their wide diversity. Compara-tively recently however results of the order of 90% sucessful cultures have been obtained (Barker and Richmond, 1971; Bishun *et al.*, 1973) which are viable over a considerable period and therefore give confidence that near normal growth rather than slow death of the cells is involved.

Having established a healthy culture, it is possible to add appropriate hormones, or indeed almost any other drug, to the culture medium and to compare the growth rate of the tumour cells under various conditions. This method of predicting hormonal response of future metastatic growth has great potential value and, although this can only be assessed by long term clinical studies, some interesting comparisons are already emerging with other predictive methods.

Methods of investigation based on the tissue culture techniques suffer from a number of disadvantages.

(1) Tumours, especially breast tumours, appear to consist of mixed popula-tion cells and are by no means homogeneous. Care must be taken to culture a representative population of cells from a particular tumour and not to select a particular clone to the exclusion of other cells. Even when this is done, however, it has been observed that some clones of cells are more readily adapted to continuous culture methods than others so that the process is itself a selective one. It has recently been noticed in our laboratory that cell clones can be separated from cultures of breast tumours, which have different genetic properties (Bishun, personal communication), and further that the separation of such clones of cells one from the other affects the growth properties of both types of cell. This suggests that specific clones of cell may affect each others' growth properties during culture; perhaps one clone could elaborate a factor (hormone?) affecting the growth of another clone. Experiments have been started to investigate this possibility.

(2) In a tissue culture system there is generally very little drug metabolism compared with the *in vivo* situation. Although steroid hormones, presumably because they are 'natural products' may be metabolized to some extent in culture the metabolic pattern is not generally that found *in vivo*. For this reason tissue culture experiments cannot adequately represent the true clinical situation. These differences can be minimized by (a) Adding known metabolites of the appropriate steroid hormone to the culture. (b) Culturing the cells in some sort of *in vivo* system. One rather ingenious means of doing this is to culture cells inside a semipermeable box which is then implanted in an animal. The animal may then be treated with the appropriate steroid so that the culture will, hopefully, come into contact with the metabolic products. Very pre-liminary experiments of this type have already been undertaken by various

groups but no evidence is yet available as to the effectiveness of this technique.

(3) It must be remembered that the tumour-host relationship plays an important part in the growth of a tumour so that it may perhaps be a mistake to grow a tumour in isolation. A more realistic system would seem to be a mixed culture between the tumour and the tissue of the host to which it metastasized. This may be even more important when the host organ itself is known to play a part in steroid metabolism or conjugation. It seems likely, now that the culturing of human tumours is reasonably well understood, that the technique of mixed cultures will prove very useful in investigating the metastatic spread of breast and other tumours.

There are two main ways in which the hormone balance can be altered in a patient with metastatic cancer of the breast.

(a) The source of endogenous hormone is removed by surgery, X-rays, or chemical treatment. This is usually referred to as ablative therapy and consists of the removal or destruction of the gonads, the adrenals, or the pituitary gland or combination of these procedures.

(b) The administration, usually in relatively large doses, of hormones which antagonize the growth of a hormone sensitive tumour. This is known as additive therapy. In practice, patients are usually treated by some combination of these two procedures.

III. ABLATION PROCEDURES

A. CASTRATION

This form of therapy has been gradually rationalized with the increasing understanding of ovarian function and of the part played by hormones in cancer therapy. The benefits which may be expected from castration in treating metastatic cancer of the breast can be considered under the following separate headings:

1. Therapeutic castration
2. Prophylactic castration
3. Prediction of future treatment

1. Therapeutic Castration

The current position of this form of therapy has been discussed by Kennedy *et al.* (1964) and by Hall and his colleagues (1963) amongst others. Some groups of workers appeared to find treatment rather more effective than others, but the data discussed by the last named group seems to be fairly typical.

They have analysed the data submitted by members of the Co-operative Breast Cancer Group from their carefully followed patients. Two groups of patients, homogeneous in their response to therapy were considered, those showing objective responses and those showing no response to castration. Each group was sub-divided according to its subsequent response to hormonal therapy. The overall response to castration (24%) is comparable to the reports of other groups. The different rate of response to hormone therapy of the groups that responded to castration (23%) and the group that did not respond to castration (7%) is significant. The response to hormonal therapy in patients in relapse after responding to castration initially, is comparable with the overall response rates for androgens and oestrogen in intact patients; while the 7% response rate in castration failure is statistically significantly lower.

Literature reviews by Lewison (1962, 1965) sets the limit of expected response to castration in pre-menopausal patients at between a quarter and a third of all cases, and the palliative benefit, although very difficult to predict, to an average duration of 10 to 14 months. These figures refer only to pre-menopausal patients who are, therefore, to this extent, selected patients. He also makes the point that the wide range of difference in response must, to some extent, be influenced by the optimism of the individual investigator.

The joint committee on Endocrine Ablative Procedures (Taylor, 1962) considered that provided the operation is performed before or within a year after the menopause, an objective regression of 29% could be expected. The average survival time is 31 months in patients who responded to ablative therapy as compared with 8.8 months for patients who did not respond. There seems, therefore, to be little doubt that therapeutic castration is of value in patients with recurrent metastatic breast cancer, especially in those who are pre- or immediately post-menopausal and in these circumstances should be performed irrespective of the stage of the disease (Raven, 1958).

2. Prophylactic Castration

Castration at the same time as initial mastectomy, has been studied as a means of preventing or delaying the appearance of metastasis. The rationale for this treatment is that if minute metastatic tumours are already established at the time of mastectomy (as is all too often the case) then it is best to remove the hormonal stimulus as early in their growth period as possible. This method of treatment has been revewed by Horsley (1962), Treves (1957a,b), Cole (1964) Eisman (1966) Lewison (1965) and others.

It appears from figures quoted by Cole, based on castration by X-ray of selected pre- or immediately post-menopausal patients, that irradiation following mastectomy gave slight benefit in increasing both five and seven year survival rates, (42.6% increased to 58.3% and 47.3% increased to 51.2%, respectively.

These results were, however, scarcely statistically significant, and McWhirter (1957) could find no significant difference of a similar group of selected Stage I and II patients, Kennedy and colleagues (1964) have shown that the interval from initial tumour therapy to recurrence is definitely increased by castration, but the survival time seems to be independent of the time of castration, so that overall survival times for therapeutic and prophylactic castration seem to be about the same. This form of therapy is still being evaluated, and it will probably be some years hence before statistically significant data becomes available.

3. Prediction of Future Treatment

The response of patients to castration is perhaps the best available single method of predicting future therapy (Kelley, 1966). If a patient shows an objective response to castration it at least indicates that the primary tumour is hormone sensitive. On the other hand, if a patient shows no response to castration, then it is probably a hormone insensitive tumour and some form of treatment other than hormone therapy must be considered. For this reason many clinicians prefer to use castration as a therapeutic rather than prophylactic treatment, so that some idea of the hormone response of the tumour can be gained. Unfortunately, however metastatic tumours derived from an apparently hormone dependent tumour are not always themselves hormone sensitive. As pointed out by Hall and his colleagues (1963), the response of patients with carcinoma of the breast to therapeutic castration can be considered as predictive in a negative sense. That is, patients who fail to respond to castration have a poor likelihood of responding to subsequent hormone therapy. Patients who respond to castration are neither more nor less likely to respond to subsequent hormone therapy. Not all workers are in complete agreement with this analysis. It has been shown (The Joint Committee on Endocrine Ablative Procedures in Disseminated Mammary Carcinoma (1962)), that about 50% of patients who have responded to castration will experience a second remission following a second ablative procedure.

B. ADRENALECTOMY

It is well known that the adrenal cortex produces both oestrogen and androgen in addition to corticosteroids. Many workers have also noticed that castration in the female is followed by an increase in size of both the pituitary and adrenal glands. It therefore follows that the removal of adrenal glands should reduce the circulating oestrogen and androgen especially in patients who have been castrated previously. However, until the availability of pure corticosteroids the maintenance of a patient after adrenalectomy was impossible. The first attempt at total adrenalectomy for the treatment of advanced cancer was by Huggins and Scott (1945) with the idea of decreasing circulating androgen in advanced cases of cancer of the prostate. With the availability of cortisone, Huggins and Bergenstal (1952) obtained promising results with adrenalectomy in prostatic cancer. There workers also applied adrenalectomy to seven patients with advanced breast cancer, and of these there was a marked regression of metastasis in three cases.

This form of treatment soon became common in most of the large treatment centres, for example, Dao and Huggins (1955), Fracchia and his colleagues (1959), Cade (1958), and many others. Bonser, Dossett and Jull (1961) have collected together figures for adrenalectomy which were published between 1955 and 1958. They obtained a total of 777 cases of which objective responses were obtained in 43%. There was considerable variation in response rates obtained from different workers, but these were probably due to the use of different criteria of response.

Dao and Huggins (1957) pointed out that although a great number of adrenalectomies had been performed this was done almost entirely as a last resort treatment for patients who had been treated with hormonal therapy until they had ceased to respond. They therefore designed experiments to determine whether it was worth while performing adrenalectomy in patients with demonstrable metastasis but who had not been previously treated with hormone therapy such as androgen or oestrogen administration. These workers randomized 95 patients suffering from metastatic cancer of the breast, 46 of these were treated with androgen and 49 by adrenalectomy, and analysis of their results showed that 9 of 44 androgen treated patients, and 23 of 47 adrenalectomized patients obtained objective regression. They also found that the duration of remission was significantly longer in patients who had had adrenalectomy than in patients treated with androgen. Their results suggested that only previous response to castration bore a significant relationship to subsequent response to adrenalectomy. The authors consider that their results provide unequivocal evidence that adrenalectomy is superior to androgen administration for the management of metastatic breast cancers.

The best method of selecting patients for this form of treatment seems to be long sustained remission after castration. There is also some reason to believe that patients who have prolonged responses to hormone therapy, particularly oestrogen therapy, may also obtain worthwhile regression from such an operation.

C. CHEMICAL INHIBITION OF THE ADRENAL CORTEX

It is well-known that cortisone exerts a feed-back mechanism on the adrenal gland which suppresses adreno-cortical secretion; this includes oestrogen and androgen. It is reasonable, therefore, to expect that this form of treatment would produce effects similar to surgical adrenalectomy. Pearson and his colleagues (1955) have shown that, in fact, remissions do occur in a considerable number of cases. However, these remissions are not of long duration and the treatment is considerably less effective than adrenalectomy.

In order to separate chemical adrenalectomy from the hormonal effects of corticosteroids, a number of other substances have been tested in an attempt to produce chemical adrenalectomy. The most effective drugs so far tested appear to be those related to the insecticide DDT. These include: DDD (1,1-Dichloro-2,2-bis-p-chlorophenyl-ethane); Perthane (1,1-Dichloro-2,2-bis(p-ethylphenyl)-ethane); o,p-DDD (1,1-Dichloro-2-(o-chlorophenyl)-2-p-chlorophenyl-ethane). These substances were carefully studied by Weisenfeld and Goldner (1962). Zimmermann and his colleagues (1956) showed that some adrenal suppression could be obtained in patients with cancer of the breast or prostate by using DDD. Bergenstal and his colleagues (1960) have obtained favourable results in adrenal cancer by using o,p-DDD and this compound was also examined in Cushing's Syndrome. It was concluded that these drugs decrease adrenal function in man, but that suppression of normal adrenal function does not occur uniformly and is not sufficient to be of value in treatment of metastatic breast or prostatic cancer.

The current position regarding chemical adrenalectomy may therefore be summed up in the following way:

Although an efficient method of chemical adrenalectomy would be very useful as a clinical tool, no method so far tried is nearly as effective or reliable as surgical adrenalectomy.

D. HYPOPHYSECTOMY

Hypophysectomy as a treatment of disseminated mammary cancer was introduced by Luft and Olivecrona (1953). Their results were so encouraging that this treatment quickly gained general acceptance and has now been used to treat a large number of cases of advanced breast cancer. The pituitary gland is a source of many hormonal factors some of which are involved in the maintenance and growth of the human breast. It is well known that castrated patients develop large pituitary and adrenal glands. It is also known that this enlargement frequently coincides with an increase in circulating hormones. Hypophysectomy may therefore exert its effect upon breast cancer either by the suppression of pituitary hormones acting directly upon the breast, such as FSH or LH, or by suppression of the hormones produced in the adrenal or other glands.

The most obvious explanation of the effect of hypophysectomy on breast cancer is perhaps the suppression of adrenal oestrogen. This effect was observed by Greenwood and Bulbrook (1959), but these authors also noticed that oestrogen levels may be elevated after hypophysectomy. It is therefore unlikely that oestrogen suppression is the only mechanism involved in the control of breast cancer by hypophysectomy. Almost certainly other factors produced by the pituitary gland also play a part in the control of breast cancer. Thus, both FSH and LH levels in circulating blood disappear shortly after operation. There is also a dramatic fall in adrenal corticoids and androgens after hypophysectomy, but these hormones do not completely disappear from the circulation,

Aldosterone, however, is affected very little by hypophysectomy, and this presumably explains why it is often easier to maintain hypophysectomized patients than to maintain those who have had adrenalectomy. Hormonal side-effects such as those produced by suppression of growth hormone, prolactin, and by diabetes insipidus can usually be successfully controlled by the administration of pituitary extracts. There are, in addition to total surgical hypophysectomy, a number of alternative ways to suppress pituitary function. These include section of the pituitary stalk, irradiation of the pituitary either from an external source, or by implantation of radioactive substances directly into the sella turcica, and the so-called chemical hypophysectomy.

Juret (1966), in his excellent review of the whole field of endocrine surgery, has collected together the results obtained by a large number of workers, of which the following are typical. Luft and his colleagues (1958) obtained 50% remission. In the collaborative study of the Joint Committee on Endocrine Ablative Procedures in Disseminated Mammary Carcinoma, 32.6% of 340 patients obtained remission. Ray and Pearson (1956) reported 42% remission, and Kennedy and French (1965), by carefully choosing patients who had previously responded to hormone therapy, obtained regressions of up to 60%. The Joint Committee obtained only 11.3% response to hypophysectomy in patients who had not responded to other endocrine procedures.

Remission times vary widely between different patients, and also from one clinician to another, depending upon the actual criteria used. As an example, Ray and Pearson quote an average remission time of 17.3 months and an average survival time of 25.8 months for patients who have responded to hormone therapy, (patients having a remission of more than six months). But the average duration of response seems to be about 12 to 15 months with a total survival time of some 18 to 20 months for patients who respond to endocrine therapy, as compared with six months, or less, for patients who do not respond. Attempts have been made to correlate the effect of hypophysectomy with the site of metastasis. Here again, it is difficult to compare regressions at different sites using varying criteria. This feat has, however, been attempted by Ray and Pearson, who suggest that the degree of remission decreases in metastatic growths in the following order of secondary site: bone (55%), lymph nodes (48%), lung (45%), skin lesions (38%), liver (30%). It is also true that some patients experience relief of bone pain, even though there is no objective remission.

Several groups of workers have attempted to compare the efficiency of hypophysectomy and adrenalectomy, but it is difficult to obtain statistically significant differences. Ray and Pearson (1956) believed that hypophysectomy was the operation of choice, as did Atkins and his colleagues (1960). Macdonald (1962), however, reported on the evidence of 690 adrenalectomies and 340 hypophysectomies that there was no significant difference in remission rate (28.4 and 32.6% respectively).

E. CHEMICAL HYPOPHYSECTOMY

In theory, any compound which exerts a feed-back mechanism on the pituitary gland will perform chemical hypophysectomy. Thus, adrenal steroids in large doses will block ACTH production, as will prednisone. In a similar way TSH can be suppressed by triiodothyronine (Gardner and his colleagues, 1962). Androgens can block gonadotrophin to some extent, as also can oestrogen administration. There also remains the possibility of suppressing pituitary function by using pituitary extracts which are deficient in the appropriate hormone, e.g. LH or FSH. None of these substances has so far shown effects to compare with surgical hypophysectomy. It would seem that the term Chemical Hypophysectomy, as currently used, is a misnomer, since apparently no chemical completely suppresses even one of the many functions of the pituitary gland.

IV. PREDICTION OF RESPONSE TO ENDOCRINE SURGERY

Since breast cancer was sometimes effectively treated, by the removal of the sources of oestrogen in the body, it seemed logical that these cases should be typified by high levels of oestrogen *in vivo*. The testing of this hypothesis awaited the development of sufficiently sensitive methods for determining oestrogen levels in both circulating blood and the tissues themselves. (Brown, 1955; Aitken and Preedy, 1956.)

Unfortunately, however the levels of circulating oestrogens in patients with breast cancer appear to bear no consistent relationship either to the hormone sensitivity of the primary tumour or to the histological or growth characteristics of a particular tumour. Even more surprisingly there was no consistent change in oestrogen levels when these patients were subjected to endocrine surgery either before or subsequent to the removal of the primary breast tumour (Forrest, 1965). It seemed therefore that there was little to be gained from the estimation of oestrogens in body fluids or tissues in so far as the prediction of the effectiveness of endocrine surgery was concerned and it was not until the discovery of specific binding sites for steroid hormones, within the cell nucleus, that interest in this technique was reawakened (see below).

A. THE DISCRIMINANT FACTOR

In the meantime another ingenious method of predicting endocrine response of tumours, the discriminant factor, was elaborated in the main by Bulbrook, Greenwood and their colleagues. This predictive method depends upon the calculation of ratios between the quantities of specific urinary steroids or groups of steroids, excreted by the cancer patient. The idea was first advanced by Allen *et al.* (1957) who observed that the ratio of the 11-deoxy-17-oxo steroids to 11-oxy-17-oxo steroids gave a prediction of the response of patients to hypophysectomy and in general a ratio greater than one suggested a good prognosis. This idea was modified by Bulbrook *et al.* (1960) who proposed that the ratios of urinary aetiocholanolone to total 17-hydroxycorticosteroids gave an index of the efficacy of hypophysectomy and possibly adrenalectomy. This has been confirmed by several other groups of workers, e.g. Juret (1968) and Atkins *et al.* (1968). The latter groups analysed their results and concluded that:

(1) Hypophysectomy was four times as likely to be effective in patients with a positive discriminant than in patients with a negative discriminant and that the survival period after hypophysectomy was, on average, longer for the positive patient.

(2) The longer the period between removal of the primary tumour and the occurrence of secondary tumours the better the response to hypophysectomy of these patients with a positive discriminant.

A number of attempts have been made to improve on the effectiveness of the discriminant factory by the inclusion of other parameters, both biochemical and clinical, by Wilson and his colleagues (1967, 1968) and others. So far no clear advantage has been shown over the original factor but studies on alternative systems continue.

A further very important aspect of this work arises from the possibility that the steroid variations may well be detected before the disease can be diagnosed by conventional means. Studies of this type which are, of necessity, of a long term nature have been undertaken by several groups of workers, notably by Bulbrook and Hayward (1967), and are still in progress but no clear evidence in support of this hypothesis has so far emerged. There remains, of course, the possibility that some form of steroid imbalance may play a part in the induction of the primary tumour but experimental confirmation of this process would be an extremely laborious and long term undertaking.

Another possible method of deciding likely response of a particular tumour to steroid therapy arises from the observation by Dao that some breast tumours possess the property of conjugating steroids with sulphate. It has been suggested that those tumours possessing a high conjugation capacity give the best response, especially to adrenalectomy and that tumours in which the ratio of dehydro-epiandrosterone sulphate to oestradiol sulphate is highest give the best responses (Dao, 1971). These experiments again give rise to interesting speculation as to whether abnormal sulphate conjugation may be used as a screening technique; is this effect detectable at a premalignant level? If on the other hand steroid conjugation has a bearing on the initiation of the malignant process may not lesions in other organs, especially perhaps the liver, affect the aetiology of breast cancer?

B. THE ESTIMATION OF HORMONE BINDING SITES

One of the main disadvantages of any predictive system which is based on the cellular distribution or metabolism of steroid hormones is that, simply because the hormone is present within the cell, it does not mean that it has an influence on the growth of the cell. It therefore follows that quantitative changes in hormone levels in body fluids are unlikely to reflect cellular growth even when the tumour becomes large relative to the organ from which it was derived. The possibility of a more direct method of estimating the part played by a particular hormone in controlling cell growth processes arose with the discovery of specific sites of action of hormones within hormone sensitive cells.

Oestrogen receptors were first identified by Jensen and his colleagues (1969) in uterine and vaginal tissues and subsequently in breast and other tissues. It has been shown that there are at least two types of binding site in the cytoplasm and nucleus of the cells but so far the exact mechanism by which oestrogens react at these sites is unknown.

Oestrogen receptors have been demonstrated in experimental hormone dependent tumours by several groups of workers and such tumours appear to lose their receptor sites as they become progressively less steroid dependent. From these results it appeared likely that the presence of oestrogen receptor sites was necessary for oestrogen sensitivity of tumours so that the estimation of these sites in tumours should give a direct indication of their hormone response. Human breast tumours contain two different oestrogen receptor sites with high and low affinity for oestrogens. The high affinity sites are thought to be involved in the cellular control process whereas the low affinity sites are apparently less specific and may be involved in the steroid transport mechanism of the cell. This lack of specificity may, to some extent, explain why experiments on the hormone uptake of tumours have contributed so little to our knowledge of steroid sensitive tissues. In any event the estimation of specific high affinity oestrogen binding sites should provide a measure of the oestrogen sensitivity of cancer cells. The method of analysis involves the incubation of malignant tissues with radioactive oestrogen (usually oestradiol) of high specific activity and the subsequent separation and estimation of the oestrogen-binding site complex. Using this type of experimental system Jensen and his colleagues (in the press) have found oestrogen receptors in approximately half the primary tumours and 30% of the metastatic tumours examined. In a preliminary study Feherty and Kellie (1971) found high affinity oestradiol receptors in 11 of 15 malignant tumours but none in benign or normal tissues. In a further study Kellie and his colleagues (in the press) have shown that of the 53 biopsies classified as carcinomas, 37 contained high-affinity oestradiol receptors, 2 were borderline, and 14 did not contain any receptor. The proportion of positive results and the range of concentrations were found to be somewhat higher in postmenopausal than in premenopausal patients. Despite detailed examination, no histological feature was found which could explain the variation in receptor concentration; neither could it be accounted for by differences in the cellularity of the biopsies. Of the 41 benign breast biopsies examined only 3 contained any high-affinity oestradiol receptor and in these the concentration was very low. The receptor has not been detected in normal breast tissue. These results are in general agreement with those obtained by Jensen's group and others (including a small number of cases in our own laboratory personal communication, Dr. M. Smethurst). It would have been impressive had there been some sort of relationship between the presence of oestrogen receptors and histological type but this was, perhaps, too much to be expected. Even assuming a relationship between receptor sites and steroid activity, the many histological examinations of tumours carried out over a long period have not revealed a definite relationship between histological type and hormone sensitivity of tumours. As an extension of this approach a study is being done in our laboratory comparing the fine structure of tumours, which are being cultured with and without added hormone, using the electron microscope. It is hoped that changes in fine structure of cells in the presence of hormones can be correlated with the presence or absence of high affinity receptor sites in the tissues. The results are being compared with clinical measurements of the steroid sensitivity of these tumours *in vivo* in collaboration with Dr. G. Edelstyn.

The presence of oestradiol receptor sites in tumour tissues has not, so far, been proved to have a definite bearing on subsequent response to endocrine therapy. These studies do, however, establish a rational basis for the prediction of endocrine therapy which can only be substantiated by long term clinical observation. The main practical difficulty with this type of prediction if performed on the primary tumour is that one must assume that the endocrine response of secondary tumours is the same as that of the primary tumour from which they arise. This is certainly not always true in our experience of certain chemically induced animal tumours and clinical experience suggests that neither is it true for human breast cancer.

V. ADDITIVE THERAPY

A. OESTROGEN TREATMENT

Inoperable or disseminated cancer of the breast was first treated with large amounts of oestrogenic substances by Haddow and his colleagues (1944). This form of treatment has been used mainly for post-menopausal women, but more recently it has been found effective in a limited number of pre-menopausal cases.

1. Post-menopausal Patients

The post-menopausal patient is usually defined as one who is at least five years post-menopausal and has atrophic vaginal smears. Some of these patients obtain quite dramatic and prolonged regression when treated with relatively large quantities of oestrogen. There is apparently very little to choose between the various forms of oestrogen therapy available, but occasionally a particular patient may not tolerate one or other of the synthetic forms of oestrogen.

Assuming that vaginal smears indicate atrophy, large quantities of oestrogen may usually be given, and the longer the free interval the better the chance of successful therapy. Re-calcification of bone lesions is often observed, and lymph node involvement can also be treated by this form of therapy. Hepatic and cerebral metastases rarely respond to oestrogen therapy.

The mechanism of action of this type of therapy is not clearly understood, although it seems likely that pituitary suppression plays a considerable part. The frequency of tumour regression is comparable with that obtained by castration. In general, this form of therapy seems to be about 30 to 40% successful, but much depends on the age of the patient. The older the patient, the greater the benefit.

There has been a great deal of comparative work done on the treatment of breast cancer patients with various hormones. Many of the most convincing results have been obtained by the Co-operative Breast Cancer Group of the Cancer Chemotherapy National Service Centre. It has been the practice to compare oestrogen response with that of androgen or some other form of treatment, and these results will be discussed in the section on androgen therapy.

The administration of large doses of oestrogen can lead to a number of complications varying in seriousness. Hypercalcaemia is the most serious of these, especially in patients with osteolytic metastases. In this case, the treatment must be stopped and large doses of hydrocortisone administered until the serum calcium returns to normal. Inorganic phosphates may also be given under these circumstances. Other less important side effects may include uterine bleeding, stress, incontinence and general fluid retention.

2. Pre-menopausal Patients

In general, large doses of oestrogen are not administered to pre-menopausal patients, but it has been shown that, under appropriate circumstances, oestrogens can produce worthwhile regression in this class of patient. For example, massive doses of oestrogenic hormone were administered to 23-pre-menopausal patients with advanced breast cancer by Kennedy (1962). Seven of these patients showed evidence of a decreased rate of tumour growth. It is suggested that oestrogenic hormones may have a dual action: stimulation of cancer cell growth by small doses of oestrogen, and a more potent inhibitory effect with large doses. Although these effects may exist simultaneously, in some patients the inhibitory effect may predominate and result in tumour regression. In post-menopausal women the inhibitory effects predominate even at moderate doses.

B. ANDROGEN THERAPY

The anti-cancer activity of testosterone was first demonstrated by Loeser in 1938. Since that time this hormone has been widely used for treatment of advanced metastases, and many related compounds have been developed for the same use.

The effectiveness of testosterone propionate on metastatic breast cancer was carefully examined by the Co-operative Breast Cancer Group of the Cancer Chemotherapy National Service Centre (1964a). Patients were chosen who had advancing metastatic breast cancer which had not been previously treated by hormone therapy. All patients were post-menopausal and classified into groups according to their menopausal age. The criterion of objective regression was a 50% decrease in size of lesions at any site in the absence of progression of other lesions. The overall regression rate was 21% and it was shown that patients with breast lesions had a regression rate significantly superior to that of patients with osseous or visceral lesions. There was no difference in the regression rate of patients in the last two groups. There was, however, evidence of the linear trend in regression rate with increasing menopausal age for patients with breast or visceral lesions, but not in patients with osseous metastases. The estimated percentage of survival at twelve months of patients in different categories is: visceral (29%), breast (45%) and osseous (51%). These results are broadly similar to those obtained by several other groups of workers. The most impressive effect of androgen treatment is the recalcification of osteolytic lesions which also gives marked relief of pain to the patient. Local soft tissue lesions and glandular involvement are also effectively treated.

The undesirable side effects of androgens are, again, hypercalcaemia and fluid retention, as in oestrogen treatment. Erythrocythemia is also produced since androgens increase erythropoiesis. Another undesirable side effect is virilization and much work has been done in the hope of discovering a non-virilizing androgen which has comparable therapeutic effects to testosterone.

In order to try to separate the beneficial effects on breast cancer from these regrettable side effects, the Co-operative Breast Cancer Group (1964b) has undertaken a wide screening programme in which some 35 different androstan, androstene, or pregnane derivatives were clinically tested for their therapeutic and non-virilizing properties. They were also compared with a small number of oestrogenic substances. Among the most effective anti-cancer substances tested were: Δ^1 Testoloactone(17-Oxa-D-homoandrosta-1,4-diene-3,17-dione), Fluoxymesterone (Androst-4-en-3-one, 9-fluro-11,17-dihydroxy-17 methyl) and the corresponding 3-one-4,5-Dihydro-2-methyltestosterone or its propionate and several other testosterone derivatives. These compounds at optimal doses appear to have comparable activity against breast cancer. The overall regression rate irrespective of metastatic site was about 20-25%, nor does any particular drug appear to offer any advantage at any one site. However, they have the considerable advantage of being appreciably less virilizing than testosterone. Testololactone in particular has been widely investigated, For example, the European Breast Cancer Group (1962), Segaloff and his colleagues (1962), and it appears to be a most interesting compound for future study. It is also significant that when comparisons were made between these drugs and oestrogenic substances or adrenalectomy, the response to androgen was inferior to either of the other two.

C. ADRENAL CORTICOSTEROIDS

Mention has already been made of the so-called 'medical adrenalectomy' by using large doses of cortisone to suppress adrenal function. Although this treatment is never as effective as adrenalectomy, it is sometimes used after castration to depress the usual adrenal hypertrophy. The drug also has a place in treating patients who suffer from hypercalcaemia and certain other conditions which are less often met with. The use of cortisone itself has been largely superseded by its derivatives hydrocortisone and prednisone or prednisolone.

A study of the long term results of treating patients with advanced breast cancer by using corticosteroids was made by Van Gilse (1962) in an attempt to clarify the effects of treatment which appeared to give clinical responses varying from zero to 50% depending on the individual worker. This author points out that the results so far obtained do not provide proof that corticosteroid therapy can be regarded as 'medical adrenalectomy'. None of the 30 patients with a good response to previous endocrine therapy and remissions which compared to those to be expected from adrenalectomy. There appeared to be no correlation between previous hormone responses and those to corticosteroids. These considerations led the author to conclude the corticosteroids are worthwhile for treatment when other forms of endocrine treatment have been exhausted, or are contra-indicated. They provide comfort in some 80% of patients (40% objective improvement and an equal number of subjective). In 30% objective improvements occurred with regression of more than 6 months, and the longest was a regression of 2 years. For patients not thoroughly treated by other endocrine therapy, corticosteroids may prolong the life of the patient in hypercalcaemic syndrome. This calcium lowering effect must, however, not be confused with the healing of bone lesions.

Although several other studies have been undertaken since, they seem to have added little to the above conclusions. It is possible that such treatments may have special significance in metastasizing tumours of certain specific sites, such as lung and brain.

The main problem in treating patients with corticosteroids is the development of a Cushings syndrome and other effects of hypercorticism. There is also the real danger of irreversible depression of the adrenal cortex or even of the pituitary by prolonged treatment with large quantities of adrenal hormone.

D. PROGESTOGENS

There is considerable evidence that progesterone exerts some control over the growth rate of certain experimental tumours in animals, especially in rat tumours induced by 7,12-dimethyl-α-benzanthracene by the technique of Huggins. There have been a few reports of treating patients with progesterone itself, but there is scant evidence of therapeutic advantage. Some progestogens were tested by the much quoted Co-operative Breast Cancer Group (1964a,b). This group found that progesterone does not cause regression in advancing breast cancer, even though oral doses of 2 g per day were given. This is a very high dose indeed. However, the highly potent agents 17-ethyl-19-nortestosterone and 17-ethynyl-17-hydroxy-estr-5,10-en-3-one at 40 mg/day produced essentially the same rate of objective regression as testosterone propionate, the reference standard. This was so whether the results from testosterone propionate were reported separately by each investigator, or reported by the group as a whole. Because of these regression rates other progestational hormones were studied: 17-acetoxy-6-methylprogesterone (medroxyprogesterone), 17-acetoxy-6-chloro-progesterone, and 17-hydroxyprogesterone caproate. The last two produced no regression.

Despite experiments which indicated that complete absorption of acetoxy-methylprogesterone did not occur when taken orally, a significant number of objective regressions were produced when this agent was tested against testoloactone. It is also interesting that hydroxylation at the 6 and 21 positions has been demonstrated for medroxyprogesterone.

Talley and his co-workers (1961) tested 6-methyl-9-fluro-17-acetoxy-21-deoxyprednisolone, which has both glucocorticoid and progestational activity. This compound has been administered to patients with progressive breast cancer, most of whom had been previously treated by other forms of hormone therapy. Five objective remissions were noticed from 20 patients, all of whom had predominantly soft-tissue metastases. The duration of this remission was from 7 to 15 months in 4 of the patients and these results were thought to be sufficiently encouraging to warrant further trials.

The probable advantage in combination therapy with the progestin and oestrogen has been suggested by Kelley (1966) who also mentioned that, in her experience, medroxyprogesterone has also been disappointing. This latter finding is in agreement with those of the Co-operative Breast Cancer Group.

VI. CANCER OF THE MALE BREAST

Carcinoma of the breast in the male is a rare form of cancer, but seems to metastasize early in the course of the disease, and is therefore a difficult form to control. Also, since the disease is uncommon, it is often difficult to obtain statistically significant results. In general, cancer of the male breast appears in rather older patients than is the case for female breast cancer.

The initial treatment of choice appears to be castration. There are reports of such cases given by Huggins and Taylor (1955), Hermann (1951) and Treves (1957) and by several other workers, most of whom quote only a few cases. Treves in the largest series (42 patients), obtained objective regression in 68% of patients which lasted for an average of 29.6 months. A very small number of adrenalectomies and hypophysectomies have been performed on male breast cancer patients and the results as far as can be judged are somewhat similar to those obtained in the female.

Treatment with large doses of oestrogen has been used by Huggins and his colleagues (1955) and several other groups subsequently, and as far as can be assessed, response seems to be similar to that which might be expected in the case of prostatic cancer. Juret (1966) concludes his interesting review of the subject by quoting the opinion of Huggins that the chances of successful bilateral adrenalectomy in male breast cancer are not far from 100% if the patient is in reasonable condition at the time of operation. This view is in agreement with results obtained by Treves, who demonstrated that hormonal dependence rate in male breast cancer seems to be at least as high as in the female. Useful parallels can be drawn from comparisons between the small number of male breast cancer cases and the much larger number of female cases.

VII. THE IMMUNOLOGICAL TREATMENT OF BREAST CANCER

Much effort has been expended with the hope of treating cancer by immunological means. There is promise in the possibility of immunological interaction in malignancy which must, paradoxically, be viewed against the overwhelming evidence that in man immunity to cancer is not clinically evident. Experiments in animals have shown that neoplastic cells are capable of evoking specific immune reactions in proven isogenic systems. Furthermore in almost all the animal models examined, and in certain human cancers, there is evidence suggesting the existence of tumour-specific antigens. Although these facts are recognized, not all tumours appear to possess specific immunogenicity. It is possible that such supposedly non-immunogenic tumours are, in fact antigenic but induce enhancing tolerogenic and resistance factors which tend to cancel each other out. It follows therefore that treatments designed to utilize a tumour's immunogenicity start with a considerable disadvantage which, although some methods of non-specific activation of the host's responsiveness to the tumour cells are showing promise, has so far proved insurmountable.

In the case of hormone sensitive tumours, however, there is a further possible mode of treatment involving immunological methods. This possibility arises from the classical work of Lieberman and his group who have shown that it is possible to immunize against steroid hormones and by this means inactivate the biological effects of these substances. In particular it has been clearly shown that both exogenous and endogenous oestrogens can be biologically inactivated by antibodies to oestradiol-17β. These workers (Ferin *et al.*, 1968) showed that ewes, immunized with conjugates of 17β-oestradiol hemisuccinate coupled to bovine serum albumin, produce antisera capable of neutralizing the hormone *in vitro* and *in vivo*. The antibodies inhibited the biological effects produced by estradiol administered to immature or mature ovariectomized rats and mice. Furthermore, they prevented uterine weight increases, endometrial stimulation and vaginal cornification due to endogenous oestrogens following treatment with human chorionic gonadrotropin. Pretreatment of intact animals with antisera inhibited the uptake by uteri, pituitaries and ovaries of tritiated oestradiol administered subcutaneously. The antibodies did not inhibit the uterine stimulation caused by administration of diethylstilboestrol. Antibodies to oestradiol did not counteract androgenic effects upon accessory sex organs produced by testosterone administered to immature male rats. Nor did antibodies elicited by testosterone-protein conjugates alter the effects of oestradiol 17β in immature rats. Contrary to anti-oestrogens which act at the target organs, the specific antibodies probably neutralize endogenous hormone in the peripheral blood, and thus provide a means of controlling endogenous hormone, outside of the target organ. The implication of this work to steroid sensitive tumours needs no underlining and techniques based on these experiments are being developed in several laboratories including our own. At present, no clinical application of this work has been forthcoming and presumably a technique having such far reaching implications will need to be approached with considerable circumspection at the human level. This method of treatment, however, if it can be applied to human hormone sensitive cancer, appears to offer an exciting possibility of treating metastatic disease by completely removing circulating steroid hormones from the blood. This might be particularly important in controlling hormones produced by non-specific cells or even perhaps ectopic hormones from the tissues themselves.

It is perhaps of interest to mention another possible method of immuno-logical treatment of invading tumours with relevance to hormone sensitive cancer. This is the technique of immunizing against enzyme systems responsible for tumour invasion. We already know that the tumour host interface is characterized by an increased level of certain hydrolytic and proteolytic enzymes the function of which appears to be the erosion of the host tissues to accommodate the invading tumour. It is possible under certain circumstances to prepare antibodies to some of these systems and preliminary results in this and other laboratories lead us to believe that the possibility exists of controlling invasion by this means (personal communication, R. G. Harris). This would be akin to encapsulating a malignant tumour and so preventing its further spread. It seems that occasionally a potentially malignant growth is naturally controlled in this way; only when the capsule is ruptured does the tumour spread (personal communication, R. W. Raven).

VIII. CONCLUSION

Steroid treatment has chiefly been of a palliative nature and for that reason steroid therapy has been applied to those patients who had already been treated by surgery and/or X-ray therapy, or else those patients with advanced metastatic disease at diagnosis. It is, therefore, often difficult to separate hormonal effects from those of other forms of treatment. Steroid therapy has often been applied only after other curative forms of therapy have failed and frequently disappointing results must also be related to this fact.

In many cases, hormonal treatment can offer increased palliation used in conjunction with potentially curative methods, such as surgery. Sequential steroid treatment of tumours in combination with cytotoxic drugs can often give more marked palliation than when administered simultaneously.

The availability of an increasing number of powerful synthetic substances, which do not have the often distressing side affects of the older hormonal preparations, should allow more effective long-term regimes of treatment to be evolved. The use of such substances will also lead to an improvement in our knowledge of the control mechanisms exerted within the cell nucleus and hence, perhaps, give the key to the hormonal control of cancer. Although steroid therapy is well established in clinical practice the fundamental mechanism by which these hormones exert their effect is still not completely understood. Recent discoveries, such as the recognition of specific hormone binding sites within the cell nucleus have given a new impetus to research on this subject which should in turn lead to a more rational approach to this form of treatment.

REFERENCES

Aitken, E. H. and Preedy, J. R. K. (1956). *Biochem. J.*, **62**, 15p.

Allen, B. J., Hayward, J. L. and Merivale, W. H. H. (1957). *Lancet* **I**, 496.

Atkins, H., Bulbrook, R. D., Falconer, M. A., Hayward, J. L., McLean, K. S. and Schurr, P. H. (1968). *Lancet* **II**, 1255.

Atkins, H. J. B., Falconer, M. A. Hayward, J. L. McLean, K. S., Schurr, P. H. and Armitage, P. (1960). *Lancet* **I**, 1148.

Barker, J. R., Richmond, C. (1971). *Brit. J. Surg.* 58, No. 10, 732-734.

Beatson, G. T. (1896). *Lancet* 2, 162.

Bergenstal, D. M., Hertz, R., Lipsett, M. B. and Moy, R. H. (1960). *Ann. Int. Med.* **53**, 672.

Bishun, N. P., Mills, J. Raven, R. W. and Williams, D. C. (1973). *Acta Cytologia.* **38**, 443.

Bonser, G. M., Dossett, J. A. and Jull, J. W. (1961). Human and Experimental Breast Cancer, Thomas, Springfield.

Brown, J. B. (1955). *Biochem. J.* **60**, 185.

Bulbrook, R. D., Greenwood, F. C. and Hayward, J. L. (1960). *Lancet* I, 1154.

Bulbrook, R. D. and Hayward, J. L. (1967). *Lancet* I, 519.

C.C.N.S.C., Breast Cancer Group (1964a). *Cancer Chemother. Rep.* **41**, Supp. 1.

C.C.N.S.C., Breast Cancer Group (1964b). *J. Amer. Med. Ass.* **188**, 1069.

Cade, S. (1958). *In* 'Endocrine Aspects of Breast Cancer' (A. R. Currie, ed.) p. 2, Livingstone.

Cole, M. P. (1964). *Brit. J. Surg.* **51**, 216.

Dao, T. L. Y. (1957). *Proc. Nat. Cancer Conf. 3rd, 1956*, p. 282. Lippencott, Philadelphia.

Dao, T. L. Y. (1971). *In* 'Proceedings of a Breast Cancer Workshop', (T. L. Y. Dao, ed.), Chicago.

Dao, T. L. Y. and Huggins, C. (1955). *Arch. Surg.* **71**, 645.

Dao, T. L. Y. and Huggins, C. (1957). *J. Amer. Pharm. Assoc.* **165**, 1793.

Eisman, S. H. (1966). *Med. Clin.* **50**, 1457.

European Breast Cancer Group (1962). *Rev. Fr. Etud. Clin. Biol.* **7**, 1067.

Feherty, P. and Kellie, A. E. (1971). *In* 'Some Implications of Steroid Hormones in Cancer' (D. C. Williams and M. H. Briggs, eds.), Heinemann, London.

Ferin, M., Zimmering, P. E., Lieberman, S. and Vandewiele, R. L. (1968). *Endocrinology* **83**, 565.

Forrest, A. P. M. (1965). *In* 'The Scientific Basis of Surgery' (W. I. Irving, ed.). Livingstone, London.

Fracchia, A. A., Holleb, A. E., Farrow, J. H., Treves, M. E., Randell, H. T., Fintbeiner, A. Jr. and Whitmore, W. F. Jr. (1959). *Cancer* **12**, 58.

Gardner, W. U. (1962). *In* 'Biological Interactions in Normal and Neoplastic Growth' (Brennan, M. H. and Simpson, W. L., eds.), p. 391. Little Brown & Co., Boston.

Gardner, B., Thomas, A. N. and Gordon, G. S. (1962). *Cancer* **15**, 334.

Greenwood, F. C. and Bulbrook, R. D. (1959). *J. Endocr.* **13**, 33.

Haddow, A., Watkinson, J. M., Paterson, E. and Koller, P. (1944). *Brit. Med. J.* **II**, 393.

Hall, T. C., Dederick, M. M., Nevinny, H. B. and Meunch, H. (1963). *Cancer Chemother. Rep.* **31**, 47.

Horsley, J. S. and Horsley, G. W. (1962). *Ann. Surg.* **155**, 935.

Hermann, J. B. (1951). *Ann. Surg.* **133**, 191.

Huggins, C. and Bergenstal, D. M. (1951). *J. Amer. Med. Ass.* **147**, 101.

Huggins, C. and Bergenstal, D. M. (1952). *Cancer Res.* **12**, 134.

Huggins, C. and Taylor, G. W. (1955). *Arch. Surg.* **70**, 303.

Huggins, C. and Scott, W. W. (1945). *Ann. Surg.* **122**, 1031.

Jensen, E. V., Suzuki, T., Nimmata, M., Smith, S. and De Sombre, E. R. (1969). *Steroids* **13**, 417.

Joint Committee on Endocrine Ablative Procedures Report, 1, Taylor (1962).

Joint Committee, reported by McDonald (1962).

Juret, P. (1966). Endocrine Surgery in Human Cancers. Thomas, Springfield.

Juret, P. (1968). *In* 'Prognostic Factors in Breast Cancer' (A. P. M. Forrest and P. B. Kunkler, eds.). p. 393, Livingstone, London.

Kelley, R. M. (1966). *Modern Treatment* 4, 778.

Kennedy, B. J. (1962). *Cancer* 15, 641.

Kennedy, B. J. and French, L. (1965). *Amer. J. Surg.* 110, 411.

Kennedy, B. J., Mielke, P. J. and Fortuny, I. E. (1964). *Surg. Gynecol. Obstet.* 118, 524.

Lewison, E. F. (1962). *Obstet. Gynecol. Scand.* 17, 769.

Lewison, E. F. (1965). *Cancer,* 18, 1558.

Loeser, A. A. (1938). *Lancet* I, 373.

Luft, R. and Olivecrona, H. (1953). *J. Neurosurg.* 10, 301.

Luft, R. Olivecrona, H. Ikkos, D. Nilsson, L. B. and Massberg, H. (1958). *In* 'Endocrine Aspects of Breast Cancer' (A. R. Currie, ed.), p. 27, Livingstone, Edinburgh.

MacDonald, I. (1962). *Surg. Gynecol. Obstet.* 115, 215.

McWhirter, R. (1957). *J. Fac. Radiol.* 8, 220.

Pearson, O. H., Limc, McLean, J. P., Lipsett, M. B. and West, C. D. (1955). *Ann. N.Y. Acad. Sci.* 61, 393.

Raven, R. W. (1958). *In* 'Cancer' (R. W. Raven, ed.). Vol. VI, p. 295. Butterworth, London.

Ray, B. S. and Pearson, O. H. (1956). *Ann. Surg.* 144, 394.

Segaloff, A., Weeth, J. B., Meyer, K. K., Rongone, E. L. and Cunningham, M. E. G. (1962). *Cancer* 15, 633.

Talley, R. W., Kelly, J. E., Brennan, M. J. and Vautkevicius, V. K. (1961). *Cancer Chemother. Rep.* 12, 59.

Taylor, S. G. (1962). *Surg. Gynecol. Obstet.* 15, 443.

Treves, M. (1957). *Cancer* 10, 393.

Treves, N. (1957). *Cancer* 12, 821.

Van Gilse, N. A. (1962). *Cancer Chemother. Rep.* 16, 293.

Weisenfeld, S., and Goldner, M. G. (1962). *Cancer Chemother. Rep.* 16, 335.

Williams, D. C. (1965). *Europ. J. Cancer* I, 115.

Wilson, R. E., Crocker, D. W. Fairgrieve, J., Bartholomay, A. F., Emerson, K. and Moore, F. D. (1967). *J. Amer. Med. Ass.* 199, 474.

Wilson, R. E. and Moore, F. D. (1968). *In* 'Prognostic Factors in Breast Cancer' (A. P. M. Forrest and P. B. Kunkler, eds.), p. 399.

Zimmermann, B., Block, H. S., Wiliams, W. L., Hitchcock, C. R. and Hoelscher, B. (1956). *Cancer* 9, 940.

ADRENOCORTICOTROPHIC HORMONE AND THE CONTROL OF ADRENAL CORTICOSTEROIDOGENESIS*

DENNIS SCHULSTER

School of Biological Sciences, University of Sussex, Falmer, Brighton, Sussex, England

1. INTRODUCTION

The functioning of the adrenal cortex and its control by Adrenocorticotrophic hormone (ACTH) is a subject which has attracted a great deal of attention in recent years and many aspects have been reviewed comprehensively. Mention must be made of 'The Adrenal Cortex' edited by Eisenstein (1967) and 'Functions of the Adrenal Cortex' edited by McKerns (1968) both of which contain reviews by many eminent researchers in the field, and document progress up to that time. Articles by Sayers (1967), Garren (1968) and Bransome (1968) are also valuable summaries, while more recent accounts

* Submitted February 1972

(Garren *et al.*, 1971; Gill, 1972) detail important contributions from one laboratory. This current presentation is an attempt to draw together some of the complexities and different ideas relating to ACTH and its acute steroidogenic action, and is not intended to provide a comprehensive survey of the literature. Reference to much important work has undoubtedly been omitted and little coverage of publications after January 1972 has been included (see Note added in proof).

Table 1. *Comparison of structures of adrenocorticotrophins from four different species[a].*

ACTH	H-Ser-Tyr-Ser-Met-Glu-His-Phe-Arg-Trp-Gly-Lys-Pro-Val-Gly-Lys-Lys-Arg
	1 2 3 4 5 6 7 8 9 10 11 12 13 14 15 16 17
	Arg-Pro-Val-Lys-Val-Tyr-Pro(——)Ala-Phe-Pro-Leu-Glu-Phe-OH
	18 19 20 21 22 23 24 34 35 36 37 38 39
	25 26 27 28 29 30 31 32 33
	NH$_2$
	$\mid$
Pig ACTH[b]	Asp-Gly-Ala-Glu-Asp-Glu-Leu-Ala-Glu
	NH$_2$
	$\mid$
Sheep ACTH	Ala-Gly-Glu-Asp-Asp-Glu-Ala-Ser-Glu
	NH$_2$
	$\mid$
Beef ACTH	Asp-Gly-Glu-Ala-Glu-Asp-Ser-Ala-Glu
	NH$_2$
	$\mid$
Human ACTH[b]	Asp-Gly-Ala-Glu-Asp-Glu-Ser-Ala-Glu

[a] From Sayers (1967)

[b] As modified by Riniker *et al.* (1972)

ACTH is the protein hormone having a specific stimulating effect on adrenal corticosteroidogenesis. It is a relatively small protein comprising 39 amino acids (M.W. of porcine ACTH is 4567). The biological activity of the hormone is barely affected by removal of amino acids from the C-terminal end of the molecule numbers 20 through to 39, although loss of even one amino acid residue from the N-terminal end results in virtually complete loss of the hormonal activity. The structures of adrenocorticotrophins from several species (Table 1) have been determined and found to be identical except for a small region of the chain from amino acid number 25 to 33. ACTH is synthesized, stored and released only by the adenohypophysis (although the placenta has also been suggested as a source of ACTH-like protein).

The plasma concentrations of ACTH under a variety of conditions have been evaluated and the data from a considerable number of laboratories have been summarized (Sayers, 1967). The most reliable estimates (Ney et al., 1963) range from 0.04-0.59 mU ACTH/100 ml plasma for normal humans under normal conditions, and in subjects undergoing surgery the level increased to 0.42-1.16 mU ACTH/100 ml plasma. Comparisons of plasma ACTH concentrations in man and rat show that they are quantitatively very similar under a variety of circumstances. The concentration of ACTH in the normal rat under normal circumstances is less than 0.5 mU/100 ml bood and rises to 1 mU/100 ml blood a few minutes after ether anaesthesia and scalding. Even one week after adrenalectomy the ACTH concentration in the rat (maintained on saline without steroid replacement therapy) only increased to 3.2 mU/100 ml blood, and this value was maximally elevated to 10 mU/100 ml blood following ether inhalation and scalding.

Blood-borne ACTH is rapidly inactivated, and in the rat the half-life of endogenous ACTH has been reported as 1 min (Snydor and Sayers, 1953). About 20% of injected ACTH is taken up by the rat kidney, and the liver is another organ that may be responsible for the rapid degradation of the hormone. Because of its short life-span in the circulation and the ability of adrenal tissue to concentrate the hormone, ACTH concentrations found in blood unfortunately give little indication as to the level of ACTH present at its site of action within the adrenal gland.

The adrenal gland has been shown to respond to ACTH in a variety of different ways. Thus ACTH:

(i)   stimulates adrenal corticosteroid formation and content
(ii) increases blood flow-rate through the adrenal
(iii) has a trophic effect and increases adrenal weight
(iv) accelerates adrenal phosphate turnover and hydrolysis of cholesterol esters
(v)   stimulates glycogenolysis and glucose oxidation in the adrenal
(vi) decreases adrenal ascorbic acid, lipid and cholesterol content.

One of the fundamental problems is to what degree these apparently quite different effects are inter-related. In particular when studying the steroidogenic effect of ACTH, it is problematical to what extent this may be dissociated from the other adrenal effects of ACTH. This becomes apparent when data obtained from in vivo studies is compared with that derived by in vitro techniques. The in vivo action of ACTH includes its effect in stimulating blood flow through the gland—an effect which results both in an increased supply of blood-borne components such as steroid precursors, cofactors and oxygen, and in an increased rate of removal of secretion products from the gland. When adrenal tissue or isolated cells are studied using *in vitro* systems, this particular effect of ACTH on blood flow rate is lacking.

The difficulties associated with the complex milieu of the *in vivo* situation may be overcome to a large extent by a variety of *in vitro* procedures. However, it is just this diversity of *in vitro* systems with their wide variation in response, which has led to some confusion in interpreting results obtained with the different *in vitro* procedures. The superfusion system of continuous incubation has been used as a closer approach to the dynamic *in vivo* situation than conventional static *in vitro* incubation procedures, and the characteristics of the adrenal response in the static *in vitro* system have exhibited important differences from those obtained using flowing *in vitro* incubation methods (Saffran *et al.*, 1971; Tait *et al.*, 1970; Schulster *et al.*, 1970).

Although it has proved difficult to obtain an adrenal cell-free system that shows steroidogenic responsiveness to ACTH or adenosine $3'5'$-cyclic monophosphate (cyclic AMP), the adaption by Sato and co-workers of ACTH-responsive murine adrenal cortex tumours to tissue cultures has made a useful system available for examining the effects of ACTH on whole cells (Buonassisi *et al.*, 1962). Several groups have utilized these cells derived from cultured adrenal tumours, in important studies into the biochemistry of ACTH action (Schimmer *et al.*, 1968; Kowal, 1970; Lefkowitz *et al.*, 1970a,b,c; Grower and Bransome, 1970). In recent years techniques have been developed for the preparation of isolated adrenal cells from normal (as opposed to tumour) tissue, using several different enzymic disaggregation procedures (Halkerston, 1968; Kloppenborg *et al.*, 1968; Swallow and Sayers, 1969; Haning *et al.*, 1970; Richardson and Schulster, 1970; Sayers *et al.*, 1971a,b) and these cell suspensions should prove to be a powerful tool in future studies of this nature.

The vascular system of the adrenal gland in man has been elucidated by Dobbie *et al.* (1968) and the following description derives from their studies. The mammalian adrenal is noted for its exceptionally high blood flow rate, and the large volume of blood regularly passing through the gland is carried in numerous small branching arteries that invest and penetrate the capsule. The zona glomerulosa is well endowed with a rich blood supply from a thin sub-capsular plexus and blood passes from this through parallel capillaries between the columns of cells in the zona fasciculata to the plexus reticularis. This latter plexus ends sharply and blood drains by relatively few channels into the sinusoids of the medulla, thence emerging from the gland. The cells of the adrenal cortex in man are plentifully supplied with a fast flowing stream of blood by this fine network of capillaries. By contrast, *in vitro* incubations of adrenal bisects or slices, where medium merely bathes the outer surface of the tissue fragment, are poor substitutes for this *in vivo* situation.

One characteristic of the conventional *in vitro* incubation system is the relatively low corticosteroid output rate observed following ACTH stimulation. This low steroid response, normally not more than 20% of the *in vivo* secretion rate (Tait *et al.*, 1970), may be due to an impaired capacity to remove metabolic products from the tissue fragments, with the consequent accumulation of corticosteroids within the tissue leading to feedback inhibitory effects (Clayman *et al.*, 1970). In addition components of the *in vitro* incubation medium are likely to be relatively inaccessible to the adrenocortical cells within pieces of tissue, again giving rise to a limitation of the steroid response to ACTH. Isolated adrenal cell suspensions, in which medium components are immediately available to every cell, have been used in an attempt to overcome these problems. The sensitivity and magnitude of the response elicited by ACTH in the isolated cell suspension, is particularly noteworthy. Median effective doses for ACTH of 6-120 μU/ml and maximal stimulations of up to 100 times the incubated control values have been reported (Swallow and Sayers, 1969; Sayers *et al.*, 1971a,b; Kitabchi and Sharma, 1971; Haning *et al.*, 1970; Richardson and Schulster, 1970).

II. ACTH RECEPTOR

The concept of receptors originated with pharmacological studies into the selective toxicity of various drugs, and has been developed to explain the specificity of the hormone—target cell interaction. A *receptor site* is visualized as a locus at which a hormone acts on its target cell to effect its particular response(s), and may be regarded as a pattern of forces forming a part of some structural system of the cell. The strength of this force field is such that an interaction (or 'binding') may be envisaged to take place between it and a corresponding pattern of forces associated with the hormone molecule. It is held that during, or as a consequence of, this initial binding, a stimulus results that can ultimately manifest itself as one or more of the hormonal responses. These concepts have been discussed at length by Clark (1937), Scheuler (1960) and Ariens (1966).

As described in the introduction the adrenal cell responds to ACTH in a wide variety of different ways, and a fundamental consideration is whether all these responses derive from a single hormone—target cell interaction or whether there are different ACTH receptors for different responses. Many alternative schemes may be postulated and an interesting discussion of this topic (related to the receptors for sex steroid hormones) has been provided by Baulieu *et al.* (1971).

Using extracts of adrenal tumour cells Lefkowitz *et al.* (1970c) have demonstrated the direct binding of iodinated ACTH to its biologically significant site. Pure monoiodo [^{125}I] ACTH was prepared that was biologically active and free of non-radioactive ACTH, and it was shown that purified extracts of adrenal cells containing ACTH-sensitive adenyl cyclase, also bound [^{125}I] ACTH. The intimate relationship between ACTH-binding and the activation of adenyl cyclase was clearly exhibited during this study, and this is further discussed in Section IV B.

That calcium is required somewhere between the binding of ACTH and the hormone activation of adenyl cyclase, has been demonstrated by Lefkowitz *et al.* (1970b). In the absence of calcium, subcellular cell membrane particles derived from adrenal tumours, were unaffected in their ability to bind ACTH, whereas the ACTH activation of adenyl cyclase was totally inhibited. Following the exogenous addition of high calcium concentrations (2 mM) both ACTH activation of adenyl cyclase and ACTH binding were similarly inhibited. Although the details of the inhibitory action of exogenous calcium have not been elucidated, it has been suggested that as well as affecting adenyl cyclase and its substrate interaction, calcium also acts directly in the interaction between ACTH and its receptor.

Further studies by Lefkowitz *et al.* (1970a) have provided the details for a rapid and sensitive assay for ACTH utilizing a purified extract of adrenal ACTH receptor protein(s) and biologically active [^{125}I] ACTH of very high specific radioactivity. The radioreceptor assay method they have described, promises to be of great value since it has the advantage that, unlike radioimmunoassay procedures, it measures biologically active ACTH. These workers have reported the detection of two orders of receptors with apparent association constants of about 10^{12} and 10^7 respectively, where the high affinity sites represent only about 0.1% of the total receptor proteins. The possibility remains, however that these observations derive from the presence of only one order of receptor and more than one species of [^{125}I] ACTH molecule.

A wide variety of ACTH analogues have been synthesized, and determination of the effect of these synthetic manipulations on the steroidogenic capabilities of such molecules, has been useful in identifying molecular structural features related to particular biological functions. These structure-function studies have demonstrated that only a portion of the total ACTH molecule is essential for steroidogenic activity. Thus although ACTH comprises a single polypeptide chain of 39 amino acid residues (Bell *et al.,* 1956), nevertheless β^{1-20}-ACTH amide (corresponding to the N-terminal end of the ACTH molecule) was found to retain full *in vivo* steroidogenic potency (Hofmann *et al.,* 1962; Lebovitz and Engel, 1964). Using a particulate fraction derived from beef adrenal cortex and a synthetic [^{14}C-Phe] labelled derivative of β^{1-20}-ACTH together with a variety of synthetic ACTH analogues, Hofmann *et al.* (1970) have deduced that major binding sites are located in the C-terminal section of ACTH between positions 11-20 and moreover that the sequence Lys-Lys-Arg-Arg (positions 15-18) is an important binding site of the molecule. On the other hand the biologically active site of the ACTH molecule was attributed to the N-terminal region, between positions 1-10. It was concluded that α-MSH (corresponding to the sequence of the first 13 amino acid residues of ACTH) possesses the functionally important segment of the ACTH structure, but is incapable of stimulating adrenal steroidogenesis since it lacks the receptor binding sites. The protein nature of the ACTH receptor was further indicated by this study. Recently Schwyzer *et al.* (1971) and Seelig *et al.* (1971) have investigated the potency of various ACTH analogues, employing an isolated adrenal cell suspension system, and have concluded that the full complement of amino acids involved in the activation of the ACTH receptor, resides between positions 4-10 of the ACTH structure. A looped conformation for ACTH was postulated with Lys-Val (positions 21 and 22) crossing over Phe-Arg-Trp (positions 7-9).

The ACTH molecule may be coupled to inert polymers such as cellulose, agarose and polyacrylamide and the complex thus produced found to retain the steroidogenic potency of the free hormone. Schimmer *et al.* (1968) have reported that a β^{1-20}-ACTH analogue diazotized to cellulose can stimulate steroidogenesis, following overnight incubations with cultures of adrenal tumours. Similarly a complex of β^{1-39}-ACTH-argarose was found capable of stimulating steroidogenesis in an isolated adrenal cell suspension (Selinger and Civen, 1971). Only in the former study was data provided demonstrating that the biological activity of the complex was not attributable to free peptides liberated from the ACTH polymer; nevertheless the possibility that the free eicosapeptide (β^{1-20}-ACTH) was being released intact from the complex was however not eliminated. Using an isolated adrenal cell suspension prepared by collagenase disaggregation, it has been shown that β^{1-24}-ACTH diazotized to polyacrylamide can stimulate steroidogenesis, and that this biological activity is not due to cleavage of peptides from the complex (Richardson and Schulster, 1971, 1972). These studies demonstrate that ACTH can effect its corticosteroid-ogenic response without entering the adrenal cell, and support the concept of specific receptor(s) for ACTH located on the outer surface of the cell membrane.

The prostaglandins have recently been implicated as playing a role in the mechanism of action of a variety of different hormones (Ramwell and Shaw, 1970). Measurements *in vitro* (Flack *et al.*, 1969) using superfused rat adrenals, showed that prostaglandins could mimic the effect of ACTH in stimulating steroidogenesis. A dose-response relationship has been established between prostaglandins and cyclic AMP formation in the mouse ovary (Kuehl *et al.*, 1970) and kinetic studies suggested the presence in mouse ovary of a single prostaglandin receptor related to luteinizing hormone. The data indicated that activation of this prostaglandin receptor is an essential requirement in the stimulation of cyclic AMP formation by luteinizing hormone, and the possibility that a similar relationship may exist between ACTH and prostaglandin was indicated.

III. CHOLESTEROL METABOLISM IN THE ADRENAL CORTEX

Mammalian adrenal tissue has a well documented ability to synthesize cholesterol from acetate. Nevertheless in some species (e.g. rat and dog) it is clear that blood-borne cholesterol (of hepatic or dietary origin) plays a major precursor role for corticosteroid biosynthesis. Such comparative aspects of the steroidogenic capabilities of the adrenal cortex have been reviewed recently (Vinson and Whitehouse, 1970).

The major pathways and subcellular localization of the enzymes involved in the biosynthesis of adrenal corticosteroids from cholesterol are outlined in Fig. 1. Further details and the various alternative schemes that have been reported, are described in several reviews (Samuels and Uchikawa, 1967; Tchen, 1968; Grant, 1968; Griffiths and Cameron, 1970) and studies involving inhibition of the adrenal steroidogenic pathways have been recently reviewed (Temple and Liddle, 1970).

That the rate limiting step in ACTH stimulated corticosteroidogenesis lies somewhere between the conversion of cholesterol into pregnenolone, was first suggested by Stone and Hechter (1954). However the exact identity of the intermediates involved in the conversion of cholesterol to pregnenolone is still somewhat uncertain. Early work suggested the hydroxylation of cholesterol, firstly at the 20α- and then at the C-22 position, followed by cleavage between C-20 and C-22 to give rise to pregnenolone and isocaproaldehyde (Solomon *et al.*, 1956; Shimizu *et al.*, 1962; Constantopoulos *et al.*, 1966). These studies have been briefly reviewed by Roberts *et al.* (1969) who, using double isotope dilution techniques, have reported the isolation of slightly over 0.5 mg of free and esterified 20α-hydroxycholesterol from 5 kg of bovine adrenal tissue.

Although Koritz and Hall (1964b) were able to confirm the transformation of 20α-hydroxycholesterol into pregnenolone by bovine adrenal acetone powder preparations, they found no accumulation of either 20α-hydroxycholesterol or 20α,22ξ-dihydroxycholesterol following incubation with [^{14}C]cholesterol. Moreover a thorough search (Simpson and Boyd, 1967) failed to prove an intermediary role for 20α-hydroxycholesterol or 20α,22ξ-dihydroxycholesterol.

Recently however Dixon *et al.* (1970) have described the isolation of crystalline 22R-hydroxycholesterol and 20α, 22R-dihydroxycholesterol (1.5 and 2.2 mg/kg of bovine adrenal, respectively). Burstein *et al.* (1970a,b) have established the conversion of cholesterol to 22R-hydroxycholesterol and 20α, 22R-dihydroxycholesterol (without resorting to the use of 'trapping agents') by acetone-dried powder preparations of human, bovine and guinea pig adrenals. Under the *in vitro* incubation conditions used for the conversion of radioactive cholesterol, the production of 22R-hydroxycholesterol was at least 3- to 20-fold greater than that of 20α-hydroxycholesterol and the amount of radioactivity appearing in 20α-hydroxycholesterol was exceedingly small. The detailed kinetic studies on these possible intermediates in the transformation of cholesterol to pregnenolone, have been reviewed (Burstein and Gut, 1971).

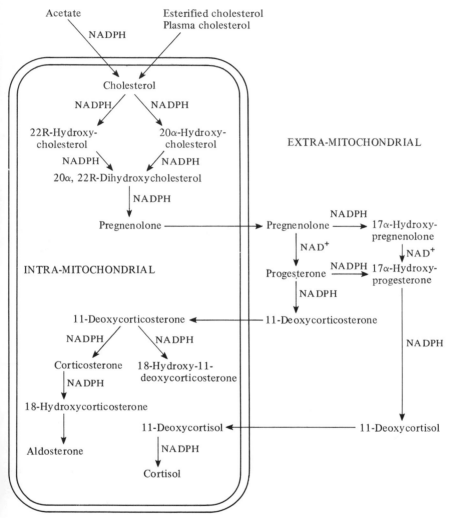

Fig. 1. Major pathways for the biosynthesis of adrenal corticosteroids.

The cholesterol side-chain desmolase activity of the rat adrenal has been measured (Kimura, 1969; Doering and Clayton, 1969) and shown to decline 7–9 days after hypophysectomy to a final level of about 10% of its normal activity. However, the level of the desmolase was observed to fall by only 25% one day after hypophysectomy, whereas the corticosteroid output rate has been shown to decrease two hours after hypophysectomy to about 10% of the ACTH stimulated rate (Garren *et al.*, 1965). It has therefore been concluded that the side-chain cleavage enzyme is not the 'labile protein' postulated by Garren as the mediator of the ACTH response (see Section VII).

As shown in Fig. 1 the cholesterol side-chain cleavage enzyme system and the 11β- and 18-hydroxylases have all been localized within the mitochondria (Halkerston *et al.*, 1961). These enzymes require NADPH and oxygen and have been shown to utilize cytochrome P_{450} as a terminal oxidase (Simpson and Boyd, 1967). The cytochrome P_{450} associated with the side-chain cleavage system has been found to exist predominantly in a high-spin state which may be converted to a low-spin state by pregnenolone (Whysner *et al.*, 1970). The transfer of

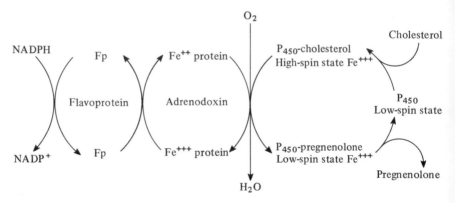

Fig. 2. Possible role of cytochrome P_{450} in the mitochondrial conversion of cholesterol to pregnenolone.

electrons via the NADPH-linked reductase system to the cytochrome P_{450} associated with side-chain cleavage, has been shown to induce a rapid change from high-spin to low-spin states (Simpson *et al.*, 1971). These concepts are outlined in Fig. 2. The change in spin state was attributed to a lower rate of cholesterol transport to the cytochrome P_{450} involved in side-chain cleavage, compared with a relatively fast rate for the oxidation of cholesterol in the high-spin complex.

Boyd *et al.* (1971) have compared the cholesterol side-chain cleavage activity in intact adrenal mitochondria from rats that were either quiescent, or stressed with ether to increase *in vivo* ACTH secretion, and from rats in which ACTH action was inhibited by cycloheximide treatment (see Section VII A). Stress was found to increase the initial rate of pregnenolone formation by a factor of two or three, and the rat adrenal mitochondrial content of high-spin cytochrome P_{450} associated with the cholesterol side-chain cleavage system, was similarly increased. Moreover in the adrenal mitochondria isolated from stressed rats, the initial cholesterol content was lower and more cholesterol was metabolized. On the other hand, 25-hydroxycholesterol (a derivative considerably more hydrophilic than cholesterol itself) was shown to be converted into pregnenolone at a similar rate by adrenal mitochondria from both stressed and cycloheximide treated rats. It was suggested that these data reflect activation of specific steps in cholesterol re-distribution, induced by ACTH.

Shima and Pincus (1969) have examined the role of cholesterol in the biogenesis of corticosteroid by the rat adrenal *in vivo*. Their results suggest that corticosterone is formed rapidly from circulating cholesterol and secreted instantaneously. The data further suggested that the precursor pool may be divided into two compartments, only one of which is dependent upon ACTH, and that ACTH could either increase the availability of sterol precursors to the mitochondrial side-chain cleavage enzyme or expand the size of this precursor pool.

The cells of the zona fasciculata are particularly rich in lipid droplets and the autoradiographic-electron microscopic studies of Moses *et al.* (1969) have demonstrated that the majority of the adrenal cholesterol resides in lipid droplets. When [^{3}H]cholesterol was exchanged with adrenal cholesterol as described in Table 2 and the glands subsequently homogenized and separated by centrifugation into subcellular fractions, most of the cholesterol was detected in the lipid layer, largely in the esterified form. In the mitochondria, microsomes and soluble cytoplasmic fraction (lipid-free) only relatively minor amounts of cholesterol were found, predominantly as the free compound (Table 2). It was further shown in these studies (Garren *et al.*, 1971) that the decrease in adrenal cholesterol content observed following ACTH injection, was explicable in terms of cholesterol ester depletion from the lipid droplet only—no other subcellular fraction exhibited diminished cholesterol content. The prior injection of cycloheximide (an inhibitor of protein synthesis, see Section VII A) has been found to block the ACTH-stimulated decrease in adrenal cholesterol (Davis and Garren, 1968), and as shown in Table 2 (line 8), a significant increase in free cholesterol was found only in the lipid droplets under these circumstances. In further studies that extend these observations, it was reported that the hydrolysis of cholesterol esters to free cholesterol was similarly enhanced by ACTH or dibutyryl cyclic AMP in adrenal gland perfusions (Davis, 1969). Moreover Ichii *et al.* (1970) have reported that in glands from ACTH-stimulated rats the rate of hydrolysis of esterified cholesterol was elevated and that this increase was unaffected by the prior administration of cycloheximide. Adrenals from ACTH-treated rats also showed a decreased rate of esterification of free cholesterol, and the hydrolysed cholesterol was found to be incorporated into the mitochondrial pool of free cholesterol, which was used in corticosteroidogenesis.

These studies from a variety of laboratories thus indicate that ACTH stimulates the production of free cholesterol from the stores of esterified cholesterol within the lipid droplets by a process that is independent of continuing protein synthesis. The locus of cycloheximide action has been defined as lying somewhere in the conversion of cholesterol to pregnenolone (see Section VII A) and Garren has suggested that because cycloheximide allows

Table 2. *Distribution of cholesterol in adrenal glands as determined by differential centrifugation*[a]

Experimental	Cell fraction			
	Homogenate	Lipid droplet	Mitochondria	Soluble
Esterified cholesterol				
Control (12)	696 ± 20	651 ± 30	4 ± 1.0	3.0 ± 1.1
Cycloheximide (6)	706 ± 30	690 ± 25	1.0 ± 0.5	2.0 ± 1.0
ACTH (14)	480 ± 38	430 ± 20	1.0 ± 0.9	3.6 ± 1.1
ACTH + cycloheximide (14)	506 ± 38	480 ± 20	0.6 ± 0.4	2.0 ± 0.9
Free cholesterol				
Control (12)	46 ± 5	7.5 ± 2.0	6.0 ± 2.0	1.2 ± 0.3
Cycloheximide (6)	46 ± 6	6.8 ± 1.0	10.0 ± 2.0	2.0 ± 0.4
ACTH (14)	40 ± 4	4.0 ± 2.0	6.4 ± 2.0	4.0 ± 1.0
ACTH + cycloheximide (14)	124 ± 11	29 ± 2.0	7.5 ± 2.0	2.9 ± 0.4

[a] Values are expressed as micrograms per 25 mg of adrenal. Number of rats is given in parentheses. The rats were hypophysectomized 8–12 hours prior to use. Cholesterol-^{3}H was injected intravenously at least 24 hours prior to performing the experiments in order to radioactively label the adrenal cholesterol. Where indicated ACTH (500 mU) was injected intravenously 90 minutes before the animals were killed. Cycloheximide (10 mg), when used, was injected intraperitoneally 100 minutes before the animals were killed.

After the indicated treatment, the animals were anesthetized with Nembutal the adrenal glands were removed and homogenized. For further details see Garren *et al.* (1971). Copyright by Academic Press. Reprinted by permission of the copyright owner.

accumulation of free cholesterol within the lipid droplets, then synthesis of some protein regulator (or another step inhibited by cycloheximide) is involved in the translocation of cholesterol to the mitochondrion from the lipid droplet. In this respect the presence of a cholesterol-binding protein has recently been demonstrated in heated extracts of acetone dried bovine adrenal mitochondria (Kan *et al.*, 1972). Moreover cholesterol side-chain cleavage in acetone dried bovine adrenal mitochondria was reported to be stimulated by this factor.

IV. ADENOSINE 3'5'-CYCLIC MONOPHOSPHATE (CYCLIC AMP)

There is a considerable body of evidence establishing adenosine 3'5'-cyclic monophosphate (or *cyclic AMP*) as an intracellular *secondary messenger* mediating the actions of a variety of different hormones (Robison *et al.*, 1971). According to this *secondary messenger* concept a hormone is initially secreted by one type of cell and travels to the cells of its target tissue. When contact with these cells is made, it stimulates the internal formation of a secondary messenger. This change in the information content of the target cells is proposed as the essential function of hormones. So far the only secondary messenger that has been identified is cyclic AMP—although others may exist, they have yet to be identified. In addition to the excellent monograph on cyclic AMP by Robison *et al.* (1971) there is also a valuable review by Jost and Rickenberg (1971) covering recent work in this field.

A. HAYNES–BERTHET HYPOTHESIS

The suggestion for involvement of cyclic AMP in the ACTH stimulation of corticosteroidogenesis was prompted initially by the studies of Haynes and Berthet (1957). Their data strongly implied that this effect of ACTH involved phosphorylase activation. Fumarate and $NADP^+$ both stimulated corticosteroidogenesis in homogenates of bovine adrenal cortex. The biosynthesis of corticosteroids requires NADPH at several points in the pathway and Haynes' studies with homogenates suggested that NADPH availability played a key role in steroidogenesis. In the adrenal cortex the enzymes of the pentose phosphate pathway play an active role, and since these enzymes are more abundant than those of glycolysis, Haynes suggested that $NADP^+$ reduction (and hence NADPH availability and steroidogenesis) followed metabolism of glucose-6-phosphate via the pentose phosphate pathway (see Fig. 3). Indications that phosphorylase played a regulatory role came from studies in which it was shown that glucose-6-phosphate and glucose-1-phosphate both stimulated corticosteroid synthesis in homogenates whereas glycogen did not. If however the adrenal homogenates were supplied with exogenously added phosphorylase, then addition of glycogen was found to stimulate steroidogenesis. Credence was given to the importance of phosphorylase when it was further shown that incubation with ACTH increased the activity of phosphorylase contained in bovine adrenal slices, in a manner that correlated entirely with the specificity of the ACTH stimulation of steroidogenesis. At this stage, cyclic AMP had been shown to be involved in the stimulation of liver phosphorylase by glucagon and adrenalin, both of which responses remarkably resembled the activation of adrenal phosphorylase by ACTH. For this reason it was suggested that cyclic AMP might be involved in the ACTH effect. This prediction was supported by studies (Haynes, 1958; Haynes *et al.*, 1959) which showed that ACTH incubated with adrenal slices increased their cyclic AMP content and moreover that cyclic AMP

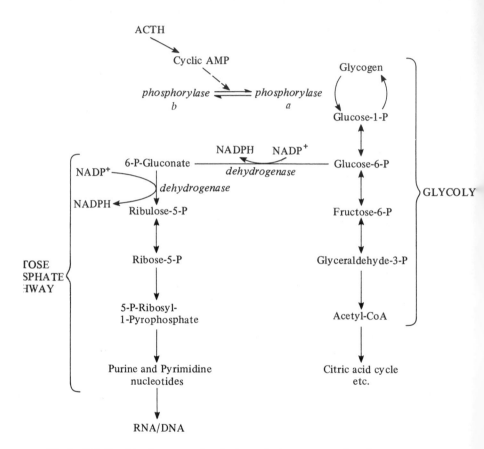

Fig. 3. Relationship between glycolysis and the pentose phosphate pathway. Key regulatory enzymes for the provision of both NADPH and RNA and DNA precursors have been postulated to function in the ACTH steroidogenic response. Such a regulatory role has been suggested both for phosphorylase by Haynes and Berthet (1957), and for glucose-6-phosphate dehydrogenase by McKerns (1968).

incubated *in vitro* with rat adrenal tissue stimulated steroid production. Glucagon and adrenalin were without effect on both adrenal steroidogenesis and cyclic AMP content, although the presence of adenyl cyclase in adrenal homogenates was clearly demonstrated. In this way the adrenal cyclic AMP response showed a specificity similar to that of its steroid synthesizing capacity.

The scheme which evolved from these experiments between 1957 and 1960 is outlined in Fig. 3. It visualized that the presence of ACTH stimulated adenyl cyclase to increase cyclic AMP production which in turn activated phosphorylase and thereby generated more glucose-1-phosphate and glucose-6-phosphate via glycogenolysis. The oxidation of this latter by glucose-6-phosphate dehydrogenase to 6-phosphogluconate, and the subsequent production of ribulose-5-phosphate would give rise to NADPH—the postulated rate-limiting factor necessary for steroid hydroxylation. However this admittedly neat scheme did not withstand the further critical experiments to which it was subjected and subsequent studies have suggested that ACTH and NADPH act to stimulate adrenal steroidogenesis by totally different and independent mechanisms (see Section V).

It was found for example that adrenal tissue maximally stimulated by incubation with ACTH showed an additional increase in corticoid production when glucose-6-P and $NADP^+$ (a NADPH generating system) was added (Koritz and Péron, 1958). Conversely, adrenals maximally stimulated by incubation with glucose-6-P and $NADP^+$, showed a further increase in corticoid production after ACTH addition. Moreover, tissue which had been frozen and was no longer capable of responding to ACTH could be stimulated to increase its steroid production by glucose-6-P and $NADP^+$, a response that was potentiated by Ca^{++}. This stimulation by Ca^{++} or by freezing, however, did not alter the phosphorylase activity of the tissue. It was subsequently shown that ACTH did not actually stimulate phosphorylase activity in the incubated adrenal gland, but merely decreased the inactivation of the enzyme (Kobayashi et al., 1963)—a finding that threw doubt on any obligatory relationship between phosphorylase and steroid synthesis. At the present time, therefore, it appears that although the concept of an intermediary role for cyclic AMP has been given much corroborative evidence, the remainder of the Haynes–Berthet scheme involving stimulation of phosphorylase and provision of NADPH is seen to be inadequate.

B. ADENYL CYCLASE

The level of cyclic AMP within a cell at any particular time is regulated by the activities of at least two enzymes: adenyl cyclase and a specific cyclic AMP phosphodiesterase. The formation of cyclic AMP from ATP is catalysed by adenyl cyclase whilst its breakdown to $5'$-AMP is regulated by phosphodiesterase.

It has been found that the methods used for the homogenization and fractionation of various tissues (e.g. liver and erythrocytes) influenced the sedimentation properties of the adenyl cyclase preparation (Davoren and Sutherland, 1963). The data obtained from these and other studies (Rodbell, 1967; Rosen and Rosen, 1969; Pohl et al., 1971; Cuatrecasas, 1971) have ascertained that for fat cells, rat liver and dog and pigeon erythrocytes, adenyl cyclase is located in the cell membrane.

There is however some doubt as to the cellular location of adenyl cyclase of the adrenal cortex, and to some extent it has been suggested that it occurs at the level of the cell membrane by inference with work on other, more extensively studied tissues. Studies on mouse adrenal tumour cells (Taunton *et al.*, 1969) support this idea since the ACTH responsive adenyl cyclase of these cells was found associated only with particulate fractions. The presence of adenyl cyclase has been found in the low speed centrifugate ('membrane-nuclear' fraction) obtained from homogenates of beef adrenal (Reddy and Streeto, 1968). Similarly in all the crude particulate fractions derived from homogenates of bovine adrenal cortex, adenyl cyclase activity was found (Satre et al., 1971) and purification of the crude mitochondrial fraction was paralleled by a decrease in the activity of associated adenyl cyclase. However this observation was contrary to that of Hechter *et al.* (1969), who found a high adenyl cyclase activity in adrenal cortex mitochondria. Although Satre *et al.* (1971) concluded from their study that the microsomal fraction of bovine adrenal homogenates exhibits the highest adenyl cyclase activity, under the homogenization and centrifugation conditions used, this fraction also contained the highest specific activity of $5'$-nucleotidase (the most commonly accepted marker enzyme for the plasma membrane fraction, cf. Touster *et al.*, 1970), and this data is therefore consistent with a localization at the cell membrane for adenyl cyclase. Further data in accord with this suggestion was provided by Kelly and Koritz (1971) working with bovine adrenal homogenates. The majority of the adenyl cyclase was found in the low speed ($2000 \times g$) pellet and it was shown that the presence of intact cells and nuclei were unlikely sources of this activity.

Considerable use has been made of the adrenal tumour cells originating from Sato's laboratory and Lefkowitz *et al.* (1970c) have used these cells and a disruption procedure under high pressure to prepare a 'solubilized extract' of ACTH-sensitive adenyl cyclase. This extract was further fractionated without separation of its ACTH-binding capacity and its ACTH-responsive adenyl cyclase activity. There was an impressive relationship between ACTH-binding and biological activity for this preparation, from which it was concluded that the binding of ACTH to its biologically significant site had been demonstrated. This study emphasized the particularly close connection between adenyl cyclase and the ACTH-receptor site.

C. PHOSPHODIESTERASE

The methylxanthines such as theophylline and caffeine are noted for their inhibitory effect on cyclic AMP phosphodiesterase, the enzyme that inactivates cyclic AMP by converting it to $5'$-AMP. For many hormones, the potentiation of their effects by theophylline and other methylxanthines has been used as good circumstantial evidence that these hormones exert their effects via adenyl cyclase (cf. Robison *et al.,* 1971, p. 41). In the adrenal, however, previous workers have found difficulty in establishing such an effect on the stimulation of steroidogenesis by ACTH, either in the quartered gland (Halkerston *et al.,* 1966) or in isolated adrenal cells prepared using trypsin and treated with caffeine (Kitabchi *et al.,* 1971) or theophylline (Sayers *et al.,* 1971a). In this latter study it was noted that, in contrast to its effect on ACTH activity, theophylline enhanced the steroidogenic effect of exogenously added cyclic AMP. These studies place some doubt on the hypothesis that cyclic AMP is the sole mediator of ACTH action.

The methylxanthines however have a wide variety of effects other than the inhibition of phosphodiesterase (which inhibition itself requires rather high concentrations). Thus methylxanthines stimulate glycogen synthetase (De Wulf and Hers, 1968), inhibit the adenosine stimulation of cyclic AMP production by guinea pig brain tissue (Kakiuchi *et al.,* 1969; Sattin and Rall, 1970) as well as inhibit adrenal protein synthesis (Halkerston *et al.,* 1966). The latter workers suggested that it was because of its inhibitory effect on protein synthesis that they had found that most concentrations of theophylline inhibited rather than potentiated the ACTH effect on steroidogenesis. This study was confirmed and extended (Bieck *et al.,* 1968) in that the steroidogenic response to cyclic AMP and dibutyryl cyclic AMP was also found to be inhibited by theophylline, again implicating a locus for theophylline action other than at phosphodiesterase. The activity of phosphodiesterase has recently been measured in isolated adrenal cells prepared by trypsin digestion, and found to be very much lower than that in whole adrenal homogenate (Kitabchi *et al.,* 1971). This may in part explain the lack of a stimulatory effect of methylxanthines on the ACTH steroidogenic response of trypsin prepared isolated cells (Sayers *et al.,* 1971a; Kitabchi *et al.,* 1971). It was further suggested that the high sensitivity of this isolated cell suspension to ACTH and cyclic AMP, may be due partly to the low activity of phosphodiesterase in this preparation. It therefore seems that for a variety of reasons these studies do not on the whole provide serious evidence *against* the concept of cyclic AMP involvement.

In other studies it has been reported (Leier and Jungmann, 1971) that cholesterol side-chain cleavage activity was increased after pre-incubation of adrenal halves with theophylline. This stimulation was observed in the absence of added ACTH or cyclic AMP and under incubation conditions during which protein synthesis was not inhibited. Studies *in vivo* (Marton *et al.,* 1971) have demonstrated that in the hypophysectomized rat, both the basal and the ACTH stimulated corticosterone secretion was increased by acute theophylline administration. However Carchman *et al.* (1971) have reported that the isolated cat adrenal perfused *in situ* responded to theophylline (0.5 mM) with increases in both basal and ACTH stimulated adrenal cyclic AMP levels, but corticosteroid release itself, was not further enhanced. In such *in vivo* studies however, which examine the responses of the whole adrenal gland incorporating a heterogeneous cell population, it is possible that cells uninvolved in the ACTH steroidogenic response contribute to the changes in cyclic AMP levels. *In vitro* studies by Szeberenyi and Fekete (1966) reported that theophylline increased the steroidogenic action of ACTH and cyclic AMP. Using isolated cells prepared by collagenase dispersion of rat adrenals, the *in vitro* theophylline potentiation of the ACTH corticosteroidogenic response has recently been demonstrated (Mackie and Schulster, 1973). Employing a dose of theophylline (10^{-3} M) which was without effect on protein synthesis in this system a consistent potentiation of the ACTH effect was found for ACTH doses submaximal for steroidogenesis. Again using collagenase disaggregated adrenal cells, Free *et al.* (1971b) have reported that various phosphodiesterase inhibitors potentiated the stimulation by ACTH or cyclic AMP. The data presented in these studies support the idea that the potentiating effect of theophylline is due (at least partly) to the endogenous accumulation of cyclic AMP.

As a further facet of this tenet, phosphodiesterase activity can be stimulated *in vitro* by imidazole. Moreover since this takes place in whole cells, those hormones which exert their effect via cyclic AMP, should be inhibited by imidazole. Such an inhibitory effect has been shown for a variety of hormonally responsive systems (cf. Robison *et al.,* 1971) and Linarelli and Farese (1970) have shown that the ACTH steroidogenic response of rat adrenal quarters is indeed antagonized by imidazole. However in this study it was found that other processes such as precursor incorporation into protein and RNA were also inhibited, and imidazole must clearly be regarded as a non-specific inhibitor.

Cyclic nucleotide phosphodiesterase from rat adrenals has recently been partially purified (Klotz *et al.*, 1972). Under the experimental conditions employed the phosphodiesterase activity was found predominantly in the 100,000 x g supernatant fraction.

D. EVIDENCE FOR THE INTERMEDIARY ROLE OF CYCLIC AMP

Many workers have now shown that cyclic AMP or dibutyryl cyclic AMP added to the adrenal tissue of various species is able to enhance corticosteroid synthesis in a manner similar to that of ACTH itself (Birmingham *et al.*, 1960; Studzinski and Grant, 1962; Ferguson, 1963; Imura *et al.*, 1965; Karaboyas and Koritz, 1965). The latter study is of importance in that it determined the site in the steroidogenic pathway at which exogenously added cyclic AMP was acting. It was found that this site was at a point between cholesterol and pregnenolone, the same as that previously defined by Stone and Hechter (1954) as the locus of the ACTH effect.

Table 3. *The Effect of ACTH and 3',5'-AMP on the transformation of corticoid precursors to corticoids by rat adrenal and beef adrenal cortex slices.*

Tissue	Precursor	Product isolated	Corrected cpm[a] in product			Ratios	
			Control	+ ACTH	+ 3',5'-AMP	ACTH/ Control	3',5'- AMP/ Control
Rat adrenal	[1-^{14}C]Acetate	Corticosterone	1,000	2,400	2,300	2.4	2.3
	[7α-^{3}H]Cholesterol	Corticosterone	1,330		3,580		2.7
	[7α-^{3}H]Cholesterol	Corticosterone	840	1,880		2.3	
	[7α-^{3}H]Δ^5-Pregnenolone	Corticosterone	2,420,000	2,650,000	3,380,000	1.1	1.4
	[7-^{3}H]Progesterone	Corticosterone	3,900,000	3,900,000	4,380,000	1.0	1.1
Beef adrenal	[1-^{14}C]Acetate	Cortisol	9,600	62,000	83,000	6.5	8.7
	[7α-^{3}H]Cholesterol	Cortisol	3,500	29,200	31,700	8.4	9.0
	[7α-^{3}H]Δ^5-Pregnenolone	Cortisol	770,000	760,000	850,000	1.0	1.1
	[7-^{3}H]Progesterone	Cortisol	890,000	870,000	810,000	1.0	0.9

[a] Calculated as follows: Initial cpm × (constant specific activity/initial specific activity). This gives a measure of the radioactivity in the original sample due to corticosterone or cortisol. From Karaboyas and Koritz (1965). *Biochemistry* **4,** 462. Copyright by American Chemical Society. Reprinted by permission of the copyright owner.

The data provided in Table 3 shows the stimulation by cyclic AMP of the conversion of radioactive precursors to corticosterone or cortisol in adrenal slices from rat or beef respectively. In rat adrenals incubated with either radioactive acetate or cholesterol, the radioactivity in the resultant corticosterone was increased by a factor of about 2.5-fold over the controls, when incubated with either ACTH or cyclic AMP. Similarly in beef adrenal cortex slices, ACTH or cyclic AMP increased the radioactivity in the cortisol product, the effect in this instance being more than 6-fold greater than the corresponding control. However the further metabolism of radioactive pregnenolone or progesterone to corticoids was virtually unaffected by ACTH or cyclic AMP. When adrenals were incubated with $[1\text{-}^{14}C]$acetate the presence of either ACTH or cyclic AMP resulted in a decreased formation of $[^{14}C]$cholesterol (see Table 4), and one

Table 4. *The effect of ACTH and 3',5'-AMP on the formation of $[^{14}C]$cholesterol from $[1\text{-}^{14}C]$Acetate by rat adrenal and beef adrenal cortex slices.*[a]

Tissue	Experi-ment	Corrected cpm in cholesterol		
		Control	+ ACTH	+ 3',5'-AMP
Rat adrenal	1	2.78×10^3	1.26×10^3	0.79×10^3
Beef adrenal	2	260×10^3	63×10^3	62×10^3
	3	51×10^3	22×10^3	15×10^3

[a] From Karaboyas and Koritz (1965). See Table 3 for further details.

(but not necessarily the only) site of action of cyclic AMP was thus identified as lying somewhere between cholesterol and pregnenolone.

The important aspect of the early ideas of Haynes and Berthet is that they provided a stimulus for further experimentation and from this framework many new ideas emanated. Convincing evidence for the intermediary role of cyclic AMP in the ACTH response, has now been provided by Grahame-Smith *et al.* (1967). Using quartered rat adrenal glands it was found that increasing concentrations of ACTH produced increasing concentrations of cyclic AMP whilst steroidogenesis was proportionately stimulated (Fig. 4). Similar results were observed *in vivo* after injecting ACTH into hypophysectomized rats (Fig. 5). Another important observation by these workers was that ACTH increased the cyclic AMP content of adrenal quarters *in vitro* within a minute, and before there was any measurable increase in ACTH-induced steroidogenesis (Fig. 6). Moreover, the relative potencies of ACTH analogues (e.g. α-melanocyte stimulating hormone and N-α-acetyl-α^{1-24}ACTH) in increasing cyclic AMP levels were reflected in their potencies as steroidogenic agents. It was not

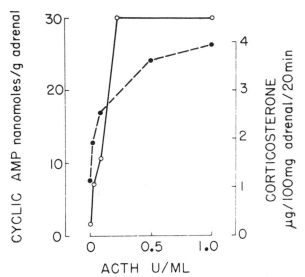

Fig. 4. The relationship between ACTH dose, adrenal cyclic AMP concentration, and rate of corticosterone synthesis *in vitro*. o——o, Adrenal cyclic AMP concentration; ●- - -●, rate of corticosterone secretion into incubation medium. Reprinted by permission of the copyright owner, from Grahame-Smith *et al.* (1967). Copyright by American Society of Biological Chemists.

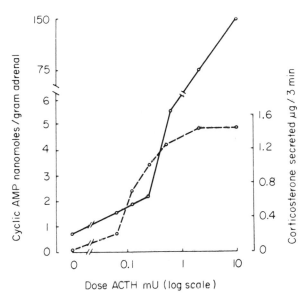

Fig. 5. The effects of various dosages of ACTH on adrenal cyclic AMP levels (o——o) and corticosterone secretion (o- - -o), in hypophysectomized rats *in vivo*. From Grahame-Smith *et al.* (1967) as modified by Robison *et al.* (1971). Copyright by Academic Press. Reprinted by permission of the copyright owner.

possible to dissociate the ability of polypeptide molecules structurally related to ACTH, to stimulate adrenal cyclic AMP, from their capacity to increase steroid synthesis. These studies further suggested that ACTH acted by increasing adenyl cyclase activity rather than by inhibiting the phosphodiesterase.

A system that has provided valuable information on the control of adrenal function is the *in vitro* superfusion technique (Orti *et al.*, 1965, Tait *et al.*, 1967

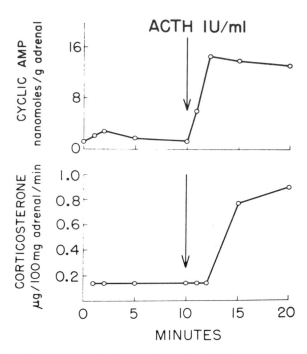

Fig. 6. The time course of changes in cyclic AMP concentration and rate of corticosterone synthesis in rat adrenal, when ACTH is added to the incubation at the point indicated by the arrow to give a final concentration of 1 unit per ml of incubation medium. Reprinted by permission of the copyright owner from Grahame-Smith *et al.* (1967). Copyright by American Society of Biological Chemists.

and Saffran *et al.*, 1967). In this system for continuous incubation, adrenal glands are incubated in medium that is continuously infused and withdrawn, allowing dynamic study of the factors regulating *in vitro* adrenal corticosteroidogenesis. Conventional static *in vitro* incubation procedures, allow the accumulation in the medium of metabolic products with the consequent possibility of feedback effects. Thus corticosterone inhibits protein synthesis in the adrenal gland (Morrow *et al.*, 1967). Ferguson *et al.* (1967) have shown that *in vitro* incorporation of precursors into rat adrenal protein and RNA fractions was inhibited by corticosterone (30 μM) and build up of this product in the medium

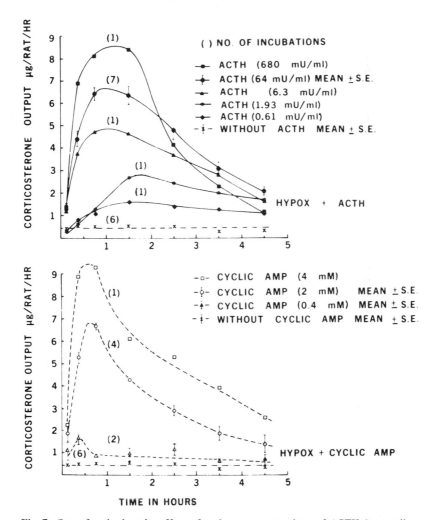

Fig. 7. Superfused adrenals: effect of various concentrations of ACTH (upper diagram: 0.61-680 mU/ml medium) and cyclic AMP (lower diagram 0.4-4.0 mM) on corticosterone output rate by decapsulated adrenals from rats 3 hr. after hypophysectomy. From Schulster *et al.* (1970). Reproduced by permission of the copyright owner.

may well affect the ACTH control processes. Dynamic *in vivo* studies avoid this particular problem. Nevertheless the complexity of the *in vivo* situation allows feedback inhibitory effects via the pituitary-adrenal endocrine system, and other side-effects such as the established influence of ACTH on adrenal blood flow (Porter and Klaiber, 1964, 1965) may confuse the picture. Moreover since it is only possible to examine the whole gland, responses of different adrenal zones or cell types cannot be studied *in vivo*. The *in vitro* continuous superfusion system overcomes these limitations and although several modifications to the original apparatus have been described (Schulster *et al.*, 1970; Pearlmutter *et al.*, 1971) the basic concept remains that of bathing the tissue in a flowing stream of oxygenated buffer solution, that continuously removes the metabolic products. Various stimulants or inhibitors etc. may be infused into the medium and these additional infusions may be started or stopped at any time during superfusion.

Continuous infusions of different doses of cyclic AMP and ACTH to superfused adrenal tissue resulted in the corticosterone output curves depicted in Fig. 7. In this study decapsulated adrenals were used, consisting of zona fasciculata-reticularis and medulla, from rats hypophysectomized 3-4 hours previously, several observations may be made from these data. Firstly, although these were all *continuous* infusions of ACTH or cyclic AMP, the corticosterone output rate rose rapidly to a maximum and then declined for all doses used. This characteristic output curve obtained by continuous ACTH infusion was reproduced by continuous infusion of cyclic AMP. For example the decay half-life of the output curve after the early maximum point was calculated to be 102 minutes for ACTH (64 mU/ml), compared with 106 minutes for cyclic AMP (2 mM). It was apparent that continuous infusion of ACTH was capable of sustaining its effect for a rather longer period of time than an equipotent dose of cyclic AMP. Nevertheless the rates of decline were virtually the same after the first hour of these doses of ACTH and cyclic AMP and this implies that the factor(s) regulating the declining corticosterone output during later time periods of superfusion are similar for both stimulators (see Section VII C). Another important aspect that may be observed from these data (Fig. 7) is that cyclic AMP, at each dose studied, exerted its maximum steroidogenic effect earlier than an equivalent dose of ACTH. If the ACTH steroidogenic effect is indeed mediated via the obligatory involvement of cyclic AMP, then it is essential to demonstrate that the kinetics of the response accord with this concept. It was found that 2 mM cyclic AMP elicited the same maximum steroidogenic response rate as 64 mU ACTH/ml, and the same total corticosterone output as 6.3 mU ACTH/ml. From the data given in Fig. 8, it may be seen that at the earlier time intervals the superfused adrenal shows a greater response to this dose of cyclic AMP than to either of the above ACTH concentrations. It should be noted that the concentration of ACTH or cyclic AMP in the medium was rapidly elevated to the required value by the addition of appropriate quantities of these compounds at the beginning of the superfusion. The results obtained from this study of the dynamic characteristics of the adrenal response are consistent with the concept of an intermediary role for cyclic AMP in the ACTH effect, and therefore provide additional strong support to the evidence in favour of this idea.

Other studies using the superfused adrenal, have described the effect of cycloheximide—a known protein synthesis inhibitor (Fig. 18, for details see

Section VII) on the ACTH or cyclic AMP induced response. For a variety of circumstances, it was shown that the dynamics of the ACTH and the cyclic AMP response, were both affected in a very similar fashion by infusions of cycloheximide. Again it was found that exogenously added cyclic AMP mimicked the characteristics of the steroidogenic stimulation by ACTH, and that the data supported the idea of a steroidogenic response to ACTH regulated via cyclic AMP.

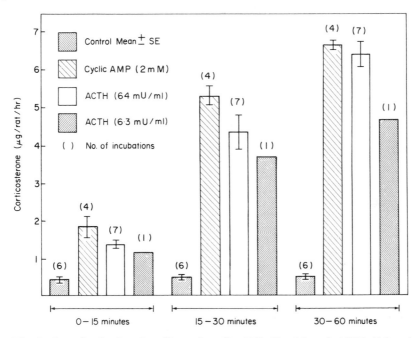

Fig. 8. Superfused adrenals: effect of cyclic AMP (2 mM) and ACTH (6.3 and 64 mU/ml) on corticosterone output rate by decapsulated adrenals from rats 3 hr after hypophysectomy. Corticosterone was assayed in superfusate collected over 0–15, 15–30 and 30–60 min. (For experimental details confer Fig. 7.)

In accord wth the earlier observation by Birmingham and Kurlents (1958), superfusion studies by Pearlmutter et al. (1971), have shown that it is the total dose of ACTH presented to the adrenal, rather than the concentration of the hormone that modulates its response. This observation is consistent with the tenet of an adrenal cell receptor as the initial site of action of ACTH, since effectively all available molecules of the hormone would be bound by a receptor protein of high binding-affinity, until saturation of all the available receptor sites. The response to N^6, O^2-dibutyryl adenosine $3',5'$-cyclic monophosphate (dibutyryl cyclic AMP) was, like that to ACTH, dependent upon the total dose.

In contrast, the overall steroidogenic response of the superfused adrenal to cyclic AMP was concentration dependent. Dibutyryl cyclic AMP is noted for its ability to stimulate adrenal steroidogenesis at 30- to 50-fold lower concentrations than cyclic AMP itself (Sayers *et al.*, 1971a; Kitabchi and Sharma, 1971; Free *et al.*, 1971a, see Fig. 9). This has been ascribed to a decrease in the permeability barriers of the adrenal cell membrane by this lipophilic derivative of cyclic AMP, so that more of the added dibutyryl cyclic AMP actually enters the cell. Alternatively, since cyclic AMP phosphodiesterase does not hydrolyse the dibutyryl derivative, all of the latter which actually manages to penetrate into

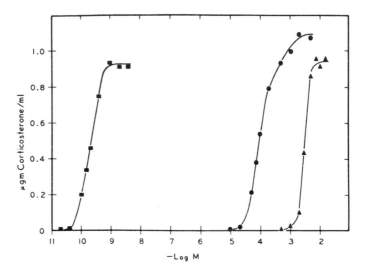

Fig. 9. Corticosterone secretion by isolated rat adrenal cells in response to ACTH (■), dibutyryl-cAMP (●) and cAMP (▲). All points represent individual incubations within a single experiment. Reprinted by permission of the copyright owner from Free *et al.* (1971a). Copyright by the American Chemical Society.

the cell, is at liberty to affect the steroidogenic control system. Regardless of whether both or either of these explanations is true, it follows that the concentration of dibutyryl cyclic AMP inside the cells will eventually approach that in the extracellular medium, thus neither explanation satisfactorily accounts for the observed adrenal response to dibutyryl cyclic AMP being dependent upon the total dose as opposed to the concentration. It has been suggested instead, that the dibutyryl cyclic AMP penetrating into the adrenal cells remains trapped inside, possibly by conversion to a (protein-bound?) form that is unable to leak out of the cell. The consequent intracellular binding of dibutyryl cyclic AMP would account for the similarity of its dose-response characteristics to those of ACTH. (Pearlmutter *et al.*, 1971.)

As noted previously, the *in vitro* cyclic AMP response was dependent upon the concentration of this nucleotide, rather than upon the total dose as was found for ACTH (Saffran *et al.*, 1971). It has been suggested that this discrepancy between the behaviour of ACTH and cyclic AMP arises from the binding capabilities of the adrenal cell, in that whereas ACTH is bound with high affinity (Lefkowitz *et al.*, 1970a) and the cell is efficiently able to take up all the available hormone, cyclic AMP is not bound and penetrates adrenal cells with difficulty. In this case, the rate of penetration of cyclic AMP into the cell and its consequent steroidogenic potency would be proportional to its concentration in the surrounding medium.

The potency of exogenously added cyclic AMP may be compared with the effect of ACTH on cyclic AMP production by isolated cells prepared by collagenase disaggregation of decapsulated rat adrenal glands. For the cells equivalent to one adrenal (contained in 1 ml of medium), ACTH (10 mU) stimulated the production of about 10^{-10} moles of cyclic AMP (Mackie *et al.*, 1972) and was comparable in steroidogenic capacity with 5×10^{-6} moles of exogenously added cyclic AMP (Richardson and Schulster, 1972). Even when allowance is made for the minute volume in which intracellular cyclic AMP is contained there is still a large discrepancy between the effectiveness of endogenously produced and exogenously added nucleotide. This could be a reflection of the impermeability of the adrenal cell membrane to cyclic AMP.

Careful studies using isolated adrenal cells prepared using trypsin (Beall and Sayers, 1972) and more recently those prepared via a collagenase disaggregation procedure (Mackie *et al.*, 1972) have examined both the dose-response characteristics and the time-course relationships following ACTH addition and the consequent cyclic AMP and corticosterone accumulation. Whereas corticosterone accumulation showed a time-lag of 3 minutes, cyclic AMP levels increased within 1 minute of adding ACTH. The data from these studies using isolated cells are entirely consistent with the contention that cyclic AMP is a mediator of ACTH stimulated steroidogenesis in the adrenal.

E. CYCLIC AMP RECEPTOR PROTEIN AND CYCLIC AMP-DEPENDENT PROTEIN PHOSPHOKINASE

The existence in adrenal cells of a cyclic AMP binding compound, has been demonstrated by the studies of Gill and Garren (1969). Subcellular fractions obtained from bovine adrenal cortex, were examined for binding of tritiated cyclic AMP, using equilibrium dialysis to separate the unbound from the bound material. The microsomal fraction and the soluble cytoplasm showed the greatest binding of radioactivity per ng protein, although binding activity was observed in all subcellular fractions. Further fractionation of the microsomes has shown that the microsomal cyclic AMP binding activity is associated predominantly with the endoplasmic reticulum rather than with free ribosomes (Table 5: Walton *et al.*, 1971). Trypsin, protease and heating to 50°C all inactivated the [^{3}H] cyclic AMP binding substance found in the microsomes and soluble cytoplasm, whereas ribonuclease and deoxyribonuclease were without effect. The protein nature of the cyclic AMP binding material indicated by these studies, has been confirmed following its purification (Gill and Garren, 1971).

The binding affinity of the receptor has been examined (Gill and Garren, 1969). A plot of cyclic AMP bound against the ratio of bound over unbound cyclic AMP exhibited a linear relationship, and a single type of noninteracting

Table 5. *Protein kinase and cAMP binding in adrenal cortex fractions*[a]

Fraction	RNA/ protein ratio	^{32}P Incorporation (nmol/mg per min.)	cAMP binding (pmol/mg)
Postmitochondrial supernatant	–	0.48	2.9
Soluble	–	0.25	2.7
Microsomes, 1st wash	–	0.43	2.5
Microsomes, 2nd wash	–	0.37	2.1
Microsomes, 3rd wash	–	0.36	2.0
Smooth membrane	0.06	0.73	3.2
Rough membrane	0.16	0.46	1.7
Free ribosomes	0.56	0.09	0.5

[a]From Walton *et al.* (1971). *Proc. Nat. Acad. Sci.* **68**, 880. Reprinted with permission.

binding site was suggested. The measured binding constant K_a was approximately 5×10^{-8} and the molarity of the binding sites was estimated at 1×10^{-7}. However at high concentrations of cyclic AMP (10^{-4} M), additional binding sites were demonstrable.

Receptor bound [^{3}H] cyclic AMP was released following trichloroacetic acid precipitation or boiling, and all the unbound radioactive material thus obtained, behaved chromatographically like cyclic AMP. It was concluded that the cyclic AMP was not metabolized or covalently associated with the receptor protein. Further studies have characterized the specificity of the receptor protein for cyclic AMP by determining the ability of several nucleotides to compete with [^{3}H] cyclic AMP for binding sites on the protein. Other cyclic 3'5'-nucleotides (cyclic IMP, cyclic GMP and cyclic CMP) were found to be very much less efficient than cyclic AMP in competing for binding sites on the receptor although they did definitely bind (Walton and Garren, 1970).

Associated with cyclic AMP receptor protein, a protein kinase has been found in the soluble cytoplasmic fraction derived from adrenal cortex tissue. The enzymic activity of this protein kinase was stimulated by cyclic AMP, and the enzyme catalyzed the phosphorylation of exogenously added histone, protamine and phosphorylase kinase, as evidenced by the incorporation of $[^{32}P]$ into protein, using $[\gamma\text{-}^{32}P]$ ATP as substrate (Gill and Garren, 1970). That this type of cyclic AMP dependent protein kinase activity was not restricted to the adrenal cell, had been previously demonstrated by studies on skeletal muscle (Walsh *et al.,* 1968) and liver (Langan, 1968) employing similar protein substrates. It was found using saturating concentrations of histone as the exogenously added substrate, that increasing concentrations of cyclic AMP stimulated the protein kinase activity with a half maximum stimulation (K_m) of 1.4 $\times$ 10^{-8} M cyclic AMP, and that saturating levels of the nucleotide stimulated kinase activity about 4-fold above the control value observed in the absence of cyclic AMP.

In both its subcellular distribution and nucleotide specificity, the cyclic AMP-dependent protein kinase has been shown to be very similar to the cyclic AMP-receptor protein (Walton *et al.,* 1971, Gill and Garren, 1970). As previously described for the receptor protein, protein kinase activity was located in adrenal microsomes as well as the soluble cytoplasmic fraction of the cell. Further fractionation of the microsomes also demonstrated that the endoplasmic reticulum, as opposed to the free ribosomes, retained most of the cyclic AMP dependent protein kinase (Table 5). Despite repeated washing both cyclic AMP-receptor and protein kinase activities remained in the microsomal fraction. Moreover treatment of the endoplasmic reticulum with sodium deoxycholate (0.25%) concomitantly solubilized cyclic AMP-receptor and protein kinase activities, and at 0.5% concentration the detergent inhibited 72% and 24% of the kinase and receptor activities respectively. As a consequence of this observed association of both receptor and kinase activities in the endoplasmic reticulum, it has been suggested that they exist together in this organelle in a unified regulatory complex.

Examination of a partially purified preparation of protein kinase from the soluble fraction has revealed the same nucleotide specificity as was found for the cyclic AMP-receptor (Gill and Garren, 1970). Furthermore, when the activities of receptor protein and protein kinase were compared during the course of a variety of protein purification procedures, including pH precipitation, calcium phosphate gel absorption, precipitation with ammonium sulphate and sedimentation in a sucrose gradient, it was found that both activities were enriched in parallel.

That the cyclic AMP-receptor and protein phosphokinase exist together in a

complex has been demonstrated by its sedimentation as a single front in the
analytical ultracentrifuge, as well as by its migration as a single band containing
both activities after polyacrylamide gel electrophoresis (Gill and Garren, 1971).
The incubation of receptor-kinase complex with cyclic AMP prior to electrophoresis caused dissociation of the cyclic AMP-bound receptor from the
activated kinase. This dissociated cyclic AMP-bound receptor migrated identi-
cally with purified receptor (obtained following chromatography on DEAE-
cellulose) instead of migrating with the protein kinase as before. The kinase thus
activated was shown to be free of cyclic AMP-receptor activity and no longer

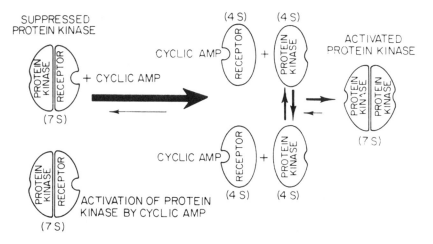

Fig. 10. Hypothetical model for the activation of protein kinase by cyclic AMP. Cyclic
AMP in binding to the receptor caused an allosteric change in the protein that results in the
dissociation of the receptor moiety from the protein kinase, thereby activating the enzyme.
The protein kinase-receptor complex sedimented at 7S; the binding of cyclic AMP to the
receptor resulted in the sedimentation of the receptor at 4S. When protein kinase is not
observed at 4S, even after the addition of cyclic AMP, it is proposed that protein kinase
molecules, in the active state, associated in a 7S complex. (From Garren *et al.,* 1971).
Reproduced with permission. Copyright by Academic Press.

responded to the nucleotide. The phosphokinase was similarly activated when
the receptor protein was differentially denatured by heating. Moreover, addition
of increasing amounts of purified receptor protein to protein kinase was found
increasingly to suppress the kinase activity, while cyclic AMP completely
overcame the suppression. From these studies the model depicted in Fig. 10, was
suggested as an explanation for the cyclic AMP stimulation of protein kinase
activity. The cyclic AMP receptor protein is envisaged as a repressor of the
protein kinase; when complexed with the kinase it inhibits the activity of the
enzyme. Cyclic AMP in binding to the receptor protein, causes the receptor to
release the kinase which is thereby fully activated.

One difficulty in interpreting this data arises from the observation by Butcher that control cyclic AMP levels in adrenal tissue are about 10^{-6} M (Grahame-Smith *et al.*, 1967) with K_a for the receptor protein and K_m of the phospho-kinase both about 10^{-8} M (Gill and Garren, 1970). The endogenous levels of adrenal cyclic AMP are therefore 100 times higher than the K_a and K_m values of the receptor and the kinase. Consequently the receptor should be fully saturated

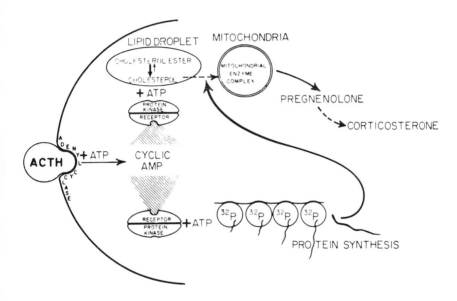

Fig. 11. Hypothetical model of the mechanism of action of ACTH in the adrenal cortical cell (from Garren *et al.*, 1971). ACTH activates adenyl cyclase on the plasma membrane, catalysing the formation of cyclic AMP. The nucleotide becomes bound to the receptor and activates protein kinase which catalyses the phosphorylation of a ribosomal moiety, thereby modulating the translation of stable mRNA(s). This results in the induction of the regulator-protein which, by an unknown mechanism, facilitates the translocation of cholesterol from the lipid droplet to the mitochondrion. Cyclic AMP is also postulated to activate the hydrolysis of cholesterol esters to free cholesterol by a mechanism involving the activation of protein kinase. Reproduced with permission. Copyright by Academic Press.

with cyclic AMP and the phosphokinase fully active, all the time. One explanation of this dilemma is that there are different pools of cyclic AMP with compartmentalization within the cell.

Recently Walton *et al.* (1971) have demonstrated that the cyclic AMP dependent phosphokinase described above catalysed the incorporation of $[^{32}P]$ from $[\gamma-^{32}P]$ ATP into protein tightly associated with ribosomes. This ribosomal phosphorylation was postulated to modulate the translation of stable mRNA as described in Fig. 11.

V. THE INVOLVEMENT OF NADPH IN ACTH ACTION

A. GLUCOSE-6-PHOSPHATE DEHYDROGENASE

The early work related to this aspect has been reviewed by Hilf (1965) and although the bulk of currently available evidence is against the original scheme of Haynes and Berthet involving activation of phosphorylase, nevertheless, some workers still maintain that NADPH availability is a rate limiting factor for steroidogenesis. A very large number of the enzymes involved in steroidogenic pathways are known preferentially to require NADPH as a cofactor and therefore at least on the face of it, this seems a very reasonable supposition. McKerns (1964) has suggested that ACTH itself binds to a receptor site(s) on the glucose-6-phosphate dehydrogenase molecule contained within adrenal cells, causing a conformational change in the enzyme and thereby leading to enhanced $NADP^+$ reduction. Using a crystalline preparation of glucose-6-phosphate dehydrogenase obtained from bovine adrenal cortex Criss and McKerns (1968) have found that ACTH reduces the apparent K_m for both $NADP^+$ and glucose-6-phosphate. From his studies McKerns visualizes a central role for glucose-6-phosphate dehydrogenase in steroidogenesis whereby ACTH activates this enzyme to increase production of not only NADPH but also pentose phosphates which may function as precursors of nucleotides for RNA and DNA synthesis (see Fig. 3).

This concept of ACTH action is difficult to accept. The experimental methods available are limited and difficult to duplicate. Measurements of the activities of the enzymes in the pentose phosphate pathway following ACTH stimulation have produced conflicting results depending upon the methods used. Later studies do not support the concept of NADPH or $NADP^+$ direct involvement in the ACTH steroidogenic effect. Although the rat adrenal cortex contains large amounts of pyridine nucleotides, it was found (Harding and Nelson, 1964a) that there was no alteration in NADPH or $NADP^+$ content several days after hypophysectomy, even though adrenal steroid output was dramatically reduced within minutes. Moreover although a variety of enzymes which might be involved in NADPH generation were studied (e.g. glucose-6-phosphate dehydrogenase, 6-phosphogluconic dehydrogenase, isocitric dehydrogenase, pyridine nucleotide transhydrogenases etc.) none of their activities showed any significant early decline (Harding and Nelson, 1964b). Neither did ACTH exhibit any effect on glucose-6-phosphate dehydrogenase nor 6-phosphogluconic dehydrogenase (Kuhn and Kissane, 1964). Examination of adrenal mitochondria obtained from normal, hypohysectomized and ACTH-treated rats has revealed similar ratios for the pyridine nucleotide content of the various cell fractions (Péron and McCarthy, 1968).

These studies suggest that NADPH is not a rate-limiting factor for steroid hydroxylation and corticosteroidogenesis, since no significant change in the extra- or intramitochondrial NADPH levels was detected.

B. EXOGENOUS NADPH

As far as the ACTH control system is concerned, the relevance of experiments demonstrating the steroidogenic effect of exogenously added NADPH is now entirely questionable. Intact cells are likely to be impermeable to such a polar compound (Lehninger, 1951) and Tsang and Carballeira (1966) have shown that enzymes leak into the medium during *in vitro* incubation of adrenal tissue. It was indicated that the effect of exogenous NADPH was upon these liberated enzymes. Furthermore, Halkerston (1968) has incubated adrenal slice preparations with trypsin and found that the steroidogenic effect of NADPH was markedly reduced, whereas the tissue remained fully responsive to ACTH. (The ACTH responsiveness of trypsinized adrenal tissue was if anything enhanced.) It has been concluded that NADPH stimulated the activity of the damaged cells only and that these cells were eliminated by the proteolytic enzyme, leaving only the ACTH responsive cells. Consequently if the stimulation of steroidogenesis by NADPH occurs only in damaged cells, it would therefore seem to have little or no bearing on the physiological mechanism of action of ACTH *in vivo*.

Nevertheless, the role of NADPH is still in some respects an open question. Although it has not been possible to show an increase in NADPH levels in response to ACTH, it could be that a steroidogenically important increase in intramitochondrial NADPH may represent an insignificant net change in total cellular $NADP^+/NADPH$ ratios. It has been proposed that ACTH may be stimulating the malate shunt and thereby affecting the overall transport of reducing equivalents from the cytoplasm into the mitochondrion. Although this concept may be feasible for the bovine adrenal where the existence of the malate shunt has been substantiated (Simpson and Estabrook, 1968), this mechanism would not appear to be feasible for the rat adrenal where the malate shunt is absent (Péron and Tsang, 1969).

Using the trypsinized adrenal tissue preparation described by Halkerston (1968), Garren *et al.* (1969) have found that when the ACTH stimulated steroidogenesis was inhibited by cycloheximide, a noted protein synthesis inhibitor, (see Section VII A) then the addition of NADPH had no effect. However if the trypsinized tissue was briefly sonicated, then NADPH markedly stimulated corticosterone synthesis and this stimulation was not affected by the presence of cycloheximide. On the other hand the ACTH-responsiveness and attendant sensitivity to cycloheximide of these cells was abolished. Again it may be concluded that the effect of exogenous NADPH is unrelated to the control system regulated by ACTH.

VI. THE REGULATION OF PREGNENOLONE SYNTHESIS

A. KORITZ-HALL HYPOTHESIS

In recent years the concept has gained support that ACTH controls steroid-ogenesis (via the intermediary action of cyclic AMP) by affecting the permeability of the mitochondrial membrane. The enzymes concerned in corticosteroid biosynthesis are found partly inside and partly outside the mitochondrion (Fig. 1). In particular the enzymes involved in the conversion of cholesterol to pregnenolone are intramitochondrial, whereas those involved in the further conversion of pregnenolone to 11-deoxycortisol or 11-deoxycorticosterone are cytoplasmic. Hence it would seem that pregnenolone synthesized inside the mitochondria must traverse the mitochondrial membrane before it can be further utilized as a corticosteroid precursor. Studies on isolated mitochondria (Koritz, 1968) have suggested that ACTH (via cyclic AMP) has its

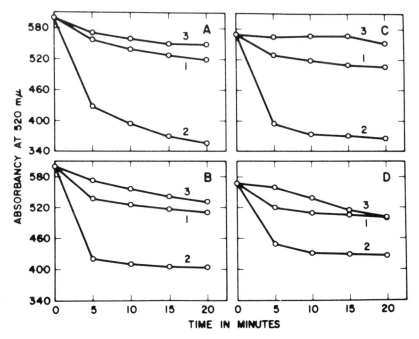

Fig. 12. ATP inhibition of swelling of adrenal mitochondria induced by several agents. In all cases curve 1 is the control and curve 2 represents the action of the swelling agents alone. These agents are: A, pronase, 2 mg; b, sodium lauryl sulfate, 1×10^{-4} M; C, palmitic acid, 1×10^{-4} M; D, myristic acid, 1×10^{-4} M. Curve 3 represents the swelling agent + ATP at a concentration of 2.4×10^{-2} M in A, and 3.6×10^{-2} M in the remaining experiments. Reproduced from Hirshfield and Koritz (1964). Copyright by the American Chemical Society. Reprinted by permission of the copyright owner.

effect at the level of the mitochondrial membrane thereby facilitating exit of pregnenolone. It may be seen from the data given in Table 6 and Figs 12 and 13, that a variety of agents such as Ca^{++}, myristic, oleic and palmitic acids, cause swelling of isolated mitochondria and that those agents capable of causing mitochondrial swelling also stimulate pregnenolone synthesis. Furthermore it was shown that if the mitochondrial swelling was inhibited by ATP, there was

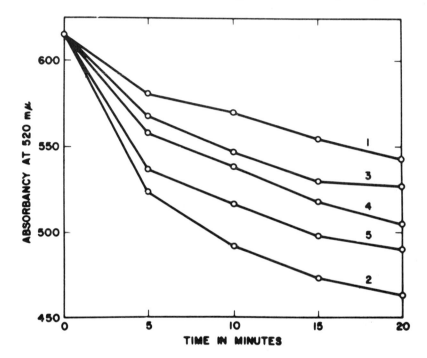

Fig. 13. Induction of swelling in adrenal mitochondria by Ca^{2+} and its inhibition by adenine nucleotides. The curves are as follows: 1, control; 2, Ca^{2+}; 3, Ca^{2+} + ATP; 4, Ca^{2+} + ADP; 5, Ca^{2+} + AMP. Swelling was induced by 11 mM Ca^{2+}. The nucleotides, which were present at the beginning of the experiment, were at a concentration of 5 mM. Reproduced from Hirshfield and Koritz (1964). Copyright by the American Chemical Society. Reprinted by permission of the copyright owner.

concomitant inhibition of pregnenolone synthesis. From these results it was suggested that a modification in mitochondrial membrane structure was a critical factor in the stimulation of pregnenolone synthesis.

A change in the permeability properties of the mitochondrial membrane could affect pregnenolone synthesis in at least two ways. It would enhance the entry of NADPH synthesized outside the mitochondria, or it could allow the exit of pregnenolone formed inside the mitochondria. Koritz and Hirshfield (1966) have shown, by two methods, that increased entry of NADPH into the

Table 6. *Inhibition by nucleotides of the stimulation of pregnenolone synthesis*[a]

Stimulatory agent	Nucleotide	Final concentration of nucleotide, M	μg Pregnenolone/mg protein			Inhibition by nucleotide, %
			Control	+ Stimulatory agent	+ Stimulatory agent and nucleotide	
Calcium	ATP	4.6×10^{-3}	0.55	2.82	0.39	100
Calcium	ADP	5.0×10^{-3}	0.46	4.73	0.78	92
Calcium	AMP	5.0×10^{-3}	0.61	5.10	4.86	5
Calcium	CTP	5.0×10^{-3}	0.43	6.74	4.56	31
Calcium	GTP	5.0×10^{-3}	0.43	6.74	6.48	4
Na lauryl sulfate	ATP	3.7×10^{-2}	0.73	2.80	0.67	100
Myristic acid	ATP	4.6×10^{-2}	0.97	3.45	1.60	75
Palmitic acid	ATP	4.6×10^{-2}	0.97	2.66	1.20	87
Oleic acid	ATP	3.7×10^{-2}	0.67	2.24	1.18	68
Pronase	ATP	2.0×10^{-2}	0.63	3.21	1.57	63

[a]Hirshfield and Koritz (1964). *Biochemistry* 3, 1994. Copyright by American Chemical Society. Reprinted by permission of the copyright owner.

mitochondria is unlikely to be an important factor in the stimulation of pregnenolone synthesis by these swelling agents. On the other hand the suggestion involving increased exit of pregnenolone is quite an attractive one. Using an acetone powder of adrenal mitochondria it has been found that pregnenolone itself inhibits conversion of cholesterol to pregnenolone and that this inhibition by pregnenolone is allosteric in nature (Koritz and Hall 1964a,b).

This observation that pregnenolone can act as an end product inhibitor of its own synthesis, provided the basis for the Koritz and Hall model to describe the action of ACTH (Fig. 14). It is postulated that ACTH acting via cyclic AMP

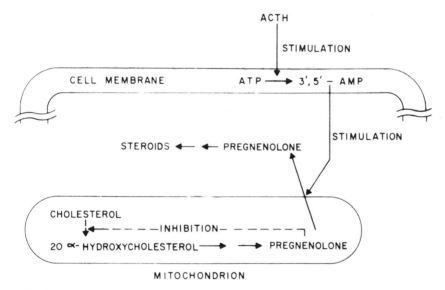

Fig. 14. A model to describe the action of ACTH proposed by Koritz (1968). Reproduced with permission.

affects the mitochondrial membrane so that exit of pregnenolone from within the mitochondria is enhanced. Increased rate of removal of pregnenolone is then thought to relieve the inhibition of its own synthesis and result in an overall increase in the rate of steroidogenesis.

The model proposed by Koritz and Hall for the ACTH mechanism is supported by the work of Urquhart and co-workers who have observed the dynamics of adrenocorticoid secretion of dog adrenals *in vivo* following ACTH infusion (Urquhart and Li, 1968). They found that there was a rapid increase in corticoid output up to a maximum with a subsequent decline back to a steady-state level (Fig. 15). When the ACTH infusion was stopped the corticoid output rapidly fell to a constant basal level. Reinfusion of ACTH could repeat this characteristic overshoot phenomenon. This dynamic pattern of *in vivo*

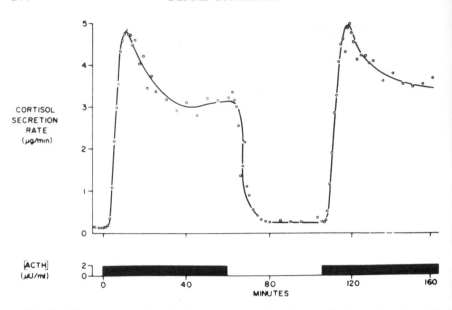

Fig. 15. Time course of cortisol secretion rate by the perfused canine adrenal in response to stepwise changes in ACTH concentration between 0 and 2 μU/ml. Reproduced with permission from Urquhart and Li (1968).

adrenal corticosteroid secretion has been subjected to an extensive mathematical analysis (Urquhart *et al.*, 1968; Urquhart and Li, 1969) and it has been shown that the Koritz and Hall model, involving the mitochondrial permeability of pregnenolone with feedback inhibition is *one* type of model that can give rise to such a characteristic dynamic output curve with an overshoot phenomenon of this type. It has been pointed out that this is not proof that the theory is correct—it merely shows that rigorous analysis of the experimental data does not conflict with this theory.

B. MITOCHONDRIAL PERMEABILITY

It has been pointed out that for the stimulation of pregnenolone biosynthesis this hypothesis predicts an increase in the activity, but not the amount, of an enzyme or enzymes involved in cholesterol conversion to pregnenolone. Experiments using a reconstituted system which included rat adrenal mitochondria and microsomes, indicated that this was indeed so (Koritz and Kumar, 1970). Mitochondria prepared from the adrenal glands of ACTH treated rats, when included in this system, gave rise to a 2- to 3-fold increase in the initial rate of corticosteroidogenesis compared with those from the adrenals of non-ACTH treated animals. On the other hand the microsomal fractions from ACTH treated and control animals were identical in their activity. It was found that, of the various enzymic steps involved in corticosterone synthesis only the synthesis of pregnenolone was increased by ACTH, and moreover that even after ACTH stimulation, the rate of pregnenolone synthesis was still the slowest step. In further experiments, when mitochondria were subjected to treatments designed to reduce permeability barriers, a requirement for exogenous NADPH emerged. From studies with such 'pretreated' mitochondria, obtained from adrenals of cycloheximide treated rats, it was concluded that the ACTH stimulation of pregnenolone synthesis involved an increase in the activity of an enzyme participating directly in pregnenolone synthesis. It was suggested that the cycloheximide-sensitive step (i.e. one involving a rapidly synthesized and labile protein—see Section VII) in the steroidogenic pathway was connected with the permeability properties of the mitochondrion, and that ACTH functioned by controlling the efflux of mitochondrial pregnenolone.

This latter concept is however not in accord with recent findings of Davis and Garren (Garren *et al.*, 1971, p. 440). Hypophysectomized rats were injected with [H^3]cholesterol, cycloheximide and ACTH as described in the legend of Table 2, and it may be seen from this data that, cycloheximide treatment results in the accumulation of free cholesterol in the lipid droplet fraction (29 μg cholesterol compared with 7.5 μg/25 mg adrenal for the control), but not in the mitochondria (7.5 μg cholesterol compared with 6.0 μg/25 mg adrenal). It may be argued that if, as suggested, cycloheximide inhibits efflux of pregnenolone by affecting mitochondrial permeability, and pregnenolone has a feedback inhibitory effect on cholesterol metabolism, then one would expect to observe accumulation of cholesterol and its metabolite(s) in the mitochondrion. Since this was not observed, Garren has suggested that cycloheximide (via its effect on protein synthesis) inhibits the ACTH response by blocking the transport of precursor cholesterol from its storage site in the lipid droplet, to the enzyme system form side-chain cleavage of cholesterol that is located in the mitochondrion.

A central facet of the Koritz-Hall concept is that ACTH stimulates steroidogenesis by removing pregnenolone feedback inhibition. However, Farese (1971a) has provided evidence that the ACTH effect is not appreciably influenced by the total intra-adrenal pregnenolone concentration. Cyanoketone has been shown to inhibit the conversion of pregnenolone to progesterone and incubation of rat adrenal sections in the presence of this compound, led to the accumulation of pregnenolone within the tissue. In the presence of cyanoketone, ACTH and cyclic AMP both stimulated pregnenolone synthesis to an equal or greater extent than corticosteroid synthesis. There was no apparent decrease in pregnenolone synthesis despite its accumulation within the gland. It would appear therefore that either the feedback inhibitory effect of pregnenolone on metabolism of cholesterol to pregnenolone (observed using an acetone powder of adrenal mitochondria) does not pertain to the intact tissue, or alternatively pregnenolone is removed from its inhibitory site within the cell, regardless of its overall accumulation within the tissue.

VII. THE ROLE OF PROTEIN AND RNA SYNTHESIS

A. STUDIES INVOLVING ANTIBIOTIC INHIBITORS OF PROTEIN SYNTHESIS

There is now a considerable amount of evidence indicating that the mechanism whereby ACTH stimulates corticosteroid synthesis, involves the translation of stable messenger RNA. The bulk of this evidence lies with investigations in which antibiotic inhibitors of protein synthesis have been used. These studies are necessarily dependent upon the assumption that these inhibitors block steroidogenesis by their established effect on protein synthesis, rather than by some generalized toxic action or unknown side effect. Nevertheless, data supporting this concept is accumulating from a wide variety of experiments, including a growing number that do not depend upon the use of antibiotics for their conclusions.

The possible involvement of a labile or short-lived protein in the ACTH response, arose with the observation (Ferguson, 1962) that puromycin—an antibiotic known to inhibit protein synthesis—also inhibited the steroidogenic effect of ACTH on rat adrenals *in vitro*. The effect of cyclic AMP was similarly inhibited. Other antibiotics noted as effective protein synthesis inhibitors such as chloramphenicol and cycloheximide, although structurally unrelated to puromycin, have also been found to inhibit the ACTH steroidogenic effect (cf. Ferguson, 1968). However, it was recognized that these antibiotics have a variety of effects on cells besides their established effect on protein synthesis, and that to *prove* a causal relationship between inhibition of protein synthesis by an antibiotic and its inhibition of the ACTH effect, was virtually impossible. For this reason Ferguson undertook a series of experiments attempting to *disprove* an obligatory involvement of protein synthesis in the stimulation of steroidogenesis by ACTH. He showed that structural analogues of puromycin correlated in their ability to inhibit protein synthesis and the ACTH steroidogenic response. Thus the aminonucleoside derivative and the D-phenylalanyl derivative of puromycin inhibited neither amino acid incorporation into adrenal protein nor ACTH steroidogenic responsiveness. On the other hand L-phenylalanyl puromycin, an analogue which did inhibit amino acid incorporation also eliminated the ACTH response.

The effect of puromycin on protein synthesis is reversible and recovery requires a finite time. When incorporation of radioactive amino acids and the steroidogenic responsiveness to ACTH were studied, both were found to return at a similar slow rate after the removal of puromycin. Furthermore, it is evident from the data in Fig. 16(a) that both inhibition of protein synthesis and inhibition of ACTH responsiveness were half maximal at the same dose of puromycin (about 10 μM). Other antibiotics, chemically and structurally unrelated to puromycin have also been examined. Chloramphenicol is a potent inhibitor of protein synthesis in bacteria, but mammalian cells appear relatively resistant to it and about 1 mM chloramphenicol was required for half maximal inhibition of both [^{14}C]leucine incorporation into protein and ACTH responsiveness (Fig. 16(b)). Similarly, using an isolated adrenal cell suspension (Richardson and Schulster, 1970) it has been shown that 1 μM cycloheximide has a half maximal inhibitory effect on ACTH stimulated steroidogenesis—the same dose that was observed to inhibit amino acid incorporation into protein by half (Fig. 16(c)).

If there had been a significant difference for any of these inhibitors in the concentration required to inhibit these two effects, then the existence of a causal relationship between them would have been dubious. Since *none* of these experiments were able to disprove the idea, Ferguson appears justified in suggesting that protein synthesis may be intimately involved in the ACTH steroidogenic effect.

The effect of cycloheximide upon cyclic AMP concentrations in rat adrenal glands incubated *in vitro* with ACTH has also been investigated (Grahame-Smith et al., 1967). It was shown that doses of cycloheximide sufficient to block steroidogenesis did not inhibit the increase in adrenal cyclic AMP concentration induced by ACTH.

The dynamics of corticosterone secretion *in vivo* after ACTH infusion and the effects of a protein synthesis inhibitor have also been studied by Garren et al. (1965). The intravenous injection of ACTH to an hypophysectomized rat resulted in a rapid rise in corticosterone output which was maintained for some time. From the data in Fig. 17, it may be seen that if cycloheximide was administered intraperitoneally 10 minutes after the injection of ACTH, when the corticosterone secretion rate had almost reached its maximum, then there was a rapid decline in the rate of steroid synthesis.

If the data from Fig. 17 is plotted semilogarithmically it may be seen that the rate of decline in steroidogenesis decreased linearly with time after cycloheximide administration. The half-life for this *in vivo* decay was calculated to be about 10 minutes.

These classic *in vivo* experiments have provided valuable data, but no allowance was made for the known influence of both ACTH and cycloheximide on adrenal blood flow rate (Stark and Varga, 1968). The possibility that the cycloheximide inhibition of ACTH induced steroidogenesis *in vivo*, may be due to effects on adrenal blood flow rate, was eliminated by the use of an *in vitro*

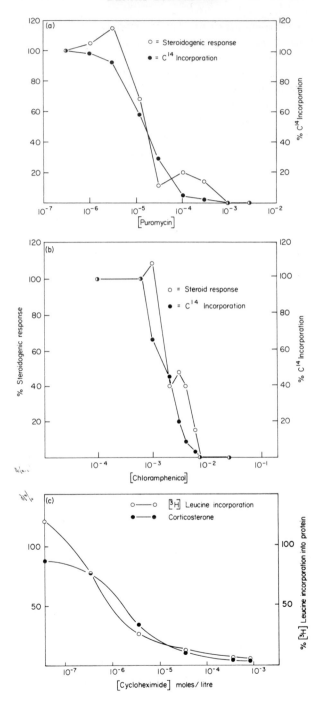

superfusion system (Schulster *et al.*, 1970). Decapsulated adrenals from acutely hypophysectomized rats were superfused in a continuous *in vitro* incubation system, and as shown in Fig. 18 the continuous infusion of ACTH or cyclic AMP elicited a rapid stimulation of corticosterone output rate, which reached a maximum within 30 minutes of infusing ACTH or cyclic AMP. Other studies on the superfused adrenal (Pearlmutter *et al.*, 1971) have reported that maximum corticosteroid production rate was reached in 20 minutes. This compares with the peak corticosteroid output rates found 8-16 minutes after ACTH infusion during *in vivo* adrenal perfusion studies in the rat (Fig. 17) and dog (Fig. 15).

The *in vitro* data given in Fig. 19 using the superfused adrenal, shows the effect obtained when cycloheximide was continuously infused 30 minutes or 2 hours after the glands had been stimulated *in vitro* by continuous infusions of either ACTH or cyclic AMP. Cycloheximide was found to have an immediate inhibitory effect and the *in vitro* decline exhibited an exponential decay with a half-life of 45-49 minutes regardless of when the cycloheximide was infused and whether ACTH or cyclic AMP was the stimulant. This may be compared with the half-life of 10 minutes observed *in vivo* following cycloheximide inhibition (Fig. 17). The effects of ACTH, cyclic AMP and cycloheximide, show that the adrenal in the *in vitro* superfusion system exhibits characteristic dynamic responses similar to, albeit less rapid than, those observed using the *in vivo* perfusion technique. The relative sluggishness of the *in vitro* superfused gland when compared with the *in vivo* perfused adrenal, may well be a function of the relative inaccessibility of cells within the tissue to essential components provided in the medium, and possibly also to the manner in which steroid products are eliminated from the tissue. In *in vitro* incubations with pieces of adrenal, only the outer cell layers are in direct contact with the medium and thus diffusion through the tissue will affect the supply of nutrients and stimulants to, and removal of steroid products from most of the adrenal cells. Analysis of the vascular architecture of the adrenal cortex suggests that it is designed to provide the cortical cells with an extremely rich arterial blood supply (Dobbie *et al.*, 1968), and thus *in vivo* the adrenal blood supply not only maintains an adequate provision of blood-borne components to each and every cell, but also facilitates removal of steroid products. Moreover the blood flow rate through the adrenal is stimulated by ACTH and the differences between these *in vitro* and *in vivo* systems may be partly attributed to this effect, since the flow rate of the

---

Fig. 16. Dose response plots for antibiotic inhibitors of protein synthesis and steroid-ogenesis. [^{14}C] Leucine and ACTH was present during the incubation period. Amino acid incorporation expressed as percentage of control (without antibiotic) incorporation. Corticosteroid production expressed as percentage of control (without antibiotic, but with ACTH). (a) Puromycin: rat adrenal quarters preincubated and incubated with puromycin in the medium (From Ferguson, 1968). (b) Chloramphenicol: conditions as for (a). (c) Cycloheximide: Isolated cell suspensions of rat adrenals, preincubated and incubated with cycloheximide in the medium. (Schulster and Richardson: unpublished observations.)

superfusion medium *in vitro* is independent of ACTH concentration. The *in vitro* incubation problems associated with the permeability of chunks of tissue may perhaps be overcome by adapting the system for the superfusion of isolated cell suspensions. (Schulster, 1973.)

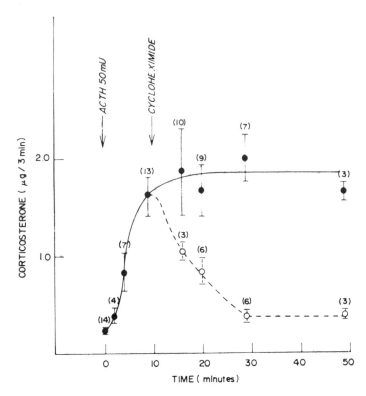

Fig. 17. Effect of cycloheximide on ACTH-stimulated steroidogenesis by the rat *in vivo*. The solid line indicates the rate of corticosterone secretion, at each point in time, following the administration of ACTH intravenously; the broken line represents the time-course of corticosterone secretion following the intraperitoneal injection of cycloheximide, 10 min after ACTH is injected intravenously. The number of rats used at each point in time is represented in parentheses. The standard error is also indicated. From Garren *et al* (1965). Reproduced with permission.

Previous *in vitro* studies (Ferguson, 1963; Maier and Staehelin, 1968) using static incubation procedures were unable to demonstrate an inhibition of the ACTH response following the late addition of puromycin or cycloheximide, although these inhibitors were effective in abolishing any stimulation of steroidogenesis by simultaneously added ACTH. The static *in vitro* incubation procedure entails assay of the total corticosteroid produced throughout the

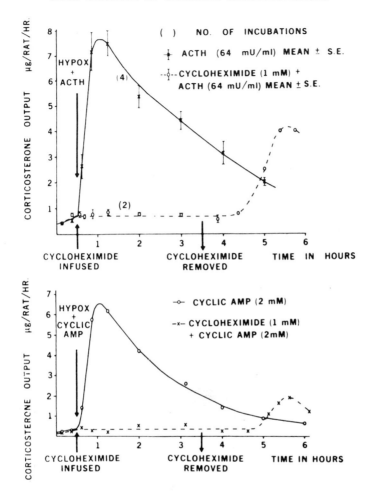

Fig. 18. Superfused adrenals: effect of continuous infusions of cycloheximide (1 mM), begun simultaneously with continuous infusions of either ACTH (upper diagram; 64 mU/ml medium) or cyclic AMP (lower diagram; 2 mM), on corticosterone output rate by decapsulated glands from hypophysectomized rats. All infusions were begun 30 min after the start of the incubation; cycloheximide infusion was ceased after a further 3 hr, while ACTH or cyclic AMP infusion continued uninterrupted. From Schulster et al. (1970). Reproduced by permission of the copyright owner.

incubation period and this accounts for the apparent lack of effect following the late addition of puromycin or cycloheximide. If the total steroid output over a set time period is used to assess adrenal functioning, then even clearly discernible changes in steroid output rates will be obscured when total steroid outputs are high. From the data in Fig. 19, where total steroid output over any given period is represented by the area under the curve for that period, it is clear that after cycloheximide infusion the rate of steroid output is markedly reduced. However, that the area under the curve (with ACTH only) is different from that under the curve (with ACTH and cycloheximide) is only clearly evident after relatively long incubation periods.

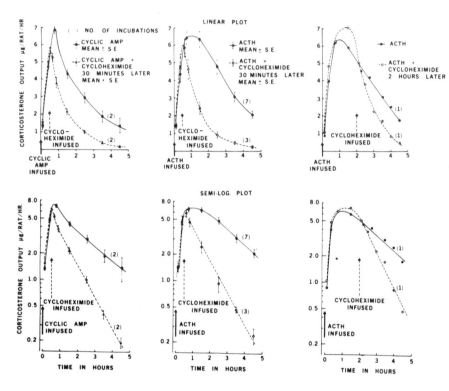

Fig. 19. Superfused adrenals: effect of continuously infused cycloheximide (1 mM), either 30 min after continuous cyclic AMP infusion (2 mM) or 2 hr after continuous ACTH infusion (64 mU/ml medium). The resulting corticosterone output rates by decapsulated adrenals from rats 3 hr after hypophysectomy are plotted both linearly (upper diagrams) and semilogarithmically (lower diagrams). From Schulster et al. (1970). Reproduced by permission of the copyright owner.

The almost immediate and total effect of cycloheximide in inhibiting the steroidogenic response to either ACTH or cyclic AMP is evident from the data shown in Fig. 18. In these experiments the partial reversibility of this inhibition was observed following removal of cycloheximide. A similar reversibility for the inhibitory effect of puromycin on both ACTH stimulated steroidogenesis and [14C] leucine incorporation into protein (Ferguson, 1968) when recovery from both inhibitory effects occurred at about the same slow rate. It is clear from these studies that a substantial part of such inhibitions by cycloheximide and puromycin are not permanent effects and that after the inhibitor is removed, the tissue is still responsive to ACTH or cyclic AMP. Therefore this inhibition of ACTH stimulated steroidogenesis can not involve a mechanism that is completely dependent upon permanent damage to the steroid responsive cells. In further experiments (Schulster et al., 1970) it was found that cycloheximide at the 1 mM level inhibited the basal corticosterone output by superfused adrenal tissue from hypophysectomized rats, by about 50%. Since the stimulation by

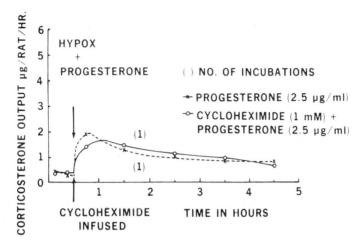

Fig. 20. Superfused adrenals: effect of simultaneous and continuous infusions of cycloheximide (1 mM) and progesterone (2.6 μg/ml medium) on corticosterone output rate by decapsulated adrenals from hypophysectomized rats. Progesterone, cycloheximide and saline infusions were all begun 30 min after the incubation started. From Schulster et al. (1970). Reproduced by permission of the copyright owner.

ACTH and cyclic AMP was totally inhibited by this dose of cycloheximide (Fig. 18), then a specific action of cycloheximide (rather than a generalized toxic effect) on the steroidogenic response, can account for at least half of this inhibition.

The conversion of progesterone to corticosterone by superfused adrenal tissue has been shown to be unaffected by 1 mM cycloheximide (Fig. 20). Thus again evidence was provided that cycloheximide did not act via a general toxic effect on the tissue, that would also include inhibition of the enzyme systems responsible for the further conversion of progesterone to corticosterone. Since this latter portion of the steroidogenic pathway remains intact in the presence of cycloheximide it was concluded that the locus of action of the antibiotic was prior to progesterone on the biosynthetic pathway.

Evidence for the specificity of the inhibitory site of cycloheximide in the steroid biosynthetic route has been provided by the *in vivo* studies of Davis and Garren (1968), from which it was concluded that cycloheximide inhibits the ACTH response by preventing the conversion of cholesterol to pregnenolone. When 10 mg cycloheximide was injected into hypophysectomized rats, the incorporation of [^{3}H] acetate into adrenal cholesterol was found to be stimulated, whereas the ACTH induced increase in corticosterone secretion was inhibited. The data obtained showed that the antibiotic did not block a step in the pathway prior to cholesterol but rather at a site subsequent to this precursor of corticosterone. The locus of antibiotic action was more precisely determined when adrenals, endogenously labelled with [^{3}H] cholesterol, were incubated *in vitro* with [^{14}C] pregnenolone. It was found that the presence of ACTH in the incubation medium increased the conversion of endogenously labelled [^{3}H]-corticosterone and that cycloheximide added to the medium blocked this stimulation. On the other hand the incorporation of [^{14}C] pregnenolone into [^{14}C] corticosterone was unaffected by the presence of either ACTH or cycloheximide.

These studies have confirmed the previous reports (Stone and Hechter, 1954; Karaboyas and Koritz, 1965) that the rate-limiting step in the steroidogenic pathway stimulated by ACTH lies in the conversion of cholesterol to pregnenolone. Furthermore they have indicated that the inhibition of protein synthesis also inhibits steroid synthesis at this site in the pathway.

Intact adrenal cells prepared by the trypsinization technique of Halkerston (1968) do not respond to NADPH, although they do respond to ACTH and this response is sensitive to cycloheximide. When these cells were broken by sonication, they were then found to respond to NADPH and cycloheximide did not block this stimulation (Garren *et al.*, 1969). It was therefore concluded that the enzymes involved in corticosterone synthesis were not themselves directly inhibited by cycloheximide. This observation is in keeping with the suggestion (see Section III) that a cycloheximide sensitive step, possibly synthesis of labile protein(s), is involved in the transport of cholesterol from its storage location in the lipid droplets to its site of further metabolism in the mitochondria.

The bulk of the current evidence would therefore support the Garren model (Fig. 11) implicating the involvement of a labile protein in the ACTH steroidogenic effect.

B. PROTEIN SYNTHESIS IN THE ABSENCE OF ANTIBIOTICS

Several valuable studies which have avoided the use of antibiotic inhibitors of protein synthesis, have been reported. These studies are not subject to the criticisms that have been levelled against the experiments involving cycloheximide and puromycin, which may exert their action by some hitherto unidentified side-effect rather than via their well known effect on protein synthesis.

Using cultures of mouse adrenocortical tumour cells Sato *et al.* (1965) found that the omission of glutamine from the tissue culture medium led to a decrease in both the steroidogenic response to ACTH and the rate of protein synthesis. Furthermore the replacement of glutamine in the medium restored the ACTH steroidogenic response as well as protein synthesis. Thus Sato was able to provide some evidence for the involvement of protein synthesis in the ACTH stimulation of steroidogenesis in tumour cell, without the use of antibiotic inhibitors.

Two factors have been isolated from supernatant fractions of adrenal homogenates and have been dubbed '*steroidogenin*' and '*steroidohibin*' (Farese, 1967). They both have the characteristics of proteins. One of these factors (steroidogenin) was found to be induced in adrenal tissue by both ACTH and cyclic AMP and this inductive process was blocked by puromycin. This factor was found to enhance corticosterone production, as well as cholesterol side chain cleavage by adrenal mitochondria. The other factor (steroidohibin) was isolated from control rat adrenal supernatant fractions and was found to inhibit cholesterol side chain cleavage by adrenal mitochondria.

Recently, Grower and Bransome (1970) have demonstrated that within 30 minutes of adding ACTH to cultures of Sato's mouse adrenal tumour cells, changes in the amount and labelling of several protein fractions were evident, following acrylamide-gel electrophoresis. These studies provided yet more circumstantial evidence that labile proteins are important in the regulation of steroid biosynthesis by ACTH.

The synthesis of protein requires a finite time, and recent data has shown that the average transit time for translation in some eukaryotic cells is about one to two minutes (Fan and Penman, 1970; Vaughan *et al.*, 1971). Using isolated adrenal cell suspensions it has been shown (Kitabchi and Sharma, 1971; Beall and Sayers, 1972; Richardson and Schulster, 1972) that after exposing the cells to ACTH a marked stimulation of steroidogenesis was apparent, only after a time lag of 3 minutes (Fig. 21). A very similar time lag has been observed following addition of cyclic AMP to these cells. Unlike studies with whole or quartered glands, the use of a suspension of cells allows immediate access of ACTH or cyclic AMP to all cells. A similar time lag is apparent in reports of studies following ACTH infusion to the canine adrenal perfused *in situ* (Urquhart and Li, 1968, Fig. 15) and the transplanted ovine perfused adrenal (Beaven *et al.*, 1964). The initial latency period before the onset of ACTH is comparable with the average transit time (1-2 minutes) required for translation in eukaryotic cells, and it is possible that this 3 minute time period largely represents the time required for synthesis of the labile protein(s) postulated to be involved in the ACTH response. That this 3 minute time lag does not incorporate any appreciable period for the intracellular accumulation of cyclic AMP, has been demonstrated using both trypsin prepared cells (Beall and Sayers, 1972) and collagenase prepared isolated adrenal cells (Mackie *et al.*, 1972). It has been found that the adrenal cyclic AMP level rises in this system in response to added ACTH, without any discernible time lag.

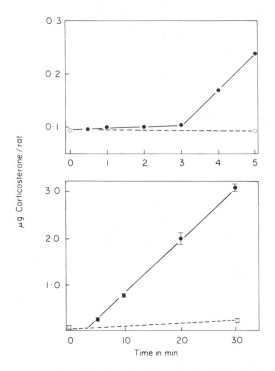

Fig. 21. Time course studies of corticosteroid production by isolated cell suspensions of rat adrenals. A 10 min preincubation period preceded the addition of ACTH at time zero. Vertical bars represent standard errors. From Richardson and Schulster (1972). Reprinted with permission by the copyright owner.

It is not possible at present to decide if the labile protein postulated as the ACTH mediator and the protein factor(s) described by Farese are one and the same. Similarly, the newly synthesized proteins apparent after acrylamide gel electrophoresis of ACTH stimulated tumour cells, are of indeterminate interest. Nevertheless a salient point is that the time interval observed for ACTH stimulation of steroidogenesis is in keeping with that for the synthesis of some adrenal proteins.

Calcium has been known to participate in the steroidogenic action of ACTH following the investigations of Birmingham *et al.* (1953) and Péron and Koritz

(1958), and the reason for the calcium requirement has since been widely studied. Farese (1971b), using incubations of rat adrenal quarters, observed a marked dependence of adrenal protein synthesis on calcium, and suggested that the maintenance of optimal adrenal protein synthesis conditions may be an explanation for the calcium requirement during the ACTH and cyclic AMP response. Rasmussen (1970) has postulated that hormonal effects in endocrine target cells may directly involve hormone or cyclic AMP induced changes in intracellular calcium. In line with this concept, ^{45}Ca uptake by the adrenal has been reported to be stimulated by ACTH (Leier and Jungmann, 1970), and Farese (1971c,d) has demonstrated that calcium directly stimulates protein synthesis in adrenal cell free systems. Moreover, in these latter studies, calcium was found to mimic the effect of ACTH on adrenal protein synthesis, by enhancing the transfer of amino acid from the amino acyl $\sim$ transfer-RNA complex to protein. Although these experiments support the idea of an important mediatory role for calcium in the effect of ACTH on protein synthesis, this appears not to be the only role of calcium, since Lefkowitz et al. (1970b) have shown that it is required during ACTH stimulation of adenyl cyclase (Section II) and Péron and McCarthy (1968) have described its direct effect on steroid hydroxylations in adrenal mitochondria.

C. RNA SYNTHESIS

The role of RNA synthesis in the acute steroidogenic effect of ACTH has been mostly studied with the aid of actinomycin D—a well documented inhibitor of RNA synthesis. Ferguson and Morita (1964) showed, using rat adrenal quarters, that addition of 10 μM actinomycin D had little or no effect on the ACTH steroidogenic response, although this dose of actinomycin D was sufficient to inhibit [^{14}C]-adenine and [^{14}C]-uridine incorporation into adrenal RNA by about 95%. Similar observations have been made (Garren et al., 1965; Ney et al., 1966) from in vivo studies on the effect of actinomycin D in the rat. From these data it has been concluded that ACTH stimulated steroidogenesis by a mechanism not involving RNA synthesis.

It is apparent that a considerable emphasis has been placed upon the ability of the adrenal to respond to ACTH after administration of actinomycin D over a narrow range of doses and time intervals. Indeed there is a considerable amount of confusion as to the effects of this antibiotic on the adrenal. Actinomycin D has been reported to elevate, lower or not affect the basal production of corticosterone by the adrenal, and the ACTH response has been found to be prevented, potentiated as well as unaffected by this antibiotic (see Bransome, 1969). The effect of actinomycin D on cyclic AMP induced steroidogenesis by a clonal epithelial culture line derived from a mouse testicular interstitial cell tumour, has also been found to be highly dependent upon the

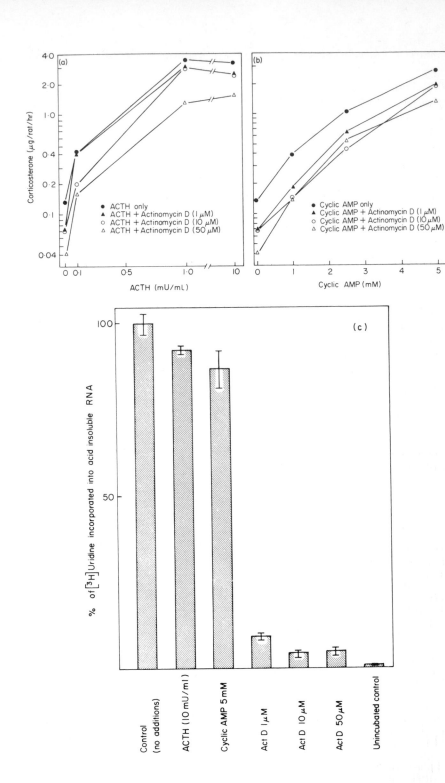

dose of actinomycin D (Shin and Sato, 1971). Actinomycin D (1.0 μg/ml) potentiated steroidogenesis at suboptimal cyclic AMP concentrations, whereas actinomycin D (4.0 μg/ml) virtually abolished the cyclic AMP induced response.

Studies employing isolated adrenal cell suspensions have demonstrated that there are conditions under which actinomycin D does have a marked inhibitory effect on the ACTH and on the cyclic AMP response. Nevertheless, at low doses of actinomycin D (e.g. 1 μM) there is an inhibition of over 95% of adrenal incorporation of [^{3}H]-uridine into acid insoluble RNA, whereas the steroidogenic responses to various doses of ACTH and cyclic AMP are largely unaffected (Fig. 22). The suggestion that the mechanism of ACTH steroidogenic action does not directly involve the initial synthesis of RNA, appears reasonably established from the studies described above.

The data previously described suggest that for both ACTH and cyclic AMP the stimulation of corticosteroid synthesis requires continuing protein synthesis but not RNA synthesis, whereas the increase in adrenal cyclic AMP concentration, effected by ACTH, does not require continuing protein synthesis (Grahame-Smith et al., 1967). Garren et al. (1971) have suggested that the mechanism by which ACTH stimulates steroidogenesis involves firstly the formation of cyclic AMP, and then the regulation by this nucleotide of adrenal protein synthesis via the translation of a stable mRNA species. The ability of the superfused adrenal to produce corticosteroids in response to continuous infusions of ACTH and cyclic AMP has been observed to decline during the later time periods (2 to 5 hours) of superfusion (Fig. 19; Schulster et al., 1968; Saffran and Rowell, 1969). This exponential decline in output had a half-life of about 100 minutes and was not attributable to irreversible changes occurring in the tissue during the course of the superfusion. Moreover it could not reasonably be attributed to any of the known factors under ACTH control. This late decline in the steroidogenic effect of ACTH under in vitro superfusion conditions has been confirmed by Mostafapour and Tchen (1972) and actinomycin D (20 μg/ml) was found to potentiate the ACTH response and delay the onset of late decline. Mostafapour and Tchen (1971) have calculated that the ability of the adrenal to respond to ACTH after hypophysectomy declines with a half-life of about 6-7 hours, and postulate that this might

---

Fig. 22. Dose response plots for actinomycin D on corticosterone production and RNA synthesis in the presence of ACTH or cyclic AMP. Isolated cell suspensions of decapsulated rat adrenal glands (Richardson and Schulster, 1972) were incubated (60 min) with actinomycin D in the medium. (a) ACTH present during the incubation period. Corticosterone production plotted on a logarithmic scale. (b) Cyclic AMP present during the incubation period. Corticosterone production plotted on a logarithmic scale. (c) [^{3}H]-Uridine present during the incubation period and its incorporation into acid insoluble RNA expressed as a percentage of control (without actinomycin D) incorporation. Vertical bars represent standard errors. (Schulster, 1974, Mol. Cell. Biol, **1**, in press.)

represent the slow decay of a RNA species involved in the synthesis of the labile protein, invoked by Garren.

The data (Schulster, 1974, in press) shown in Fig. 22, although eliminating the possibility that in stimulating steroidogenesis, ACTH acts via the synthesis of RNA, nevertheless are consistent with a permissive role for RNA synthesis. The small, but distinct inhibition (20-40%) of both the ACTH and cyclic AMP responses by low concentrations (1 μM) of actinomycin D, implies that continued synthesis of a relatively stable species of RNA (with a half-life of an hour or more is required for full continued expression of the ACTH response. The possibility of a non-specific effect of the antibiotic remains, however, and as usual the inhibitor effects are not simple to interpret. Nevertheless the available data would support the model outlined in Fig. 11.

ACKNOWLEDGEMENTS

The author gratefully acknowledges the financial support of the Wellcome Trust, the Medical Research Council and Armour Pharmaceutical Co. He would also like to thank his colleagues, Malcolm Richardson, Caroline Mackie and Jeffrey McIlhinney for helpful discussions during the preparation of the manuscript.

REFERENCES

Ariens, E. J. (1966). *Adv. Drug Res.* **3**, 235.

Baulieu, E.-E., Alberga, A., Jung, I., Lebeau, M.-C., Mercier-Bodard, C., Milgrom, E., Raynaud, J.-P., Raynaud-Jammet, C., Rochefort, H., Truong, H. and Robel, P. (1971). *Recent Progr. Horm. Res.* **27**, 351.

Beall, R. J. and Sayers, G. (1972). *Arch. Biochem. Biophys.* **148**, 70.

Beaven, D. W., Espiner, E. A. and Hart, D. S. (1964). *J. Physiol. (London).* **171**, 216.

Bell, P. H., Howard, K. S., Shepherd, R. G., Finn, B. M. and Meisenhelder, J. H. (1956). *J. Amer. Chem. Soc.* **78**, 5059.

Bieck, P., Stock, K. and Westermann, E. (1968). *Life Sci.* **7**, 1125.

Birmingham, M. K., Elliot, F. H. and Valere, P. H. L. (1953). *Endocrinology* **53**, 687.

Birmingham, M. K. and Kurlents, E. (1958). *Endocrinology* **62**, 47.

Birmingham, M. K., Kurlents, E., Lane, R., Muhlstock, B. and Traikov, H. (1960). *Can. J. Biochem. Physiol.* **38**, 1077.

Boyd, G. S., Brownie, A. C., Jefcoate, C. R. and Simpson, E. R. (1971). *Biochem. J.* **125**, 1P.

Bransome, E. D. (1968). *Ann. Rev. Physiol.* **30**, 171.

Bransome, E. D. (1969). *Endocrinology* **85**, 1114.

Buonassisi, V., Sato, G. and Cohen, A. I. (1962). *Proc. Nat. Acad. Sci. U.S.* **48**, 1184.

Burstein, S. and Gut, M. (1971). *Recent Progr. Horm. Res.* **27**, 303.

Burstein, S., Kimball, H. L. and Gut, M. (1970a). *Steroids* **15**, 809.

Burstein, S., Zamoscianyk, H., Kimball, H. L., Chaudhuri, N. K. and Gut, M. (1970b). *Steroids* **15**, 13.

Carchman, R. A., Jaanus, S. D. and Rubin, R. P. (1971). *Mol. Pharm.* **7**, 491.

Clark, A. J. (1937). *In* 'Heffter's Handbuch der Experimentellen Pharmakologie' (W. Heubner and J. Schuller, eds.), Vol. 4. Springer, Berlin.

Clayman, M., Tsang, D. and Johnstone, R. M. (1970). *Endocrinology* **86**, 931.

Constantopoulos, G., Carpenter, A., Satoh, P. S., Tchen, T. T. (1966). *Biochemistry* **5**, 1650.

Criss, W. E. and McKerns, K. W. (1968). *Biochemistry* **7**, 2364.

Cuatrecasas, P. (1971). *Proc. Nat. Acad. Sci. U.S.* **68**, 1264.

Davis W. W. (1969). *Fed. Proc.* **28**, 701.

Davis, W. W. and Garren, L. D. (1968). *J. Biol. Chem.* **243**, 5153.

Davoren, P. R. and Sutherland, E. W. (1963). *J. Biol. Chem.* **238**, 3016.

De Wulf, H. and Hers, H. G. (1968). *Eur. J. Biochem.* **6**, 552.

Dixon, R., Furutachi, T. and Lieberman, S. (1970). *Biochem. Biophys. Res. Commun.* **40**, 161.

Dobbie, J. W., Mackay, A. M. and Symington, T. (1968). *In* 'Memoirs of the Society for Endocrinology' (V. H. T. James and J. Landon, eds.), No. 1, p. 103. Cambridge University Press, London.

Doering, C. H. and Clayton, R. B. (1969). *Endocrinology* **85**, 500.

Eisenstein, A. B. (ed.) (1967). 'The Adrenal Cortex'. Little-Brown, Boston.

Fan, H. and Penman, S. (1970). *J. Mol. Biol.* **50**, 655.

Farese, R. V. (1967). *Biochemistry* **6**, 2052.

Farese, R. V. (1971a). *Endocrinology* **89**, 958.

Farese, R. V. (1971b). *Endocrinology* **89**, 1057.

Farese, R. V. (1971c). *Endocrinology* **89**, 1064.

Farese, R. V. (1971d). *Science, N.Y.* **173**, 447.

Ferguson, J. J. (1962). *Biochim. Biophys. Acta* **57**, 616.

Ferguson, J. J. (1963). *J. Biol. Chem.* **238**, 2754.

Ferguson, J. J. (1968). *In* 'Functions of the Adrenal Cortex' (K. W. McKerns ed.), Vol. 1, pp. 463–478. Appleton-Century-Crofts, New York.

Ferguson, J. J. and Morita, Y. (1964). *Biochim. Biophys. Acta* **87**, 348.

Ferguson, J. J., Morita, Y. and Mendelsohn, (1967). *Endocrinology* **80**, 521.

Flack, J. D., Jessup, R. and Ramwell, P. W. (1969). *Science, N.Y.* **163**, 691.

Free, C. A., Chasin, M., Paik, V. S. and Hess, S. M. (1971a). *Biochemistry* **10**, 3785.

Free, C. A., Chasin, M., Paik, V. S. and Hess, S. M. (1971b). *Fed. Proc. Amer. Soc. Exp. Biol.* **30**, 1268.

Garren, L. D. (1968). *Vitam. Horm.* (*New York*) **26**, 119.

Garren, L. D., Ney, R. L. and Davis, W. W. (1965). *Proc. Nat. Acad. Sci. U.S.* **53**, 1443.

Garren, L. D., Davis, W. W., Gill, G. N., Moses, H. L., Ney, R. L. and Crocco, R. M. (1969). *Proc. 3rd Int. Congr. Endocrinol. 1968* p. 102.

Garren, L. D., Gill, G. N., Masui, H. and Walton, G. M. (1971). *Recent Progr. Horm. Res.* **27**, 433.

Gill, G. N. (1972). *Metabolism* **21**, 571.

Gill, G. N. and Garren, L. D. (1969). *Proc. Nat. Acad. Sci. U.S.* **63**, 512.

Gill, G. N. and Garren, L. D. (1970). *Biochem. Biophys. Res. Commun.* **39**, 335.

Gill, G. N. and Garren, L. D. (1971). *Proc. Nat. Acad. Sci. U.S.* **68**, 786.

Grahame-Smith, D. G., Butcher, R. W., Ney, R. L. and Sutherland, E. W. (1967). *J. Biol. Chem.* **242**, 5535.

Grant, J. K. (1968). *J. Endocrinology* **41**, 111.

Griffiths, K. and Cameron, E. H. D. (1970). *In* 'Advances in Steroid

Biochemistry and Pharmacology' (M. H. Briggs, ed.), Vol. 2, pp. 223–265. Academic Press, London and New York.

Grower, M. F. and Bransome, E. D. (1970). *Science, N.Y.* **168,** 483.

Halkerston, I. D. K. (1968). *In* 'Functions of the Adrenal Cortex' (K. W. McKerns, ed.), Vol. 1, pp. 399–461. Appleton-Century-Crofts, New York.

Halkerston, I. D. K., Eichorn, J. and Hechter, O. (1961). *J. Biol. Chem.* **236,** 374.

Halkerston, I. D. K., Feinstein, M. and Hechter, O. (1966). *Proc. Soc. Exp. Biol. Med.* **122,** 896.

Haning, R., Tait, S. A. S. and Tait, J. F. (1970). *Endocrinology* **87** 1147.

Harding, B. W. and Nelson, D. H. (1964a). *Endocrinology* **75,** 501.

Harding, B. W and Nelson, D. H. (1964b). *Endocrinology* **75,** 506.

Haynes, R. C. (1958). *J. Biol. Chem.* **233,** 1220.

Haynes, R. C. and Berthet, L. (1957). *J. Biol. Chem.* **225,** 115.

Haynes, R. C., Koritz, S. B. and Péron, F. G. (1959). *J. Biol. Chem.* **234,** 1421.

Hechter, O., Bar, H. P., Matsuba, M. and Soifer, D. (1969). *Life Sci.* **8,** 935.

Hilf, R. (1965). *New England J. Med.* **273,** 798.

Hirshfield, I. N. and Koritz, S. B. (1964). *Biochemistry* **3,** 1994.

Hofmann, K., Yajima, H., Liu, T. Y., Yanaihara, N., Yanaihara, C. and Humes, J. L. (1962). *J. Amer. Chem. Soc.* **84,** 4481.

Hofmann, K., Wingender, W. and Finn, F. M. (1970). *Proc. Nat. Acad. Sci. U.S.* **67,** 829.

Ichii, S., Okada, N. and Ikeda, A. (1970). *Endocrinol. Jap.* **17,** 83.

Imura, H., Matsukura, S., Matsuyama, H., Setsuda, T. and Miyake, T. (1965). *Endocrinology* **76,** 933.

Jost, J. P. and Rickenberg, H. V. (1971). *Ann. Rev. Biochem.* **40,** 741.

Kakiuchi, S., Rall, T. W. and McIlwain, H. (1969). *J. Neurochem.* **16,** 485.

Kan, K. W., Ritter, M. C., Ungar, F. and Dempsey, M. E. (1972). *Biochem. Biophys. Res. Commun.* **48,** 423.

Karaboyas, G. C. and Koritz, S. B. (1965). *Biochemistry* **4,** 462.

Kelly, L. A. and Koritz, S. B. (1971). *Biochim. Biophys. Acta* **237,** 141.

Kimura, T. (1969). *Endocrinology* **85,** 492.

Kitabchi, A. E. and Sharma, R. K. (1971). *Endocrinology* **88,** 1109.

Kitabchi, A. E., Wilson, D. B. and Sharma, R. K. (1971). *Biochem. Biophys. Res. Commun.* **44,** 898.

Kloppenborg, P. W. C., Island, D. P., Liddle, G. W., Michelakis, A. M. and Nicholson, W. E. (1968). *Endocrinology* **82,** 1053.

Klotz, V., Vapaatalo, H. and Stock, K. (1972). *Nauyn-Schmiedebergs Arch. Pharmakol.* **273,** 376.

Kobayashi, S., Yago, N., Morisaki, M., Ichii, S. and Matsuba, M. (1963). *Steroids* **2,** 167.

Koritz, S. B. (1968). *In* 'Functions of the Adrenal Cortex' (K. W. McKerns ed.), Vol. 1, pp. 27–48. Appleton-Century-Crofts, New York.

Koritz, S. B. and Hall, P. F. (1964a). *Biochim. Biophys. Acta* **93,** 215.

Koritz, S. B. and Hall, P. F. (1964b). *Biochemistry* **3,** 1298.

Koritz, S. B. and Hirshfield, I. N. (1966). *In* 'Proc. 2nd International Congress on Hormonal Steroids', p. 404. Excerpta Medica Foundation, Amsterdam.

Koritz, S. B. and Kumar, A. M. (1970). *J. Biol. Chem.* **245,** 152.

Koritz, S. B. and Péron, F. G. (1958). *J. Biol. Chem.* **230,** 343.

Kowal, J. (1970). *Recent Progr. Horm. Res.* **26,** 623.

Kuehl, F. A., Humes, J. L., Tarnoff, J., Cirillo, V. J. and Ham, E. A. (1970). *Science, N.Y.* **169**, 883.

Kuhn, C. and Kissane, J. M. (1964). *Endocrinology* **75**, 741.

Langan, T. A. (1968). *Science, N.Y.* **162**, 579.

Lebovitz, H. E. and Engel, F. L. (1964). *Endocrinology* **75**, 831.

Lefkowitz, R. J., Roth, J. and Pastan, I. (1970a). *Science, N.Y.* **170**, 633.

Lefkowitz, R. J., Roth, J. and Pastan, I. (1970b). *Nature (London)* **228**, 864.

Lefkowitz, R. J., Roth, J., Pricer, W. and Pastan, I. (1970c). *Proc. Nat. Acad. Sci. U.S.* **65**, 745.

Lehninger, A. L. (1951). *J. Biol. Chem.* **190**, 345.

Leier, D. J. and Jungmann, R. A. (1970). Program of 52nd Meeting Endocrine Society, St. Louis, Mo., June, p. 85.

Leier, D. J. and Jungmann, R. A. (1971). *Biochim. Biophys. Acta* **239**, 320.

Linarelli, L. G. and Farese, R. V. (1970). *Pharmacology* **4**, 33.

Mackie, C. and Schulster, D. (1973). *J. Endocrinology* **57**, xx.

Mackie, C., Richardson, M. C. and Schulster, D. (1972). *FEBS Lett.* **23**, 345.

Maier, R. and Staehelin, M. (1968). *Acta Endocr. (Kbh)* **58**, 619.

Marton, J., Stark, E., Mihaly, K. and Varga, B. (1971). *Acta Physiol. Acad. Sci. Hung.* **40**, 229.

McKerns, K. W. (1964). *Biochim. Biophys. Acta* **90**, 357.

McKerns, K. W. (ed.) (1968). 'Functions of the Adrenal Cortex'. Appleton-Century-Crofts, New York.

Morrow, L. B., Burrow, G. N. and Mulrow, P. J. (1967). *Endocrinology* **80**, 883.

Moses, H. L., Davis, W. W., Rosenthal, A. S. and Garren, L. D. (1969). *Science, N.Y.* **163**, 1203.

Mostafapour, M. K. and Tchen, T. T. (1971). *Biochem. Biophys. Res. Commun.* **44**, 774.

Mostafapour, M. K. and Tchen, T. T. (1972). *Biochem. Biophys. Res. Commun.* **48**, 491.

Ney, R. L., Shimizu, N., Nicholson, W. E., Island, D. P. and Liddle, G. W. (1963). *J. Clin. Invest.* **42**, 1669.

Ney, R. L., Davis, W. W. and Garren, L. D. (1966). *Science, N.Y.* **153**, 896.

Orti, E., Barker, R. K., Lanman, J. T. and Brasch, N. (1965). *J. Lab. Clin. Med.* **66**, 973.

Pearlmutter, A. F., Rapino, E. and Saffran, M. (1971). *Endocrinology* **89**, 963.

Péron, F. G. and Koritz, S. B. (1958). *J. Biol. Chem.* **233**, 256.

Péron, F. G. and McCarthy, J. L. (1968). *In* 'Functions of the Adrenal Cortex' (K. W. McKerns ed.), Vol. 1, pp. 261–337. Appleton-Century-Crofts, New York.

Péron, F. G. and Tsang, C. P. W. (1969). *Biochim. Biophys. Acta* **180**, 445.

Pohl, S. L., Krans, M. J., Kosyreff, V., Birnbaumer, L. and Rodbell, M. (1971). *J. Biol. Chem.* **246**, 4447.

Porter, J. C. and Klaiber, M. S. (1964). *Am. J. Physiol.* **207**, 789.

Porter, J. C. and Klaiber, M. S. (1965). *Am. J. Physiol.* **209**, 811.

Ramwell, P. W. and Shaw, J. E. (1970). *Recent Progr. Horm. Res.* **26**, 139.

Rasmussen, H. (1970). *Science, N.Y.* **170**, 404.

Reddy, W. J. and Streeto, J. M. (1968). *In* 'Functions of the Adrenal Cortex' (K. W. McKerns ed.) Vol. 1, pp. 601–622. Appleton-Century-Crofts, New York.

Richardson, M. C. and Schulster, D. (1970). *Biochem. J.* **120**, 25P.

Richardson, M. C. and Schulster, D. (1971). *Biochem. J.* **125**, 60P.

Richardson, M. C. and Schulster, D. (1972). *J. Endocrinology* **55**, 127.

Riniker, B., Sieber, P., Rittel, W. and Zuber, H. (1972). *Nature New Biol.* **235**, 114.

Roberts, K. D., Bandy, L. and Lieberman, S. (1969). *Biochemistry* **8**, 1259.

Robison, G. A., Butcher, R. W. and Sutherland, E. W. (1971). 'Cyclic AMP'. Academic Press, New York and London.

Rodbell, M. (1967). *J. Biol. Chem.* **242**, 5744.

Rosen, O. M. and Rosen, S. M. (1969). *Arch. Biochem. Biophys.* **131**, 449.

Saffran, M. and Rowell, P. (1969). *Endocrinology* **85**, 652.

Saffran, M., Ford, P., Mathews, E. K., Kraml, M. and Garbaczewska, L. (1967). *Can. J. Biochem.* **45**, 1901.

Saffran, M., Mathews, E. K. and Pearlmutter, F. (1971). *Recent Progr. Horm. Res.* **27**, 607.

Samuels, L. T. and Uchikawa, T. (1967). *In* 'The Adrenal Cortex' (A. B. Eisenstein ed.), pp. 61-102. Little-Brown, Boston.

Sato, G. H., Rossman, T., Edelstein, L., Holmes, S. and Buonansisi, V. (1965). *Science, N.Y.* **148**, 1733.

Satre, M., Chambaz, E. M., Vignais, P. V. and Idelman, S. (1971). *FEBS Lett.* **12** 207.

Sattin, A. and Rall, T. W. (1970). *Mol. Pharmacol.* **6**, 13.

Sayers, G. (1967). *In* 'Hormones in Blood' (C. H. Gray, ed.), pp. 169-194. Academic Press, New York and London.

Sayers, G., Ma, R. M. and Giordano, N. D. (1971a). *Proc. Soc. Exp. Biol. Med.* **136**, 619.

Sayers, G., Swallow, R. L. and Giordano, N. D. (1971b). *Endocrinology* **88**, 1063.

Schimmer, B. P., Ueda, K. and Sato, G. H. (1968). *Biochem. Biophys. Res. Commun.* **32**, 806.

Schueler, F. W. (1960). 'Chemobiodynamics and Drug Design'. Blakiston, New York.

Schulster, D. (1973). *Endocrinology* **93**, 700.

Schulster, D., Tait, S. A. S. and Tait, J. F. (1968). *Proc. 3rd Int. Congr. Endocrinol. Mexico,* Excerpta Medica Foundation, New York, p. 31.

Schulster, D., Tait, S. A. S., Tait, J. F. and Mrotek, J. (1970). *Endocrinology* **86**, 487.

Schwyzer, R., Schiller, P., Seelig, S. and Sayers, G. (1971). *FEBS Lett.* **19**, 229.

Seelig, S., Sayers, G., Schwyzer, R. and Schiller, P. (1971). *FEBS Lett.* **19**, 232.

Selinger, R. C. L. and Civen, M. (1971). *Biochem. Biophys. Res. Commun.* **43**, 793.

Shima, S. and Pincus, G. (1969). *Endocrinology* **84**, 1048.

Shimizu, K., Gut, M. and Dorfman, R. I. (1962). *J. Biol. Chem.* **237**, 699.

Shin, S-i. and Sato, C. H. (1971). *Biochem. Biophys. Res. Commun.* **45**, 501.

Simpson, E. R. and Boyd, G. S. (1967). *Eur. J. Biochem.* **2**, 275.

Simpson, E. R. and Estabrook, R. W. (1968). *Arch. Biochem. Biophys.* **126**, 977.

Simpson, E. R., Jefcoate, C. R. and Boyd, G. S. (1971). *FEBS Lett.* **15**, 53.

Snydor, K. L. and Sayers, G. (1953). *Proc. Soc. Exp. Biol. Med.* **83**, 729.

Solomon, S., Levitan, P. and Lieberman, S. (1956). *Rev. Can. Biol.* **15**, 282.

Stark, E. and Varga, B. (1968). *Acta Med. Acad. Sci. Hung.* **25**, 367.

Stone, D. and Hechter, O. (1954). *Arch. Biochem. Biophys.* **51**, 457.

Studzinski, G. P. and Grant, J. K. (1962). *Nature (London)* **193**, 1015.
Swallow, R. L. and Sayers, G. (1969). *Proc. Soc. Exp. Biol. Med.* **131**, 1.
Szeberenyi, Sz. and Fekete, G. (1966). *Acta Physiol. Acad. Sci. Hung.* **30**, 328.
Tait, S. A. S., Tait, J. F., Okamoto, M. and Flood, C. (1967). *Endocrinology* **81**, 1213.
Tait, S. A. S., Schulster, D., Okamoto, M., Flood, C. and Tait, J. F. (1970). *Endocrinology* **86**, 360.
Taunton, O. D., Roth, J. and Pastan, I. (1969). *J. Biol. Chem.* **244**, 247.
Tchen, T. T. (1968). *In* 'Functions of the Adrenal Cortex' (K. W. McKerns, ed.), Vol. 1, pp. 3–26. Appleton-Century-Crofts, New York.
Temple, T. E. and Liddle, G. W. (1970). *Ann. Rev. Pharmol.* **10**, 199.
Touster, O., Aronson, N. N., Dulaney, J. T. and Hendrickson, H. (1970). *J. Cell Biol.* **47**, 604.
Tsang, C. P. W. and Carballeira, A. (1966). *Proc. Soc. Exp. Biol. Med.* **122**, 1031.
Urquhart, J. and Li, C. C. (1968). *Am. J. Physiol.* **214**, 73.
Urquhart, J. and Li, C. C. (1969). *Ann. N.Y. Acad. Sci.* **156**, 756.
Urquhart, J., Krall, R. L. and Li, C. C. (1968). *Endocrinology* **83**, 390.
Vaughan, M. H. Pawlowski, P. J. and Forchhammer, J. (1971). *Proc. Nat. Acad. Sci. U.S.* **68**, 2057.
Vinson, G. P. and Whitehouse, B. J. (1970). *In* 'Advances in Steroid Biochemistry and Pharmacology' (M. H. Briggs, ed.), Vol. 1, pp. 163–342. Academic Press, London and New York.
Walsh, D. A., Perkins, J. P. and Krebs, E. G. (1968). *J. Biol. Chem.* **243**, 3763.
Walton, G. M. and Garren, L. D. (1970). *Biochemistry* **2**, 4223.
Walton, G. M., Gill, G. N., Abrass, I. B. and Garren, L. D. (1971). *Proc. Nat. Acad. Sci. U.S.* **68**, 880.
Whysner, J. A., Ramseyer, J. and Harding, B. W. (1970). *J. Biol. Chem.* **245**, 5441.

NOTE ADDED IN PROOF

Since submission of this manuscript many pertinent publications have appeared. A few of particular interest include the following studies.

In plasma and in pituitary extracts 'Big ACTH' has been identified and partly characterized (Yalow and Berson, 1973) as a large protein that can release a component resembling ACTH. The data suggest that, like other peptide hormones, ACTH is synthesized and secreted in the form of a larger protein from which it may be derived. Several laboratories have further examined the effects of ACTH analogues and fragments on adenyl cyclase stimulation and corticosteroidogenesis (Ide *et al.*, 1972; Seelig and Sayers, 1973) and reported good correlation between these two effects of the analogues.

A procedure has been described for the isolation of a plasma membrane enriched fraction from bovine adrenal cortex that is suggested to contain an ACTH receptor (Finn *et al.*, 1973); it binds ACTH and ACTH analogues and fragments, and moreover contains an ACTH sensitive adenyl cyclase. The ready accessibility of this material will aid studies into receptor mechanisms and characterization of those regions of the ACTH polypeptide molecule involved in binding and those related to biological activity. This receptor preparation may moreover prove valuable for use in a radio-receptor assay for ACTH, as indeed will the development of cyclic AMP-binding protein covalently linked to

Sepharose in providing an insoluble and stable complex for use in the assay of cyclic AMP (Fisch *et al.*, 1972). The employment of endocrine tissue receptors in radioligand-receptor assays has been reviewed (Schulster, 1974). Using isolated adrenal cells, divergent effects of ACTH and its *o*-nitrophenyl sulphonyl derivative (NPS-ACTH) have been observed (Moyle *et al.*, 1973) and the data suggest that either very small amounts of cyclic AMP are involved in the steroidogenic effect of ACTH or that factor(s) other than cyclic AMP mediate this action. These studies also implied the presence of two receptors for ACTH in the adrenal cell population used—either in the same cell or different cell types. Further support for two ACTH receptors, one of high affinity present in 1000 sites/cell and the other of low affinity present in much greater concentration, derives from binding studies of purified I^{125}-labelled biologically active ACTH, to intact isolated adrenal cells (McIlhinney and Schulster, 1974).

Apart from the data of Moyle *et al.* (1973) other studies have queried the obligatory mediatory role of cyclic AMP. Sharma (1973) has proposed that the ACTH effect on the isolated adrenal cell is via two different mechanisms operating at two different steps in the conversion of cholesterol to pregnenolone: one is cyclic AMP dependent and the other mode of ACTH action is cyclic AMP independent. It is of interest that studies on isolated fat cells have shown that actinomycin D can simultaneously enhance the ACTH effect on lipolysis and suppress the increase of cyclic AMP caused by ACTH (Lang and Schwyzer, 1972). These studies indicate that in these cells cyclic AMP need not necessarily mediate all of the responses to ACTH.

Alternate sections of adrenal glands have been examined histologically and assayed for cyclic AMP (Orenberg and Glick, 1972) and this technique has revealed a sharp peak of cyclic AMP concentration in the reticular zone of the gland; ACTH caused another similar peak to appear in the outer fasciculata zone. The effect of theophylline and other methylxanthine inhibitors of phosphodiesterase, in potentiating both the cyclic AMP levels and the steroidogenic effect of submaximal concentrations of ACTH, has now been demonstrated using both *in vivo* and *in vitro* systems (Peytremann *et al.*, 1973a; Mackie and Schulster, 1973) thereby establishing one of the important criteria for a mediatory involvement of cyclic AMP in the ACTH effect. Theophylline not only inhibits phosphodiesterase but also inhibits the glycolytic action of both ACTH and exogenous steroids (Birmingham and Bartova, 1973). Protein kinase activity in homogenates of whole adrenal glands from rats treated with ACTH have been studied (Ichii, 1972). The state of activation of cyclic AMP dependent protein kinase within isolated adrenocortical cells has also been examined and ACTH found to cause a rapid and complete activation of this enzyme within two minutes of hormone addition (Richardson and Schulster, 1974); the data demonstrating a sigmoid log-dose response curve for the activation of protein kinase by ACTH and a potentiation of this effect by theophylline, implicate an important role for protein kinase in the action of ACTH.

The cytochrome P_{450} in adrenal mitochondria responsible for cholesterol side-chain cleavage, has been postulated as existing in at least two forms (Jefcoate *et al.*, 1973)—one form bound in an active high-spin enzyme-substrate complex with cholesterol, which may therefore be converted to pregnenolone, and the other form in a low-spin state not bound to cholesterol, possibly because of a restraint imposed by the mitochondrial membrane conformation. ACTH is suggested to lift this restraint, thereby enhancing the binding of cholesterol to cytochrome P_{450}. Brownie *et al.* (1973) have provided spectroscopic evidence that in adrenal mitochondria from hypophysectomized rats, ACTH increases the amount of cholesterol bound to cytochrome P_{450}. Moreover kinetic studies on the adrenal cholesterol side-chain cleavage system have revealed that access of substrate to this enzyme system appears to be the rate-limiting step (Burstein *et al.*, 1972).

The role of calcium ions has been further pursued. Leier and Jungmann (1973) have reported that increases in $^{45}Ca^{++}$ concentrations of various subcellular fractions occurred 5 minutes after addition of ACTH to adrenal bisects, and that ACTH stimulated steroidogenesis requires, at least in part, increased Ca^{++} accumulation in the gland. Similarly the absence of calcium reduced the effect of ACTH on both cyclic AMP accumulation and steroidogenesis by isolated adrenal cells (Sayers *et al.*, 1972); these workers propose from their observations that the strength of the signal generated by ACTH-receptor interaction and received by adenyl cyclase is related to the extracellular Ca^{++} concentration, but that the adenyl cyclase itself is confined to a compartment (on the inner plasma membrane) in which the Ca^{++} concentration remains similar to that of the cytosol (0.1 μM) despite wide extracellular variations. Clearly it would be valuable to establish the membranal localization of adenyl cyclase in adrenocortical cells. A cytochemical technique has been described (Howell and Whitfield, 1972) for such a localization in the A and B cells of isolated rat islets of Langerhans, and the adenyl cyclase activity was found exclusively and almost uniformly along the plasma membranes of these cells. Some precipitation was noted along the outer surface of the membrane (also by Reik *et al.*, 1970) and it was suggested that this could indicate liberation of some cyclic AMP outside of these cells. Birmingham and Bartova (1973) have also found that exogenous calcium is required for both the glycolytic and steroidogenic response to ACTH and suggest that it acts by enhancing the ACTH stimulated synthesis of cyclic AMP. From their studies on the perfused cat adrenal Rubin *et al.* (1972) and Jaanus *et al.* (1972) have proposed a model whereby ACTH-receptor interaction dissociates calcium from its adenyl cyclase binding site, thereby causing increased activity of adenyl cyclase and the redistribution of calcium to some active site within the cell—possibly the mitochondria or endoplasmic reticulum—that couples steroid production and release.

Adrenal corticosteroidogenesis is stimulated by a variety of agents other than ACTH and cyclic AMP and recent reports include that of cholera toxin (Donta *et al.*, 1973), angiotensin II—which produced an increase in cyclic AMP that correlated with and occurred prior to the stimulation of corticosteroid production (Peytremann *et al.*, 1973b) and prostaglandins E_1 and E_2 which had an effect on bovine adrenal slices that implied the existence of a common receptor site with ACTH (Saruta and Kaplan, 1972); angiotensin was found to have an additive effect with prostaglandin E_1. Using superfused rat adrenal bisects, Flack and Ramwell (1972) have reported a transient stimulation of corticosteroid synthesis by prostaglandin E_2, although it was also noted that prostaglandin E_2 did not increase cyclic AMP concentrations in rat adrenal glands *in vitro*. An increased sensitivity to ACTH was noted in isolated cells prepared from hypophysectomized rats compared with those prepared from normal rats (Sayers and Beall, 1973) and this may be attributed to a variety of possibilities including an increase in the number of receptor sites per cell following hypophysectomy.

Using superfused adrenals, Mostafapour and Tchen (1972) have observed that actinomycin D potentiates the steroidogenic effect of ACTH both as a prolongation of the duration of steroid output and as an increase in the rate of steroid output—a feature akin to the superinduction effect found by Tomkins and co-workers (1972) with corticoid stimulated HTC cells. The kinetics of incorporation of ^{3}H-uridine into total cytoplasmic RNA has been studied *in vitro* using superfused rat adrenals (Castells *et al.*, 1973) and a change in the labelling patterns of cytoplasmic RNAs separated on polyacrylamide gels has provided good evidence that ACTH induces adrenal cytoplasmic RNA synthesis within 30 minutes. As early as 15 minutes after the infusion of ACTH, an increase in ^{3}H-uridine incorporation into cytoplasmic RNA, consistent with previous *in vivo* studies, was evident. Clearly the superfusion system is of value in studying the role of RNA synthesis in the ACTH effect, and Tsang and Johnstone (1973) have shown that it is not increased steroid levels in the gland, but elevated levels of 5'-AMP (a potent inhibitor of precursor incorporation into RNA) that may have been the inhibitory factor involved in previous static *in vitro* incubations demonstrating inhibition of precursor incorporation into RNA by ACTH and cyclic AMP. The involvement of labile protein in the ACTH response has been investigated *in vitro* using isolated cells (Schulster *et al.*, 1972) and the decay half-life in this system calculated to be 2–4 minutes.

REFERENCES

Birmingham, M. K. and Bartova, A. (1973). *Endocrinology* **92**, 743–749.

Brownie, A. C., Alfano, H., Jefcoate, C. R., Orme-Johnson, W. H., Beinhert, H. and Simpson, E. R. (1973). *Ann. N.Y. Acad. Sci.* **212**, 344.

Burstein, S., Dinh, J., Co, N., Gut, M., Schleyer, H., Cooper, D. Y. and Rosenthal, O. (1972). *Biochemistry*, **11**, 2883–2890.

Castells, S., Addo, N. and Kwateng, K. (1973). *Endocrinology* **93**, 285–291.

Donta, S. T., King, M. and Sloper, K. (1973). *Nature New Biol.* **243**, 246–247.

Finn, M. F., Widnell, C. C. and Hofmann, K. (1972). *J. Biol. Chem.* **247**, 5695–5702.

Fisch, H. U., Pliska, V. and Schwyzer, R. (1972). *Eur. J. Biochem.* **30**, 1–6.

Flack, J. D. and Ramwell, P. W. (1972). *Endocrinology* **90**, 371–377.

Howell, S. L. and Whitfield, M. (1972). *J. Histochem. Cytochem.* **20**, 873–879.

Ichii, S. (1972). *Endocrinol. Jap.* **19**, 229–235.

Ide, M., Tanaka, A., Nakamura, M. and Okabayashi, T. (1972), *Arch. Biochem. Biophys.* **149**, 189–196.

Jaanus, S. D., Carchman, R. A. and Rubin, R. P. (1972). *Endocrinology* **91**, 887–895.

Jefcoate, C. R., Simpson, E. R., Boyd, G. S., Brownie, A. C. and Orme-Johnson, W. H. (1973). *Ann. N.Y. Acad. Sci.* **212**, 243.

Lang, U. and Schwyzer, R. (1972). *FEBS Lett.* **21**, 91–94.

Leier, D. J. and Jungmann, R. A. (1973). *In* 'Research on steroids. Proc. Vth International Study Group for Steroid Hormones; Rome, Dec. 1971'. Societa Editric Universo, Rome (in press).

Mackie, C. and Schulster, D. (1973). *Biochem. Biophys. Res. Commun.* **53**, 545–551.

McIlhinney, R. A. J. and Schulster, D. (1974). *J. Endocrinol.* (in press).

Mostafapour, M. K. and Tchen, T. T. (1972). *Biochem. Biophys. Res. Commun.* **48**, 491–495.

Moyle, W. R., Kong, Y. C. and Ramachandran, J. (1973). *J. Biol. Chem.* **248**, 2409-2417.

Orenberg, E. K. and Glick, D. (1972). *J. Histochem. Cytochem.* **20**, 923-928.

Peytremann, A., Nicholson, W. E., Liddle, G. W., Hardman, J. G. and Sutherland, E. W. (1973a). *Endocrinology* **92**, 525-530.

Peytremann, A., Nicholson, W. E., Brown, R. D., Liddle, G. W. and Hardman, J. G. (1973b). *J. Clin. Invest.* **52**, 835-842.

Reik, L., Petzold, G. L., Higgins, J. A., Greengard, P. and Barrnett, R. J. (1970). *Science, N.Y.* **168**, 382.

Richardson, M. C. and Schulster, D. (1974). *Biochem. J.* (in press).

Rubin, R. P., Carchman, R. A. and Jaanus, S. D. (1972). *Nature New Biol.* **240**, 150-152.

Saruta, T. and Kaplan, N. M. (1972). *J. Clin. Invest.* **51**, 2246-2251.

Sayers, G. and Beall, R. J. (1973). *Science, N.Y.* **179**, 1330-1331.

Sayers, G., Beall, R. J. and Seelig, S. (1972). *Science, N.Y.* **175**, 1131-1133.

Schulster, D. (1973). *Brit. Med. Bull.* **30** (in press).

Schulster, D., Richardson, M. C. and Mackie, C. (1972). *Biochem. J.* **129**, 8-9P.

Seelig, S. and Sayers, G. (1973). *Arch. Biochem. Biophys.* **154**, 230-239.

Sharma, R. K. (1973). *J. Biol. Chem.* **248**, 5473-5476.

Tomkins, G. M., Levinson, B. B., Baxter, J. D. and Dethlefsen, L. (1972). *Nature New Biol.* **239**, 9-14.

Tsang, D. and Johnstone, R. M. (1973). *Endocrinology* **93**, 119-126.

Yalow, R. S. and Berson, S. A. (1973). *J. Clin. Endocrinol. Metab.* **36**, 415-423.

AUTHOR INDEX

Numbers followed by an asterisk refer to the page on which the reference is listed

SUBJECT INDEX

CUMULATIVE INDEX OF TITLES

Numbers in **bold face** refer to the volume.